Therapeutics and Pharmacology

Therapeutics and Pharmacology

Edited by **Mark Avis**

SYRAWOOD
PUBLISHING HOUSE

New York

Published by Syrawood Publishing House,
750 Third Avenue, 9th Floor,
New York, NY 10017, USA
www.syrawoodpublishinghouse.com

Therapeutics and Pharmacology
Edited by Mark Avis

© 2016 Syrawood Publishing House

International Standard Book Number: 978-1-68286-166-0 (Hardback)

Printed in the United States of America.

Contents

Preface

Pharmacology is a broad field concentrating on the design and discovery of new and useful drugs. Constant research is occurring in this field across the globe. This book comprises contributions of international experts in all areas of clinical and experimental pharmacology. Also included in this book are some contemporary and progressive clinical trials. It will prove beneficial to students, academicians, pharmacologists and anyone else who wants to gain an in-depth knowledge of this field.

This book is a comprehensive compilation of works of different researchers from varied parts of the world. It includes valuable experiences of the researchers with the sole objective of providing the readers (learners) with a proper knowledge of the concerned field. This book will be beneficial in evoking inspiration and enhancing the knowledge of the interested readers.

In the end, I would like to extend my heartiest thanks to the authors who worked with great determination on their chapters. I also appreciate the publisher's support in the course of the book. I would also like to deeply acknowledge my family who stood by me as a source of inspiration during the project.

Editor

1

Prescription of antiviral drugs during the 2009 influenza pandemic: an observational study using electronic medical files of general practitioners in the Netherlands

Mariëtte Hooiveld[1*], Tine van de Groep[2], Theo JM Verheij[2], Marianne AB van der Sande[2,3], Robert A Verheij[1], Margot AJB Tacken[4] and Gerrit A van Essen[2]

Abstract

Background: After the clinical impact of the A(H1N1) pdm09 virus was considered to be mild, treatment with antiviral drugs was recommended only to patients who were at risk for severe disease or who had a complicated course of influenza. We investigated to what extent antiviral prescriptions in primary care practices were in accordance with the recommendations, what proportion of patients diagnosed with influenza had been prescribed antiviral drugs, and to what extent prescriptions related to the stated indications for antiviral treatment.

Methods: We used data from routine electronic medical records of practices participating in the Netherlands Information Network of General Practice LINH in the period August - December 2009. We considered patient and practice characteristics, clinical diagnoses and drug prescriptions of all patients who contacted their general practitioner in the given period and who had been prescribed antiviral medication (n = 351) or were diagnosed with influenza (n = 3293).

Results: Of all antiviral prescriptions, 69% were in accordance with the recommendations. Only 5% of patients diagnosed with influenza were prescribed antiviral drugs. This percentage increased to 12% among influenza patients belonging to the designated high risk groups. On the other hand, 2.5% of influenza patients not at high risk of complications received antiviral treatment. In addition to the established high risk factors, the total number of drug prescriptions for a patient in this year was a determinant of antiviral prescriptions. Information on time since onset of symptoms and the clinical presentation of patients was not available.

Conclusions: General practitioners in the Netherlands have been restrictive in prescribing antiviral drugs during the influenza pandemic, even when patients met the criteria for antiviral treatment.

Keywords: Drug prescriptions, General practice, Influenza, Human, Antivirals, Pandemics, Practice guidelines as topic

Background

On April 30th 2009, the first case of influenza A(H1N1) pdm09 was identified in the Netherlands, while it eventually caused an epidemic with influenza activity above baseline in the period 12 October through 13 December 2009 (fall season in the northern hemisphere) [1].

During the emerging pandemic, all patients suspected of influenza were indicated for treatment with antiviral drugs and their relatives (household contacts) were eligible for prophylactic antiviral drug use. Antiviral drugs were sufficiently available from the national stockpile that has been established since the H5N1 outbreak in 2003. In the beginning of August 2009, the Health Council of the Netherlands and the National Institute for Public Health and the Environment (RIVM) concluded, in concordance with WHO recommendations [2], that the impact of the H1N1 virus on morbidity and

* Correspondence: m.hooiveld@nivel.nl
[1]NIVEL, Netherlands Institute for Health Services Research, Utrecht, PO Box 1568, 3500 BN Utrecht, the Netherlands
Full list of author information is available at the end of the article

mortality appeared to be similar to seasonal influenza virus, based on its so far documented relatively mild course [3,4]. Treatment with antiviral drugs was now only recommended for patients at risk for severe disease and patients having a complicated course of influenza [5]. Prophylactic prescriptions were no longer recommended. High risk patients were defined as the same patients eligible for seasonal influenza vaccination, *i.e.* all patients of 60 years or above and patients with certain medical conditions [5,6]. In addition to that, children under two years of age, pregnant women in their third trimester, and patients having symptoms of influenza in whom the infection occurred to be unusually severe or with complications were considered [5]. In the Netherlands, oseltamivir was the drug of first choice for treatment of high risk patients suspected of influenza during the pandemic. Treatment with zanamivir was reserved for patients suspected for an infection with a resistant influenza virus. Oseltamivir was only available as a prescription drug, not over the counter, and it was in stock for approximately one third of the Dutch population (5 million doses for 16 million inhabitants).

In view of future epidemics, it is important to evaluate the implementation of and compliance to the recommended guidelines. The general aim of this study was therefore to investigate whether the prescription of oseltamivir by general practitioners (GPs) in the Netherlands was in accordance with the national guidelines described above. We used data from a large national database to estimate 1) the proportion of patients receiving oseltamivir according to the guidelines in relation to patients' and practices' characteristics, and 2) what proportion of patients diagnosed with influenza received oseltamivir and which factors determined this prescription.

Methods
Practices and patients selection
Data for this study were derived from the routine electronic medical records of GP practices that participate in the Netherlands Information Network of General Practice (LINH), a national network of around 90 general practices, who are representative of all Dutch general practices with respect to geographical distribution and degree of urbanization [7]. All Dutch citizens are enlisted as patients in a family practice, so the population listed in a general practice can be used as the denominator in epidemiological studies. The GP is the first professional to contact for health problems and a referral to the secondary health care system (hospitals and medical specialists) can only be made by the GP. The LINH practice population consists of more than 350,000 registered patients, representative of the Dutch population with respect to age and gender. The database holds longitudinal data on morbidity, prescriptions and referrals.

Clinical diagnoses are coded using the ICPC (International Classification of Primary Care) coding system [8]. Drugs are coded according to the Anatomical Therapeutic Chemical (ATC) classification [9]. GP practices were included when they provided data on the registration of claimed services, ICPC-coded diagnoses, and ATC-coded prescriptions for the full calendar year of 2009. Only patients enlisted with the general practice during the whole year 2009 were included. Data collection within the LINH network is carried our according to Dutch legislation on privacy. Each patient is coded with an anonymous administrative number. The key to this coding number is only with the general practitioner. The privacy regulation of the LINH network was approved by the Dutch Data Protection Authority. According to the Dutch Central Committee on Research Involving Human Subjects, obtaining informed consent is not obligatory for observational studies and approval by the Medical Ethical Committee was not necessary.

Data collection
All contacts (claims) of patients with the GPs were considered. First, patients having a prescription of oseltamivir (ATC-code J05AH02) between August 8 and December 31, 2009 were considered. No prescriptions of zanamivir were registered. When there was more than one oseltamivir prescription, only the first one was taken into account. We looked for all diagnoses within 7 days before or after the date of prescription, in order to take into account registration delays. However, in 88% of oseltamivir prescriptions, the diagnosis was registered at the same day. We specifically considered diagnoses of influenza (ICPC-code R80, which will be used by GPs for patients with influenza-like illness in the context of an influenza epidemic, or upon virological confirmation of an influenza virus), another acute respiratory infection (ARI, defined by ICPC-codes R74 - acute upper respiratory infection, R78 - acute bronchitis/bronchiolitis or R81 - pneumonia), and non-specified virus infection (A77, which can be used by GPs for patients with influenza-like illness outside the influenza season).

Patients who did not receive oseltamivir were evaluated for a diagnosis of influenza. When more than one episode was present, the date of the first consultation was taken. Recommended treatment of high risk patients with oseltamivir was based on age (<2 years or ≥60 years), comorbidity (cardiac disease, respiratory disease, diabetes mellitus, chronic renal insufficiency, reduced resistance against infections and children up to 18 years using salicylates), a complicated course of illness (the occurrence of pneumonia within 7 days before or after the diagnosis of influenza or ARI, or the need to prescribe antibiotics – not for urinary infections – within these days), or a third trimester pregnancy (an oseltamivir prescription or an influenza diagnosis between 20 to 34 weeks after a first contact related to pregnancy, based on the assumption that pregnant women usually have their first pregnancy-related contact with their GP between weeks 6 and 20; a contact indicating the birth of a child had to be no more than 14 weeks after oseltamivir prescription or influenza diagnosis). Details on ICPC- and ATC-codes used to classify high-risk patients have been published elsewhere [10].

Additional patient characteristics comprised gender, month of prescribing, total number of contacts with the practice in 2009, and the total number of prescriptions in 2009 besides oseltamivir. Other underlying chronic health conditions were based on a selection of diseases with a high prevalence, a long-term course and a serious illness, as used in the National Public Health Compass (www.nationaalkompas.nl). This selection is based on the list of chronic conditions from the Australian Family Medicine Research Centre (www.fmrc.org.au) and adapted from ICPC-2 to ICPC-1. Practice characteristics included practice type, dispensing practice, and level of urbanisation and geographic region of the practice location.

Statistical analysis

In the group of patients with a diagnosis of influenza, we evaluated the proportion of patients whom had been prescribed oseltamivir and whom should have been prescribed it. Univariate logistic regression analyses were performed on the association between the prescription of oseltamivir and a recommendation for a prescription, as well as other patients' and practices' characteristics. Multivariable regression analyses were performed to assess potential determinants independently associated with the prescription of oseltamivir. Likewise, we evaluated whether oseltamivir was prescribed according to the guidelines among all patients receiving oseltamivir. Because of the recommendation to prescribe oseltamivir to both very young (under two years of age) and old (60 years or above) patients, we added age-squared in the multivariable models to take into account the u-shaped association when using the continuous age variable. Only variables that significantly improved the model fit, based on Likelihood-ratio tests (p-value < 0.05), were included. Since patients were clustered within practices, we used multilevel logistic regression. All analyses were performed in Stata version 11.2 (StataCorp LP, College Station, TX, USA).

Results

We included 68 GP practices with complete and reliable data records for the year 2009. Twelve patients with missing age were excluded, leaving 260,298 enlisted patients for analyses (1.6% of the Dutch population). Of all patients, 351 (1.4 per 1,000 enlisted patients) had been prescribed oseltamivir. The total number of oseltamivir

prescriptions ranged between practices from 0 (11 practices) to 10.7 prescriptions per 1000 enlisted patients (right-skewed distribution; geometric mean = 0.9; geometric standard distribution = 3.4).

Half of the patients receiving oseltamivir had a diagnosis of influenza (n = 181; 51.6%). The most frequently registered diagnoses in 105 patients not having influenza, ARI or a non-specified viral infection were general disease (21 patients), fever (17 patients), other viral disease (12 patients), and 'no disease' (11 patients). No valid ICPC-code was recorded for 23 patients (6.6%). Of all oseltamivir prescriptions, 241 (68.7%) were to patients belonging to the designated high risk groups. Table 1 shows the distribution of the underlying reasons for qualification for oseltamivir in these patients.

Table 2 shows factors that independently influenced a prescription according to clinical guidelines among all patients who had been prescribed oseltamivir. As expected, both a very young and a higher age were associated with an increased chance of having an oseltamivir prescription according to the recommendations. Independently of age, a higher number of contacts with the GP and a higher number of prescriptions in general were positively associated with prescribing oseltamivir according to the guidelines.

A total of 3,293 patients (1.3% of the study population) were diagnosed with influenza and oseltamivir was prescribed to 181 (5.5%). The weekly number of influenza

Table 1 Characteristics of 241 patients at high risk of severe illness who had been prescribed oseltamivir

	n of patients	(%)
High risk group description		
Age only	53	(22.0)
Co-morbidity only	101	(41.9)
Complicated course of illness only	13	(5.4)
Age and co-morbidity	49	(20.3)
Age and complicated course of illness	2	(0.8)
Co-morbidity and complicated course	15	(6.2)
Age, co-morbidity and complicated course	8	(3.3)
Specific co-morbidity at risk for complications*		
Cardiac disease	60	(24.9)
Respiratory disease	106	(44.0)
Diabetes mellitus	27	(11.2)
Chronic renal insufficiency	5	(2.1)
Reduced resistance against infections	24	(10.0)
Children using salicylates	1	(0.4)
Third trimester of pregnancy	3	(1.2)

*Numbers add up above 100% because of multiple co-morbidities per patient.

Table 2 Factors influencing a prescription of oseltamivir according to clinical guidelines in 351 patients with antiviral medication

Variable	Univariate analysis		Adjusted multilevel analysis		
	OR	(95% CI)	OR	(95% CI)	P-value
Age at prescription (continuous)	0.87	(0.83 to 0.91)	0.84	(0.80 to 0.90)	<0.001
Age-squared	1.00	(1.00 to 1.00)	1.00	(1.00 to 1.00)	<0.001
Number of contacts with GP in 2009					
<6	ref	-	ref	-	
6 or more	3.00	(1.87 to 4.82)	2.19	(1.18 to 4.08)	0.014
Total number of prescriptions in 2009*					
<8	ref	-	ref	-	
8 or more	4.60	(2.80 to 7.57)	3.24	(1.63 to 6.42)	0.001

GP = general practitioner; OR = odds ratio; CI = confidence interval.
*Excluding oseltamivir prescriptions.

patients followed well the epidemiologic curve of the Dutch influenza-like illness (IAZ) surveillance (data not shown) [1]. Of all influenza patients, 1,051 (31.9%) belonged to the designated high risk groups, of whom 126 (12.0%) indeed received oseltamivir. This percentage varied from 9.5% (*n* = 16) among children aged 2 to 14 years to 18.0% (*n* = 18) among children under two years of age. On the other hand, 2,242 patients diagnosed with influenza did not belong to the high risk groups and yet 55 (2.5%) received a prescription of oseltamivir.

Univariate analyses showed that age, underlying comorbidity, the total number of contacts with the GP in 2009 and the total number of prescriptions in 2009 were determinants of the prescription of oseltamivir among influenza patients (Table 3). Patients with underlying comorbidity had the highest chance of an oseltamivir prescription. All of the designated high risk groups were statistically significantly associated with oseltamivir prescription, except children receiving chronic aspirin therapy. Taking into account specific medical conditions showed that patients with respiratory diseases and pregnant women had a higher chance of treatment, while no associations were observed for other underlying diseases. Ten percent of all influenza patients had a complicated course of illness, but this was not associated with oseltamivir treatment. Practice characteristics were not associated with oseltamivir prescriptions.

The results of the multilevel model with age, co-morbidity, complicated course of illness and number of prescriptions, are presented in Table 3 as well. After adjustment for other factors, an age of 60 years or above in itself was not associated with oseltamivir prescription.

Independently of a high risk for severe disease due to age, co-morbidity or a complicated course of illness, the total number of drug prescriptions was positively associated with the prescription of oseltamivir.

Among influenza patients who did not belong to the designated high risk groups, chronic health conditions other than those at high risk of severe illness were not associated with oseltamivir prescription, nor were age, gender, and consultation rate or practice characteristics (Table 4). The only significant determinant for oseltamivir prescriptions was the total number of drug prescriptions in 2009. The odds ratio for drug prescriptions did not change in the multilevel logistic model (OR = 2.28; 95% CI = 1.20 to 4.32).

Discussion

This study showed that general practitioners in the Netherlands have been restrained in prescribing oseltamivir during the influenza pandemic. Only 5% of all patients diagnosed with influenza were prescribed oseltamivir, and only 12% of those who were at high risk of severe illness. On the other hand, when GPs have prescribed oseltamivir, they have rather well followed the recommendations in the national guidelines. Only 2.5% of influenza patients not at high risk were prescribed oseltamivir, and of all antiviral drugs prescribed, 69% were for patients at high risk for severe disease. The total number of drug prescriptions in 2009 and the total number of GP consultations, which can be considered proxies for underlying morbidity, were determinants for oseltamivir prescription in addition to the high risk factors of co-morbidity, a very young or an older age.

Strengths and limitations of this study

This study was conducted using a large database of patients, representative for the general Dutch population, providing a complete picture of morbidity and prescriptions. A limitation of this study was the lacking information on specific details on presented symptoms. More severely ill patients could have been hospitalized, but information on care provided outside the general practice was lacking in our data. This could have resulted in an underestimation in the number of patients with a more severe illness, causing a negative association with the prescription of oseltamivir.

Co-morbidity at high risk of complications was defined by ICPC- and ATC-codes that are used in general practices to select patients eligible for influenza vaccination [10,11]. This method has been used to monitor the Dutch influenza vaccination rate in different high risk groups for several years, using the LINH database, with stable and representative results [12,13]. We assumed these patients had at least one contact (claim) with their

Table 3 Potential factors influencing the prescription of oseltamivir by general practitioners to 3,293 influenza patients

Variable	Prescription of oseltamivir, n of patients (%)				Univariate analysis		Adjusted multilevel analysis	
	No		Yes		OR	(95% CI)	OR	(95% CI)
Gender							*(not in model)*	
Male	1,477	(47.5)	88	(48.6)	*ref*	-		
Female	1,635	(52.5)	93	(51.4)	0.94	(0.70 to 1.28)		
Age at diagnosis								
< 2 yrs	82	(2.6)	18	(9.9)	3.62	(2.07 to 6.36)	5.71	(3.01 to 10.80)
2 to 14 yrs	972	(31.2)	32	(17.8)	0.54	(0.36 to 0.83)	0.70	(0.44 to 1.11)
15 to 24 yrs	469	(15.1)	20	(11.0)	0.70	(0.43 to 1.16)	0.88	(0.51 to 1.52)
25 to 59 yrs	1,321	(42.4)	80	(44.2)	*ref*	-	*ref*	-
60 yrs or older	268	(8.6)	31	(17.1)	1.84	(1.19 to 2.87)	0.96	(0.58 to 1.57)
Co-morbidity at risk for complications								
No	2,562	(82.3)	89	(49.2)	*ref*	-	*ref*	-
Yes	550	(17.7)	92	(50.8)	4.82	(3.53 to 6.57)	4.94	(3.29 to 7.40)
Number of co-morbidities at risk							*(not in model)*	
0	2,562	(82.3)	89	(49.2)	*ref*	-		
1	443	(14.2)	70	(38.7)	4.55	(3.27 to 6.32)		
2 or 3	107	(3.4)	22	(12.1)	5.92	(3.57 to 9.81)		
Specific co-morbidity at risk for complications*							*(not in model)*	
Cardiac disease	178	(5.7)	28	(15.6)	3.04	(1.97 to 4.68)		
Respiratory disease	290	(9.3)	54	(30.0)	4.17	(2.95 to 5.89)		
Diabetes mellitus	112	(3.6)	17	(9.4)	2.79	(1.64 to 4.77)		
Chronic renal insufficiency	9	(0.3)	3	(1.7)	5.84	(1.57 to 21.82)		
Reduced resistance against infections	59	(1.9)	9	(5.0)	2.72	(1.33 to 5.59)		
Children using salicylates	13	(0.4)	1	(0.6)	1.33	(0.17 to 10.24)		
Third trimester of pregnancy	12	(0.4)	3	(1.7)	4.38	(1.22 to 15.68)		
Complicated course of illness								
No	2,810	(90.3)	159	(87.8)	*ref*	-	*ref*	-
Yes	302	(9.7)	22	(12.2)	1.29	(0.81 to 2.04)	0.95	(0.57 to 1.58)
Contacts with GP in 2009						-	*(not in model)*	
<6	1,850	(59.4)	86	(47.5)	*ref*			
6 or more	1,262	(40.6)	95	(52.5)	1.62	(1.20 to 2.19)		
Prescriptions in 2009 †								
<8	2,300	(73.9)	92	(50.8)	*ref*	-	*ref*	-
8 or more	812	(26.1)	89	(49.2)	2.74	(2.03 to 3.71)	1.36	(0.89 to 2.09)

GP = general practitioner; OR = odds ratio; CI = confidence interval.
*Reference group does not have the specific co-morbidity.
†Excluding oseltamivir prescriptions.

GP, resulting in at least one record with the specified codes. We think it is very unlikely that a patient with a certain chronic condition did not contact his or her general practitioner for an entire year, nor was prescribed any medication for this chronic condition during that year. Misclassification of patients with co-morbidity is therefore unlikely.

Comparison with other studies

Our observations are in line with those from Fietjé and colleagues [14], who found that 85% of Dutch patients with an oseltamivir prescription belonged to the high risk groups. Their study was based on telephone interviews with patients who filled a prescription for oseltamivir through community pharmacists. Results from other countries on

Table 4 Potential factors influencing the prescription of oseltamivir to 2,242 influenza patients not at high risk

	Prescription of oseltamivir, *n* of patients (%)				Univariate analysis	
Variable	No		Yes		OR	(95% CI)
Patient characteristics						
Gender						
Male	1,039	(47.5)	29	(52.7)	*ref*	-
Female	1,148	(52.5)	26	(47.3)	0.81	(0.47 to 1.39)
Age at diagnosis						
2 to 14 yrs	819	(37.4)	16	(29.1)	0.69	(0.37 to 1.29)
15 to 24 yrs	411	(18.8)	12	(21.8)	1.03	(0.52 to 2.06)
25 to 59 yrs	957	(43.8)	27	(49.1)	*ref*	-
Chronic health condition not at high risk						
No	1,754	(80.2)	45	(81.8)	*ref*	-
Yes	433	(19.8)	10	(18.2)	0.90	(0.45 to 1.80)
Number of contacts with GP in 2009						
<6	1,468	(67.1)	36	(65.5)	*ref*	-
6 or more	719	(32.9)	19	(34.5)	1.08	(0.61 to 1.89)
Total number of prescriptions in 2009*						
<8	1,888	(86.3)	41	(74.5)	*ref*	-
8 or more	299	(13.7)	14	(25.5)	2.16	(1.16 to 4.00)
Practice characteristics						
Type of practice						
Solo practice	706	(32.3)	24	(43.6)	*ref*	-
Duo practice	437	(20.0)	8	(14.6)	0.54	(0.24 to 1.21)
Group practice	1,044	(47.7)	23	(41.8)	0.65	(0.36 to 1.16)
Dispensing practice	101	(4.6)	2	(3.6)	0.78	(0.19 to 3.24)
Urbanicity practice location						
(Very) strongly urban	1,116	(51.0)	27	(49.1)	0.84	(0.42 to 1.68)
Moderately urban	418	(19.1)	12	(21.8)	*ref*	-
Mildly/not urban	653	(29.9)	16	(29.1)	0.85	(0.40 to 1.82)

GP = general practitioner; OR = odds ratio; CI = confidence interval.
*Excluding oseltamivir prescriptions.

prescriptions of oseltamivir during the A(H1N1)pdm09 pandemic are scarce. In a study by Hersh and colleagues, antivirals were prescribed in 58% of influenza visits to US ambulatory physicians [15]. The prescription rate for patients younger than 2 years was 47% and 68% for patients 65 years or older. Information on underlying medical conditions was not available. A study from the UK focusing on 90 pregnant women presenting with influenza-like illness in primary care, 61% were prescribed antiviral drugs [16]. Forty-three women were in their third trimester, of whom 26 (60%) received antivirals. In a Chicago hospital, 65% of high-risk patients with influenza-like illness received oseltamivir treatment [17]. These figures are much higher than in our study.

The results of our study show that if oseltamivir was prescribed, it was in accordance with the guidelines in most cases. A study by Grol et al. showed that compliance to guidelines was rather good in Dutch primary care; recommendations were followed in, on average, 61% of the decisions [18]. Based on our research it can therefore be said that when general practitioners in the Netherlands prescribed oseltamivir, they followed the recommendations on the prescribing fairly well. But they often did not prescribe, even when oseltamivir was recommended. The availability of antiviral drugs was no problem, since they were available from the national stockpile.

A possible explanation for withholding oseltamivir to patients at higher risk of complications might have been a late presentation of the patient. From the Dutch influenza-like illness surveillance we know that patients wait on average 3 days before contacting a doctor for respiratory complaints [19], while treatment with antiviral drugs should start preferably within 48 hours of the onset of illness. We had no information on time since onset of symptoms, but awareness and anxiety about the on-going pandemic may have urged patients to contact their GP earlier than usually.

Conclusions

In conclusion, this study showed that general practitioners in the Netherlands have been very restrained in prescribing antiviral drugs during the influenza pandemic. Where GPs have used antiviral medication, they have rather well followed the recommendations in the national guidelines. To our knowledge, this is the first study in which recommendations for prescribing oseltamivir in primary care has been evaluated in detail. More information is needed on the reasons for underuse of antiviral drugs in patients belonging to the designated high risk groups. We believe it is important to evaluate the implementation of recommended guidelines. In this way, in the case of future epidemics, the recommendations may be adjusted and can be applied even more effectively.

Abbreviations
ARI: Acute respiratory infection other than influenza; ATC: Anatomical Therapeutic Chemical classification; CI: Confidence interval; GP: General practitioner; ICPC: International Classification of Primary Care; LINH: Netherlands Information Network of General Practice; OR: Odds ratio.

Competing interests
The authors declare that they have no competing interests.

Authors' contributions
MH, RV, MT and GvE contributed to conception and design. MH and TvdG acquired and analysed the data and drafted the manuscript. All authors read, contributed to and approved the final manuscript.

Acknowledgements
We would like to thank all the members of the LINH group and the practice staff of all the participating general practices for their cooperation. We would also like to thank Peter Zuithoff, data manager at the Julius Center, for his help in analysing the data.

Funding
This work was supported by the Netherlands Organisation for Health Research and Development ZonMW (grant number 125050003).

Author details
[1]NIVEL, Netherlands Institute for Health Services Research, Utrecht, PO Box 1568, 3500 BN Utrecht, the Netherlands. [2]Julius Center for Health Sciences and Primary Care, University Medical Center Utrecht, Utrecht, the Netherlands. [3]Centre for Infectious Disease Control, National Institute for Public Health and the Environment, Bilthoven, the Netherlands. [4]IQ healthcare, Scientific Institute for Quality of Healthcare, Radboud University Nijmegen Medical Centre, Nijmegen, the Netherlands.

References
1. Donker GA: *Continuous Morbidity Registration at Dutch Sentinel General Practice Network 2009*. NIVEL: Utrecht; 2011.
2. World Health Organization: *Global Alert and Respons (GAR) - Pandemic (H1N1) 2009 – full list of updates*. [http://www.who.int/csr/disease/swineflu/updates/en/index.html]
3. Wielders CC, van Lier EA, van 't Klooster TM, van Gageldonk-Lafeber AB, van den Wijngaard CC, Haagsma JA, Donker GA, Meijer A, van der Hoek W, Lugnér AK, Kretzschmar ME, van der Sande MA: **The burden of 2009 pandemic influenza A(H1N1) in the Netherlands.** *Eur J Public Health* 2012, **22:**150–157.
4. van 't Klooster TM, Wielders CC, Donker T, Isken L, Meijer A, van den Wijngaard CC, van der Sande MA, van der Hoek W: **Surveillance of hospitalisations for 2009 pandemic influenza A(H1N1) in the Netherlands, 5 June – 31 December 2009.** *Euro Surveill* 2010, **15:**pii:19461.
5. World Health Organization: *Clinical management of human infection with pandemic (H1N1) 2009: revised guidance*. Geneva: WHO; 2009.
6. Health Council of the Netherlands: *Influenza vaccination: revision of the indication. Publication no. 2007/09*. The Hague: Health Council of the Netherlands; 2007.
7. Stirbu-Wagner I, Dorsman SA, Visscher S, Davids R, Gravestein JV, Abrahamse H, van Althuis T, Jansen B, Schlief A, Tiersma W, Walk C, Wentink E, Wennekes L, Braspenning J, Korevaar JC: *The Netherlands Information Network of General Practice. Facts and numbers in primary care [in Dutch]*. Utrecht/Nijmegen: NIVEL/IQ; 2010. [http://www.linh.nl]
8. Lamberts H, Wood M (Eds): *ICPC. International Classification of Primary Care*. Oxford: Oxford University Press; 1987.
9. WHO Collaborating Centre for Drug Statistics Methodology: *Guidelines for ATC classification and DDD assignment 2010*. Oslo: Norwegian Institute of Public Health; 2009.
10. Tacken M, Mulder J, Visscher S, Tiersma W, Donkers J, Verheij R, Braspenning J: *Monitoring vaccination rate Dutch national influenza prevention program 2009 [in Dutch]*. LINH: Nijmegen/Utrecht; 2010.
11. Van Essen GA, Bueving HJ, Voordouw ACG, Berg HF, Van der Laan JR, de Jeude CP VL, Boomsma LJ, Opstelten W: **Dutch College of General Practitioners-guideline influenza and influenza vaccination (first revision) [in Dutch].** *Huisarts Wet* 2008, **51**. appendix 1–2.
12. Tacken MAJB, Braspenning JCC, Berende A, Hak E, De Bakker DH, Groenewegen PP, Grol RP: **Vaccination of high-risk patients against influenza: impact on primary care contact rates during epidemics - analysis of routinely collected data.** *Vaccine* 2004, **22:**2985–2992.
13. Tacken M, Braspenning J, Spreeuwenberg P, Van den Hoogen H, Van Essen G, De Bakker D, Grol R: **Patient characteristics determine differences in the influenza vaccination rate more so than practice features.** *Prev Med* 2002, **35:**401–406.
14. Fietjé EH, Philbert D, van Geffen EC, Winters NA, Bouvy ML: **Adherence to oseltamivir guidelines during influenza pandemic, the Netherlands.** *Emerg Infect Dis* 2012, **18:**534–535.
15. Hersh AL, Stafford RS: **Antiviral prescribing by office-based physicians during the, H1N1 pandemic.** *Ann Intern Med* 2009, **2011**(154):74–76.
16. Yates L, Pierce M, Stephens S, Mill AC, Spark P, Kurinczuk JJ, Valappil M, Brocklehurst P, Thomas SH, Knight M: **Influenza A/H1N1v in pregnancy: an investigation of the characteristics and management of affected women and the relationship to pregnancy outcomes for mother and infant.** *Health Technol Assess* 2010, **14:**109–182.
17. Aziz M, Vasoo S, Aziz Z, Patel S, Eltoukhy N, Singh K: **Oseltamivir overuse at a Chicago hospital during the 2009 influenza pandemic and the poor predictive value of influenza-like illness criteria.** *Scand J Infect Dis* 2012, **44:**306–311.
18. Grol R, Dalhuijsen J, Thomas S, in't Veld C, Rutten G, Mokkink H: **Attributes of clinical guidelines that influence use of guidelines in general practice: observational study.** *BMJ* 1998, **317:**858–861.
19. Dijkstra F, van 't Klooster TM, Brandsema P, van Gageldonk-Lafeber AB, Meijer A, van der Hoek W: *Annual report surveillance respiratory infections*. Bilthoven: RIVM; 2010 [in Dutch].

2

Suppression of eukaryotic initiation factor 4E prevents chemotherapy-induced alopecia

Zeina Nasr[1], Lukas E Dow[2], Marilene Paquet[3], Jennifer Chu[1], Kontham Ravindar[5], Ragam Somaiah[5], Pierre Deslongchamps[5], John A Porco Jr[6], Scott W Lowe[2,4] and Jerry Pelletier[1,7,8*]

Abstract

Background: Chemotherapy-induced hair loss (alopecia) (CIA) is one of the most feared side effects of chemotherapy among cancer patients. There is currently no pharmacological approach to minimize CIA, although one strategy that has been proposed involves protecting normal cells from chemotherapy by transiently inducing cell cycle arrest. Proof-of-concept for this approach, known as cyclotherapy, has been demonstrated in cell culture settings.

Methods: The eukaryotic initiation factor (eIF) 4E is a cap binding protein that stimulates ribosome recruitment to mRNA templates during the initiation phase of translation. Suppression of eIF4E is known to induce cell cycle arrest. Using a novel inducible and reversible transgenic mouse model that enables RNA$_i$-mediated suppression of eIF4E *in vivo*, we assessed the consequences of temporal eIF4E suppression on CIA.

Results: Our results demonstrate that transient inhibition of eIF4E protects against cyclophosphamide-induced alopecia at the organismal level. At the cellular level, this protection is associated with an accumulation of cells in G1, reduced apoptotic indices, and was phenocopied using small molecule inhibitors targeting the process of translation initiation.

Conclusions: Our data provide a rationale for exploring suppression of translation initiation as an approach to prevent or minimize cyclophosphamide-induced alopecia.

Keywords: Chemotherapy-induced alopecia, eIF4E, eIF4A, Translation initiation, Genetic engineered mouse model, Cyclophosphamide

Background

Chemotherapy-induced hair loss (alopecia) is an unmet challenge in clinical oncology and considered one of the most psychologically negative factors in cancer patient care. The psychological impact of chemotherapy-induced alopecia (CIA) is significant. In conjunction with vomiting and nausea, it is among the most feared side-effects of chemotherapy [1]. CIA is seen with alkylating agents (e.g., cyclophosphamide), cytotoxics (e.g., doxorubicin), antimicrotubules (e.g., paclitaxel), and topoisomerase inhibitors (e.g., etoposide) and is a consequence of perturbations of hair-follicle cycling and hair shaft production. No reliable preventative pharmacological approach for CIA is currently available [2].

Strategies aimed at protecting normal cells from chemotherapeutic agents may offer benefit to prevent CIA. One approach, known as cyclotherapy, aims to selectively and transiently induce cell cycle arrest in normal cells [3,4]. In proof of principle experiments, the MDM2 antagonist, nutlin-3a, was used to activate p53 and induce a reversible cell-cycle arrest in non-transformed cells - protecting them from S or mitotic phase inhibitors. In contrast, p53$^{-/-}$ tumor cells do not cell cycle arrest and remain susceptible to chemotherapy [5-8]. However, nutlin-3a is not clinically approved, has poor efficacy *in vivo*, requires a high working concentration (200 mg/kg) in mice [9,10], and induces cell cycle arrest within a narrow concentration window (between 2 μM and 10 μM) [11,12]. There is thus a need to identify and

* Correspondence: jerry.pelletier@mcgill.ca
[1]Departments of Biochemistry, McGill University, Montreal, Quebec H3G 1Y6, Canada
[7]Department of Oncology, McGill University, Montreal, Quebec H3G 1Y6, Canada
Full list of author information is available at the end of the article

test additional small molecules that could be used to entice a cyclotherapy response.

In eukaryotes, suppression of eukaryotic initiation factor (eIF) 4E activity slows G1 progression in yeast [13] and non-transformed mammalian cells [14,15]. eIF4E is required for ribosome recruitment during translation initiation and is thought to function through eIF4F, a heterotrimeric complex that consists of (i) eIF4E, a cap-binding protein; (ii) eIF4A, an RNA helicase required for generating a ribosome landing pad; and (iii) eIF4G, a large scaffolding protein [16]. Assembly of eIF4F is regulated by mTOR and is thought to be a nodal point mediating proliferative and survival consequences of increased signaling flux through the PI3K/mTOR pathway [17]. There is thus significant interest in identifying specific inhibitors of eIF4F for assessment as anti-neoplastic agents [17].

We have recently described the development of a novel inducible RNAi platform in the mouse that combines GFP-coupled shRNA technology with a Flp/FRT recombinase-mediated cassette exchange (RMCE) strategy to generate mice that conditionally express shRNAs [14,18]. Two strains that we generated enabled inducible and reversible suppression of eIF4E at the organismal level - the effects of which are well tolerated in the mouse [14,19]. One tissue in which this system shows high eIF4E suppression is in the skin, including hair follicle cells (this study). We therefore envisioned that this model would be useful for assessing a potential role for eIF4E suppression in CIA. Using a well-established protocol for studying CIA in mice [20], we demonstrate that transient eIF4E suppression prior to chemotherapy protects from CIA by decreasing apoptosis of hair follicle cells. These results provide genetic validation for targeting eIF4E as a mean to reduce CIA.

Methods

General reagents

Doxycycline hydrochloride (Sigma-Aldrich) was dissolved in water at 1 mg/ml with 5% sucrose and supplied to mice in their drinking water. Cyclophosphamide (Sigma-Aldrich) was resuspended in water and stored at 4°C. Nutlin-3a, paclitaxel, nocodazole, and vinorelbine were purchased from Sigma-Aldrich, resuspended in DMSO and stored at −20°C.

Cell lines

Normal human primary fibroblast BJ/TERT (obtained from Dr. Joe Teodoro, McGill University) and MRC5 lung fibroblast cells (ATCC) were cultured in Dulbecco's modified Eagle's medium. All media was supplemented with 10% Fetal Bovine Serum (FBS), 100 U/ml penicillin/streptomycin (P/S), and 100 U/ml L-Glutamine. Cells were grown at 37°C and 5% CO_2.

Targeting construct and ES cell generation

The generation of sh4E.389, sh4E.610 and shFLuc.1309 mice has been previously described [14]. CAGs-RIK mice harbor a CAGs promoter driving expression of rtTA3 and the fluorescent protein Kate2 targeted to the *Rosa26* locus (Figure 1A) (Dow, Nasr, Lowe, and Pelletier; In Preparation).

Mouse studies

All mice strains were maintained on a C57BL/6 background. CAGs-RIK mice were crossed to sh4E.389, sh4E.610 and shFLuc.1309 mice [14] to generate bi-transgenic animals. Mice harboring the shFLuc.1309 allele serve as negative controls whereas using two independent sh4E alleles controls for off-target effects. Mice were genotyped by PCR amplification using the primers for CAGs-RIK (5′-GCTTGTTCTTCACGTGCCAG-3′ and 5′-CTGCTAACCATGTTCATGC-3′), sh4E.389 (5′-AATTACTAGACAACTGGATTGCCT-3′ and 5′-GAAGAACAATCAAGGGTCC-3′), sh4E.610 (5′-GCCACAGATGTATTTAGCTCTAAC-3′ and 5′-GAAGAACAATCAAGGGTCC-3′) and shFLuc.1309 (5′-CACCCTGAAAACTTTGCCCC-3′ and 5′-AAGCCACAGATGTATTAATCAGAGA-3′). All mice strains were maintained on a C57BL/6 background. shRNAmir activation was induced in mice by supplying doxycyline in the drinking water for the indicated periods of time. Dox-supplemented water was changed every 4 days.

Cyclophosphamide (CyP)-induced alopecia

To synchronize hair growth in mice, hair was plucked from the back of mice. Nine days later (time of active hair growth at the anagen VI stage), mice were injected once with 150 mg/kg CyP by intra-peritoneal delivery. In experiments in which sheIF4E or shFLuc miRs were induced, Dox was added to the drinking water for 5 days prior to CyP delivery. Skin sections were harvested at days 12 and 21 post-depilation.

Western blot analysis

For Western blot analysis, cells were lysed in RIPA buffer (50 mM Tris–HCl [pH 7.5], 150 mM NaCl, 1 mM DTT, 0.1% SDS, 1% NP-40, 0.5% sodium deoxycholate, 0.1 mM phenylmethylsulfonyl fluoride [PMSF], 1 mg/ml each of leupeptin, pepstatin, and aprotinin). Protein lysates were quantified by the Bio-Rad protein assay and 30 μg of proteins was resolved by SDS-PAGE, transferred to PVDF membranes (Millipore), probed with the indicated antibodies, and visualized using enhanced chemiluminescence (ECL) detection (Amersham). The antibodies used for protein expression analysis were directed against eIF4E (Cell Signaling, #9742), p53 (Santa Cruz, #sc-126), and tubulin (Sigma-Aldrich, #T5268).

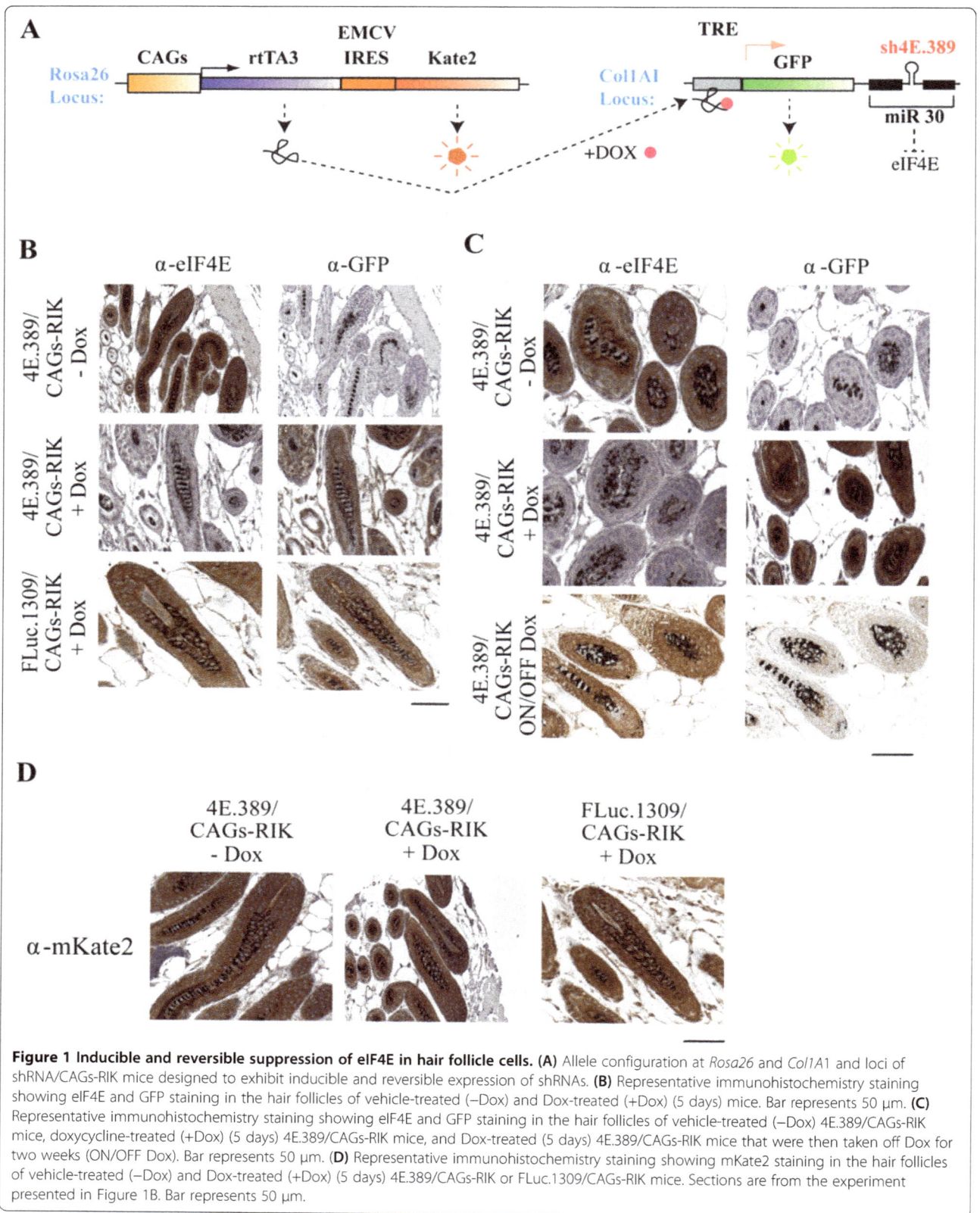

Figure 1 Inducible and reversible suppression of eIF4E in hair follicle cells. (A) Allele configuration at *Rosa26* and *Col1A*1 and loci of shRNA/CAGs-RIK mice designed to exhibit inducible and reversible expression of shRNAs. (B) Representative immunohistochemistry staining showing eIF4E and GFP staining in the hair follicles of vehicle-treated (−Dox) and Dox-treated (+Dox) (5 days) mice. Bar represents 50 μm. (C) Representative immunohistochemistry staining showing eIF4E and GFP staining in the hair follicles of vehicle-treated (−Dox) 4E.389/CAGs-RIK mice, doxycycline-treated (+Dox) (5 days) 4E.389/CAGs-RIK mice, and Dox-treated (5 days) 4E.389/CAGs-RIK mice that were then taken off Dox for two weeks (ON/OFF Dox). Bar represents 50 μm. (D) Representative immunohistochemistry staining showing mKate2 staining in the hair follicles of vehicle-treated (−Dox) and Dox-treated (+Dox) (5 days) 4E.389/CAGs-RIK or FLuc.1309/CAGs-RIK mice. Sections are from the experiment presented in Figure 1B. Bar represents 50 μm.

Ex Vivo treatment studies

Cells were cultured in triplicate in 6-well plates and pre-treated with 5 μM nutlin-3a, 40 nM hippuristanol, 40 nM Cr131-b, 10 μM 4E1RCat, or 10 μM 4E2RCat for 24 hours, followed by removal of the drug and exposure to 50 nM paclitaxel, 200 nM nocodazole, or 40 nM vinorelbine for 48 hours. The compounds were then removed and cells allowed to recover for 5 days. For eIF4E suppression, cells were transfected with siRNA against human eIF4E using Lipofectamine 2000 according to the manufacturer's recommendations (Sigma-Aldrich). Two days later, cells were exposed to chemotherapy for 48 hrs, after which they were washed and allowed to recover for 5 days. Cells were counted using a Z2 Coulter Counter (Beckman Coulter).

For Giemsa staining, cells were fixed with ice-cold methanol-acetone (1:1 mixture) for 8 min at −20°C, and left to dry at RT. Giemsa solution (Sigma-Aldrich) was diluted 1:20 in PBS buffer and put on cells for 20 min at RT, after which time they were extensively washed with water. Plates were left to dry and visualized by microscopy (AxioScope; Zeiss).

For cell cycle analysis, cells (10^6 cells/ml) were washed in PBS following compound treatment, fixed in 75% ethanol for 1 hour at 4°C, and stained with 50 mg/ml propidium iodide (Sigma-Aldrich) (containing 3.8 mM sodium citrate, and 500 mg/ml RNase A) for 3 hr at 4°C. DNA content was analyzed by FACScan (BD Biosciences).

Immunohistochemistry analysis

Tissues were fixed in 10% neutral buffered formalin for 48 hours before embedding in paraffin and sectioned at 5 μm depth. Sections were dewaxed and rehydrated in a graded series of decreasing alcohol concentrations followed by a water wash. For antigen retrieval, sections were boiled for 15 min in 10 mM citric acid buffer (pH 6.0), followed by a 1 hr incubation in blocking buffer UltraVBlock (Anti-Rabbit HRP/DAB Detection Kit, Abcam), and a 10 min incubation with 3% hydrogen peroxide. Sections were then stained with rabbit primary antibodies against eIF4E (Cell Signaling, #9742, 1:50), GFP (Cell Signaling, # 2555, 1:800), mKate2 (Evrogen, #AB233, 1:800), and cyclin D1 (Cell Signaling, # 2926, 1:100) for 24 hours at 4°C, followed by incubation with biotinylated goat anti-rabbit IgG and streptavadin peroxidase (Anti-Rabbit HRP/DAB Detection Kit, Abcam) for 30 min each. Sections were washed with TBS buffer (0.1 M Tris−HCl (pH 7.5), 0.15 M NaCl) and the signal visualized using 3,3′-diaminobenzidine chromogen. Sections were counterstained with hematoxylin, dehydrated, and mounted using permount. Slides were scanned using an Aperio ScanScope (Aperio, Vista) and signals analyzed using an Aperio ImageScope (Aperio, Vista). Apoptosis was detected by TUNEL using the DeadEnd Fluorometric TUNEL System kit according to the manufacturer's recommendations (Promega) and TUNEL positive cells were visualized using an Axio Observer fluorescent microscope (Zeiss).

Statistics

For statistical analysis, unpaired Student t-test with Welch correction was performed using GraphPad InStat version 3.10.

Study approval

All animal studies were approved by the McGill University Faculty of Medicine Animal Care Committee.

Results

Transient eIF4E suppression protects from CIA

In eukaryotes, modulation of eIF4E can lead to profound consequences on cell cycle progression [13-15]. We therefore sought to directly determine if suppression of eIF4E could protect against CIA. To this end, we took advantage of a recently developed transgenic mouse model in which we could potently suppress eIF4E in hair follicles in an inducible and reversible manner (Figure 1A, B) (Dow, Nasr, Lowe and Pelletier, In Preparation) [14]. As predicted, eIF4E was not suppressed in the hair follicle cells of FLuc.1309/CAGs-RIK mice - a control strain expressing a neutral shRNA to firefly luciferase [21] (Figure 1B). Importantly, eIF4E suppression could be reversed upon removal of doxycycline (Dox) from the drinking water (Figure 1C). Expression of Kate2 was used in all experiments as a surrogate marker to identify cells expressing rtTA3 (Figure 1D). These experiments highlight the value of CAGs-RIK mice in manipulating eIF4E levels in the hair follicle cells and in using Kate2 to track rtTA3 expression.

Hair growth in mice can be synchronized by depilation and proceeds through 3 stages − anagen (growth phase), catagen (regression phase), and telogen (resting phase) (Figure 2A). 4E.389/CAGs-RIK, 4E.610/CAGs-RIK and FLuc.1309/CAGs-RIK mice were depilated and following a four day recovery period were administered Dox or vehicle for 5 days followed by a single injection of CyP (at day 9 after depilation) (Figure 2B). Following recovery (with no Dox administered during this period) for 12 days, Dox-pretreated 4E.389/CAGs-RIK and 4E.610/CAGs-RIK mice showed full hair re-growth compared to Dox-pretreated FLuc.1309/CAGs-RIK or vehicle-treated mice (Figure 2B). These results indicate that suppression of eIF4E prior to chemotherapy delivery effectively protects against CIA.

To better understand the consequences of eIF4E suppression on the hair follicles of CyP-treated mice, sections were prepared from skin harvested 3 days post-CyP

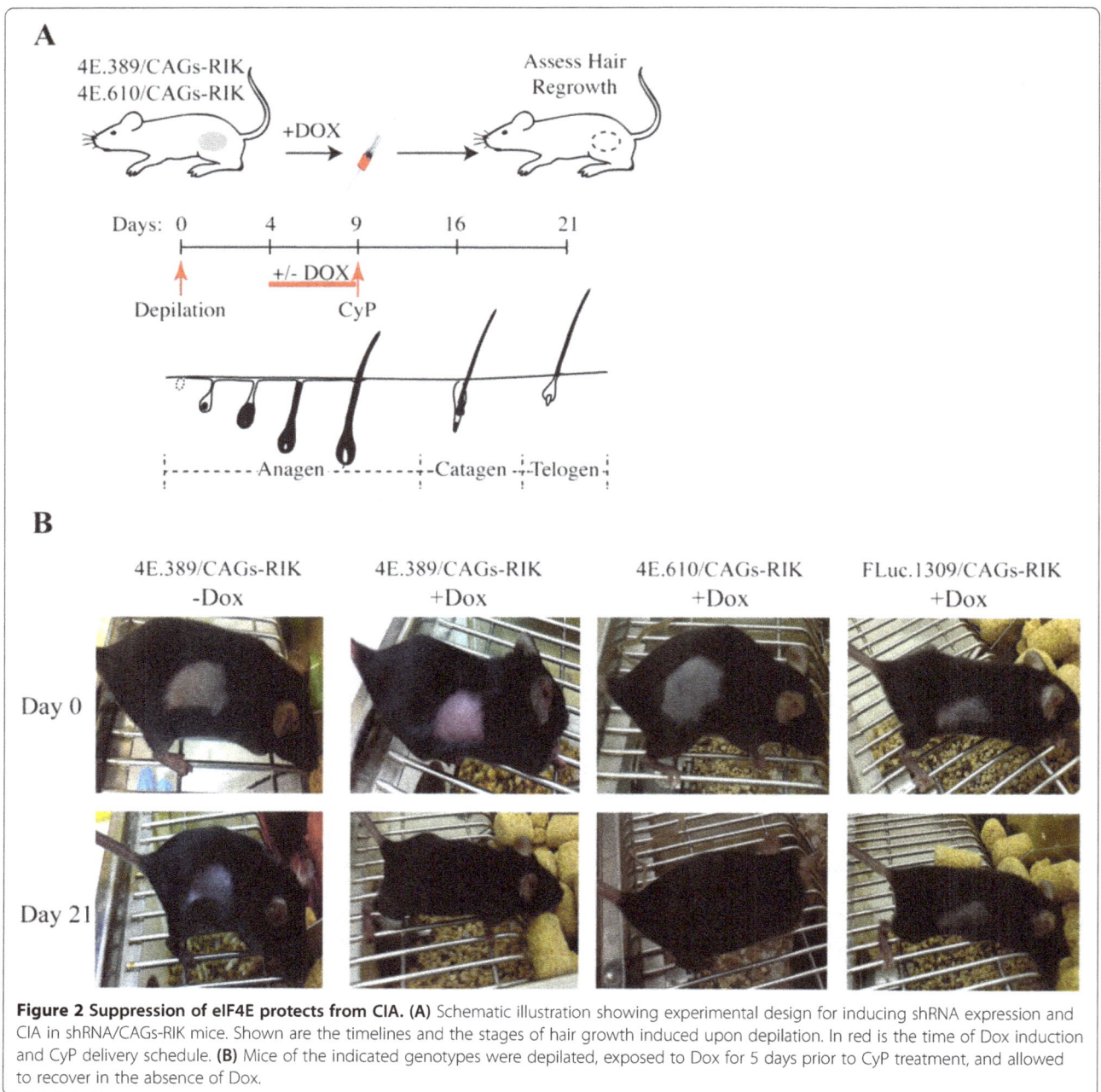

Figure 2 Suppression of eIF4E protects from CIA. (A) Schematic illustration showing experimental design for inducing shRNA expression and CIA in shRNA/CAGs-RIK mice. Shown are the timelines and the stages of hair growth induced upon depilation. In red is the time of Dox induction and CyP delivery schedule. **(B)** Mice of the indicated genotypes were depilated, exposed to Dox for 5 days prior to CyP treatment, and allowed to recover in the absence of Dox.

treatment (Figure 3A). Dox-treated FLuc.1309/CAGs-RIK mice exposed to CyP showed dystrophy of the hair follicles, whereas Dox-treated 4E.389/CAGs-RIK mice exposed to CyP had follicles in the anagen phase - similar to mice that had not been exposed to CyP (Figure 3A, B; H&E stain). eIF4E levels were suppressed in sections of 4E.389/CAGs-RIK mice (Figure 3A; eIF4E) compared to FLuc.1309/CAGs-RIK mice, and this correlated with reduced expression of cyclin D1 (Figure 3A; cyclin D1), a known eIF4E-responsive target [22]. TUNEL staining

revealed a significant proportion of apoptotic hair follicle cells in CyP-treated FLuc.1309/CAGs-RIK mice - as denoted by arrowheads (Figure 3A; TUNEL). In contrast, sections from CyP-treated 4E.389/CAGs-RIK mice in which eIF4E had been suppressed showed little evidence of apoptotic bodies (Figure 3A, C). These results demonstrate that eIF4E suppression prior to CyP treatment protects against CyP-induced apoptosis.

Histopathological examination of the hair follicles from Dox-treated FLuc.1309/CAGs-RIK mice, taken 12 days

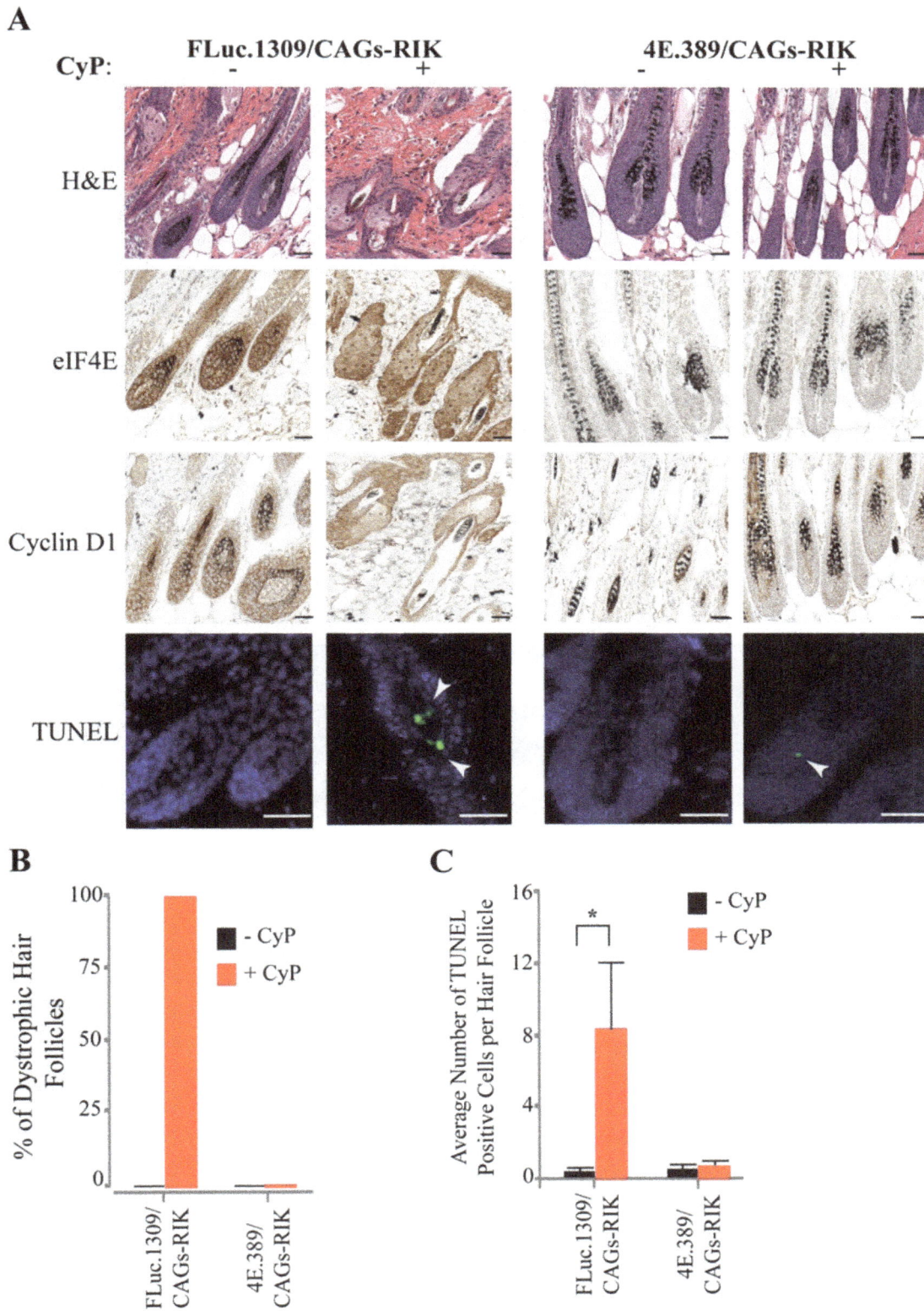

Figure 3 (See legend on next page.)

(See figure on previous page.)
Figure 3 Representative immunostaining of skin sections from Dox-treated shRNA/CAGs-RIK mice 3 days post-CyP. (A) Skin sections from mice of the indicated genotypes were processed for H&E staining, immunostained for the indicated proteins, or processed for visualization of apoptotic bodies as described in the Methods. Bars = 25 μm. **(B)** Percent of dystrophic hair follicles in mice of the indicated genotype taken 3 days after cyclophosphamide delivery. n = 3 mice. Bars denote S.E.M. **(C)** Average number of apoptotic cells per hair follicle. Five different fields (5 follicles/field) were analyzed from sections obtained from 2 different mice. Bars denote S.E.M.

after CyP administration revealed that most were in the end of anagen/early catagen phases and showed remnants of disruption of melanin accumulation (intrafollicular/perifollicular ectopic melanin granules) (Figure 4), an indication of damage-response pathways of the hair follicles after chemotherapy [23]. In contrast, hair follicles of Dox-treated 4E.389/CAGs-RIK mice taken 12 days after CyP administration were in the final catagen or telogen stages (Figure 4), indicating that these follicles had transitioned through the entire growth cycle. At this stage, eIF4E and cyclin D1 expression had returned to normal levels in Dox-treated 4E.389/CAGs-RIK mice compared to Dox-treated FLuc.1309/CAGs-RIK mice (Figure 4).

Suppression of eIF4E or eIF4A protects against chemotherapy induced cell death

To better understand the molecular basis by which suppression of eIF4E leads to protection from chemotherapy-induced damage at the cellular level, we assessed the chemotherapeutic response of non-transformed cells as a consequence of eIF4E inhibition. As a positive control, exposure of hTERT-immortalized BJ cells to nutlin-3a afforded impressive protection to the mitotic poison paclitaxel (PAC) (Figure 5A). Suppression of eIF4E by RNA Interference (RNAi) afforded protection to PAC, as did inhibition of eIF4F activity using the small molecule inhibitor CR131-b (a rocaglamide previously referred to

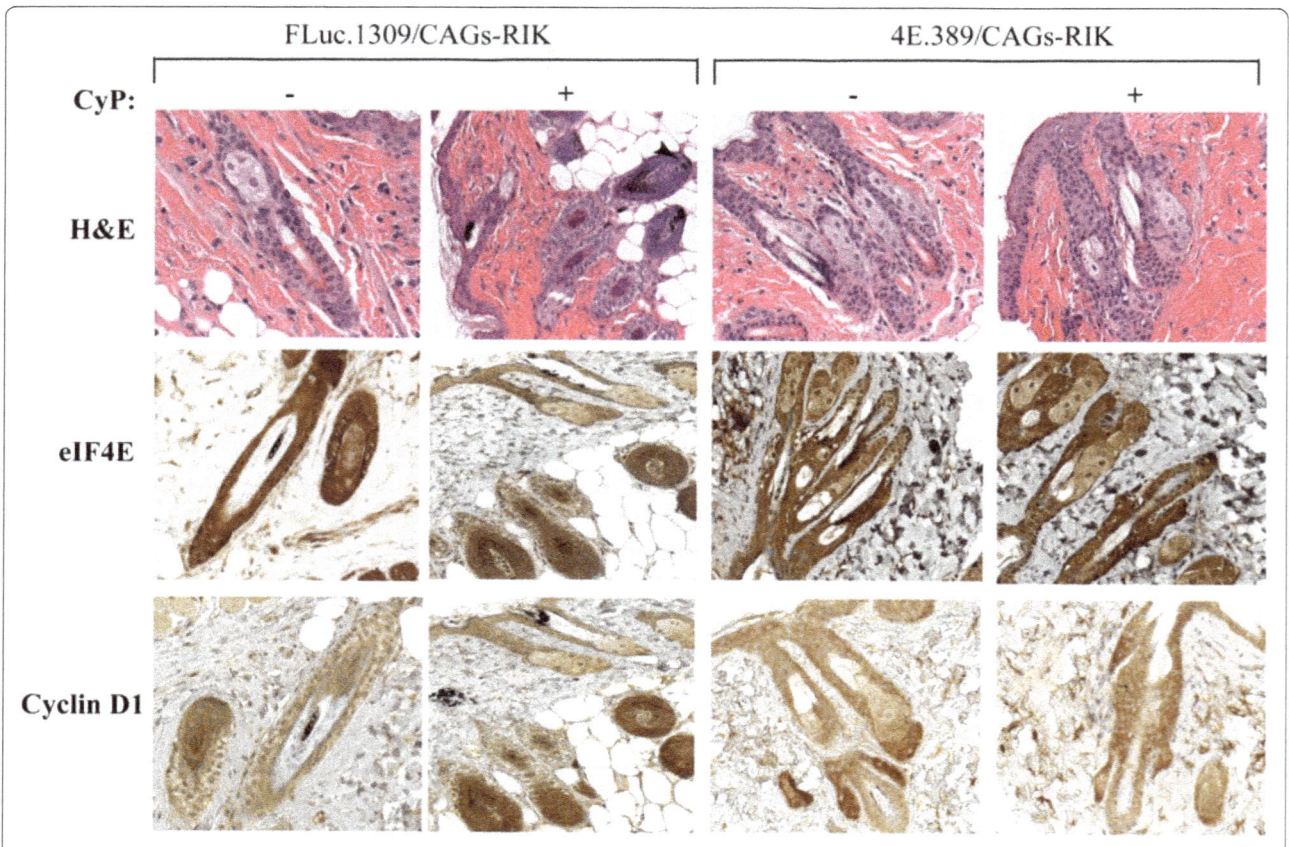

Figure 4 Representative immunostaining of skin sections from Dox-treated shRNA/CAGs-RIK mice 12 days post-CyP exposure. Representative immunostaining of skin sections from Dox-treated mice of the indicated genotype taken 12 days after cyclophosphamide delivery. Bars = 50 μm.

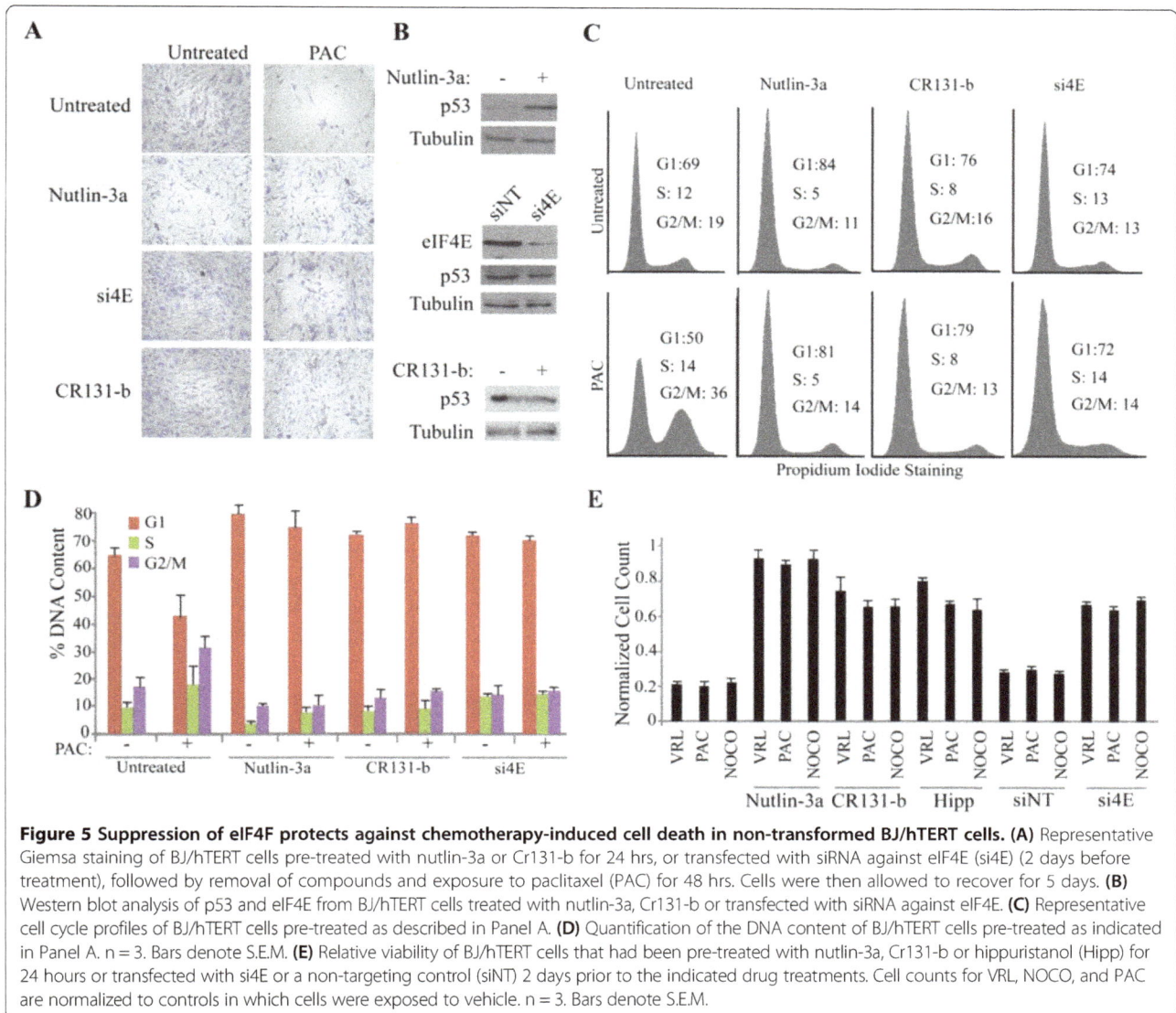

Figure 5 Suppression of eIF4F protects against chemotherapy-induced cell death in non-transformed BJ/hTERT cells. (A) Representative Giemsa staining of BJ/hTERT cells pre-treated with nutlin-3a or Cr131-b for 24 hrs, or transfected with siRNA against eIF4E (si4E) (2 days before treatment), followed by removal of compounds and exposure to paclitaxel (PAC) for 48 hrs. Cells were then allowed to recover for 5 days. **(B)** Western blot analysis of p53 and eIF4E from BJ/hTERT cells treated with nutlin-3a, Cr131-b or transfected with siRNA against eIF4E. **(C)** Representative cell cycle profiles of BJ/hTERT cells pre-treated as described in Panel A. **(D)** Quantification of the DNA content of BJ/hTERT cells pre-treated as indicated in Panel A. n = 3. Bars denote S.E.M. **(E)** Relative viability of BJ/hTERT cells that had been pre-treated with nutlin-3a, Cr131-b or hippuristanol (Hipp) for 24 hours or transfected with si4E or a non-targeting control (siNT) 2 days prior to the indicated drug treatments. Cell counts for VRL, NOCO, and PAC are normalized to controls in which cells were exposed to vehicle. n = 3. Bars denote S.E.M.

as (−)-9 in Ref [24]), which acts as a chemical inducer of dimerization and sequesters eIF4A from the eIF4F complex (Figure 5A) [25]. In these experiments, nutlin-3a induced p53 levels, whereas eIF4E suppression or CR131-b treatment did not, suggesting that the effects of eIF4E or eIF4A suppression on cell survival are not a consequence of p53 induction (Figure 5B).

We examined the cell cycle parameters of BJ/hTERT cells to characterize potential changes caused by the aforementioned treatments (Figure 5C-D). Exposure of BJ/hTERT cells to nutlin-3a or CR131-b, as well as RNAi-mediated suppression of eIF4E, caused an increase in the G1 population (Figure 5C-D). These results were not unique to PAC as these pre-treatments also protected from cell death induced by vinorelbine (VRL, a mitotic poison) and nocodazole (NOCO, a microtubule inhibitor) (Figure 5E and Additional file 1: Figure S1A).

We also tested hippuristanol [26], an eIF4A inhibitor that has a completely different scaffold and mechanism of action compared to CR-131b, and obtained similar results (Figure 5E and Additional file 1: Figure S1A). As well, the eIF4E:eIF4G interaction inhibitors [27], 4E1RCat and 4E2RCat, provided protection from PAC, NOCO and VRL (Additional file 1: Figure S1A-C). These results were recapitulated in MRC5 cells, a non-transformed lung fibroblast cell line (Figure 6) indicating that the protective effects of blocking eIF4F activity are not cell line specific.

To determine if eIF4F activity had to be inhibited prior to drug treatment to obtain the observed protection, we treated BJ/hTERT cells with nutlin-3a, an eIF4A inhibitor (CR-131-b), or eIF4E:eIF4G interaction inhibitors (4E1RCat and 4E2RCat) concomitantly with PAC, NOCO, or VRL and noticed only a weak protection from cell death (Additional file 2: Figure S2). Taken together,

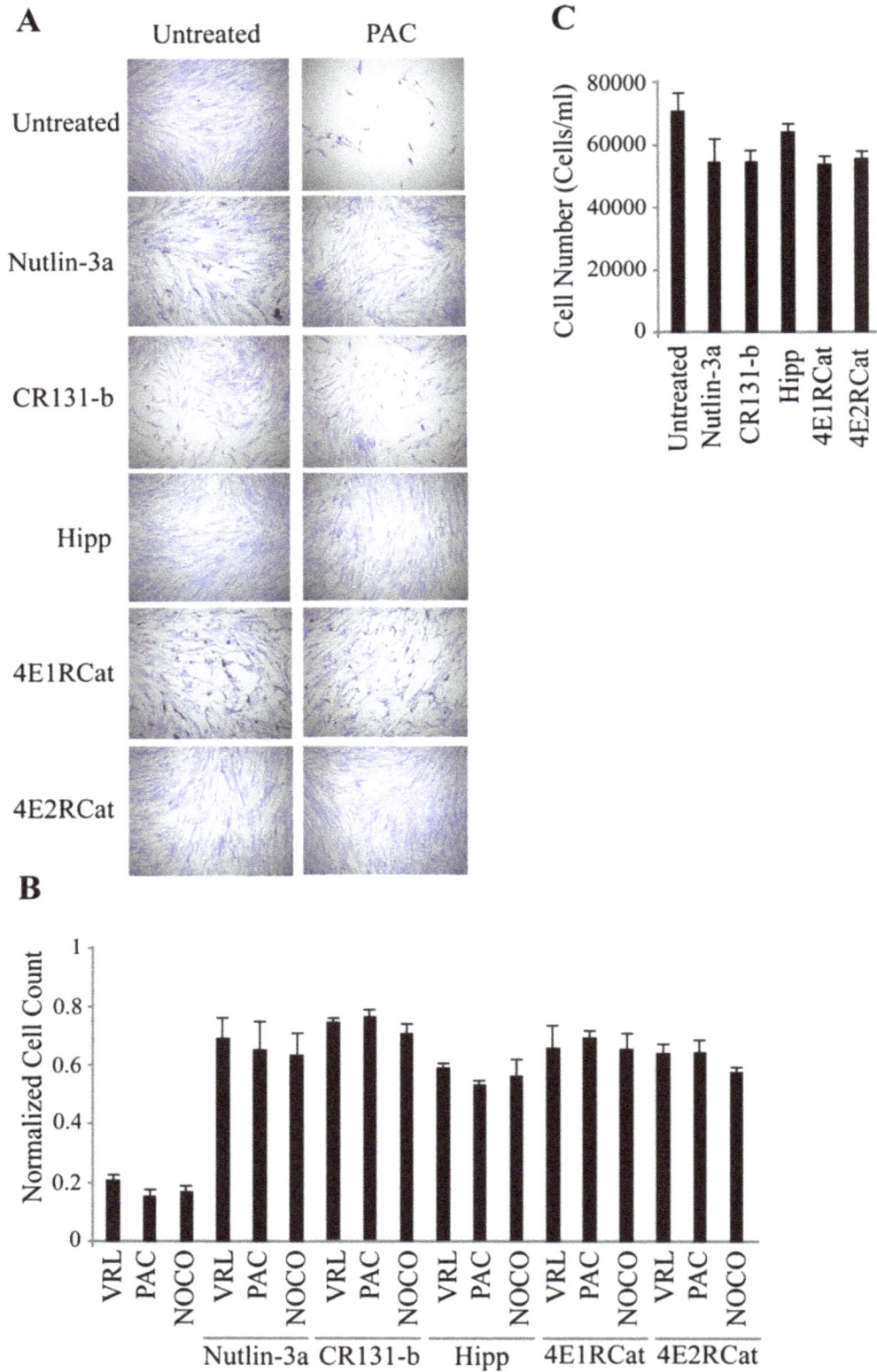

Figure 6 (See legend on next page.)

(See figure on previous page.)
Figure 6 Suppression of eIF4F protects against chemotherapy-induced cell death in non-transformed MRC5 cells. (A) Representative Giemsa staining of MRC5 cells that had been pre-treated with nutlin-3a, Cr131-b, Hipp, 4E1RCat or 4E2RCat for 24 hours , followed by exposure to paclitaxel for 48 hrs. **(B)** Relative viability of MRC5 cells that had been pre-treated with nutlin-3a, Cr131-b, hippuristanol (Hipp), 4E1RCat or 4E2RCat for 24 hours and followed by exposure to 40 nM vinorelbine (VRL), 200 nM nocodazole (NOCO), or 50 nM paclitaxel (PAC) for 48 hrs. Cell counts for VRL, NOCO, and PAC were normalized to controls that had not been pre-treated. n = 3. Bars denote S.E.M. **(C)** Cell numbers after treatment of MRC5 cells with the indicated compounds for 24 hours and left to recover for 7 days. n = 3. Bars denote S.E.M.

these results indicate that suppression of eIF4E or eIF4A, prior to exposure of cells to cytotoxic agents, affords the greatest degree of protection to chemotherapy-induced cell death.

Discussion

Alopecia is a frequent side effect of chemotherapy. Previous experiments of CIA in animal models have suggested the use of small molecule modifiers of the cell cycle to protect against chemotherapy. One example is the use of calcitriol (1,25-dihydroxyvitamin D3), known to induce G0/G1 arrest and inhibit DNA synthesis in keratinocytes [28]. Topical administration of calcitriol is able to protect from CIA in a neonatal rat model [29]. Although calcitriol did not fully protect adult mice from CIA, it facilitated hair re-growth by dampening CyP-induced apoptosis [30,31].

Using a novel transgenic model in which we could inhibit eIF4E expression using inducible shRNA technology, we demonstrated that eIF4E suppression *in vivo* afforded striking protection to CIA. We note that administration of the eIF4A inhibitor, CR131-b, by intravenous injection to depilated mice for 5 consecutive days (once a day at 0.2 mg/kg) prior to CyP delivery failed to protect against CIA (data not shown). We attribute this to inadequate delivery of the compound to the intended target cells and these experiments will require more thorough knowledge of the tissue biodistribution and resident half-life of CR131-b in cells of the hair follicles, as well as appropriate surrogate markers to optimize the *in vivo* dose required to block cell cycling of the intended target cells.

Since inhibition of translation initiation by targeting eIF4F activity leads to accumulation of cells in G1 [14,32-34], it was reasonable to test the ability of several of the current translation initiation inhibitors in cyclotherapy. To date, several small molecules have been identified that either interfere with eIF4E-cap interaction, eIF4E:eIF4G interaction, or eIF4A helicase activity [17]. We showed that suppression of eIF4E, inhibition of the eIF4A helicase, or disruption of the eIF4E:eIF4G interaction provided significant protection to several chemotherapeutics *ex vivo* (Figures 5 and 6 and Additional file 1: Figure S1).

Suppression of eIF4E does not lead to global inhibition of protein synthesis but rather to a selective block in the ribosome recruitment phase of a subset of mRNAs. This would suggest that the expression of specific mRNA transcripts is affected in cells of the hair follicles and responsible for the cell cycle and apoptotic block. One potential mechanism is through reduced expression of cyclin D1, a key cell cycle regulator and known eIF4E target [22,35,36]. We postulate that the reduction of cyclin D1 in the hair follicles during anagen phase (Figure 3) blocks the majority of cells in G1, thus minimizing cell damage by CyP. This would be consistent with the reduction in apoptosis observed (Figure 3). We have not defined the eIF4E responsive mRNAs responsible for blunting CyP-induced apoptosis but this may simply be a consequence of the G1 block imposed by reductions in cyclin D1. Identifying such transcripts would require an unbiased and genome-wide approach to determining those mRNAs whose translation become altered during eIF4E suppression in the hair follicles. Overall, our results are in line with the principles of cyclotherapy [37,38].

We do not expect that eIF4E suppression or eIF4F inhibition will interfere with the efficacy of chemotherapy agents due to the absence of effective cell cycle checkpoints in cancer cells. Indeed, in many documented cases, the opposite is observed – that is, enhanced chemotherapy efficacy (synergy) in the presence of compounds that target translation [25,39-41]. Given that suppressing translation initiation appears a promising approach for cancer therapy, by using small molecule inhibitors of eIF4A or eIF4E:eIF4G interaction or using antisense oligonucleotides (ASOs) against eIF4E [17], the current results offer an added benefit of targeting translation for chemotherapy – that of protecting against CIA.

Conclusions

In this study, we used a novel murine model that serves as a genetic approximation to drug target inhibition. Targeting the translation initiation factor, eIF4E, in non-transformed cells resulted in an accumulation of cells in G1, affording protection against chemotherapy-induced apoptosis. Suppression eIF4E in cells of the hair follicles provided profound protection against chemotherapy-induced alopecia. This correlated with a reduction in cyclin D1 levels and is consistent with a cyclotherapy response. Our results demonstrate the protective effect that inhibiting translation initiation has on minimizing CIA.

Additional files

> **Additional file 1: Figure S1.** Suppression of eIF4F protects against chemotherapy-induced cell death in non-transformed BJ/hTERT cells. **(A)** Cell count for BJ/hTERT cells treated with the indicated compounds or siRNAs for 24 hours and allowed to recover for 7 days. n = 3. Bars denote S.E.M. **(B)** Representative Giemsa staining of BJ/hTERT cells pre-treated with 4E1RCat and 4E2RCat for 24 hours followed by treatment with PAC for 48 hours and allowed to recover for 5 days. **(C)** Relative viability of BJ/hTERT cells that had been pre-treated with 4E1RCat or 4E2RCat for 24 hours followed by exposure to VRL, NOCO, or PAC for 48 hrs and allowed to recover for 5 days. Cell counts for VRL, NOCO, and PAC were normalized to cells exposure to vehicle. n = 3. Bars denote S.E.M.
>
> **Additional file 2: Figure S2.** Simultaneous inhibition of eIF4F with mitotic inhibitors does not protect against chemotherapy-induced cell death. **(A)** Representative Giemsa staining of BJ/hTERT cells treated with nutlin-3a, CR131-b, 4E1RCat or 4E2RCat in conjunction with paclitaxel for 48 hours. **(B)** Relative viability of BJ/hTERT cells that had been treated with nutlin-3a, Cr131-b, 4E1RCat or 4E2RCat and VRL, NOCO, or PAC for 48 hrs, then allowed to recover for 5 days. Cell counts for VRL, NOCO, and PAC were normalized to cells exposed to vehicle. n = 3. Bars denote S.E.M.

Abbreviations

CIA: Chemotherapy-induced alopecia; eIF: Eukaryotic initiation factor; RNA_i: RNA Interference; mTOR: Mammalian target of rapamycin; PI3K: Phosphoinositide 3-kinase; PMSF: Phenylmethylsulfonyl fluoride; FBS: Fetal bovine serum; P/S: Penicillin/Streptomycin; TBS: Tris-buffered saline; GFP: Green fluorescent protein; RMCE: Recombinase-mediated cassette exchange; shRNAs: Short hairpin RNAs; CAGS: Cytomegalovirus enhancer/chicken β-actin promoter; CAGs-RIK: Cytomegalovirus enhancer/chicken β-actin promoter–reverse tetracycline transactivator–internal ribosome entry site–Katushka 2; rtTA3: Reverse tetracycline transactivator 3; Kate2: Katushka 2; SDS: Sodium dodecyl sulfate; PAGE: Polyacrylamide gel electrophoresis; PVDF: Polyvinylidene fluoride; RT: Room temperature; PBS: Phosphate buffered saline; PCR: Polymerase chain reaction; CyP: Cyclophosphamide; Dox: Doxycycline; ECL: Enhanced chemiluminescence; hTERT: Human telomerase reverse transcriptase; PAC: Paclitaxel; VRL: Vinorelbine; NOCO: Nocodazole; Hipp: Hippuristanol; siNT: Non-targetting siRNA control; SEM: Standard error of the mean; TUNEL: Terminal deoxynucleotidyl transferase dUTP nick end labeling.

Competing interests

SWL is founder on the scientific advisory board of Mirimus, Inc., a company that has licensed technology related to the mice used in this lab. All other authors declare they have no competing interests.

Authors' contributions

ZN performed genetic crosses, tissue preparation, immunohistochemical analysis of tissues, cell viability assays, cell cycle analysis, Western blot analysis, and drafted the manuscript. LED designed and characterized the CAGs-RIK mice. MP analyzed all tissue sections and provided expert advice on interpretation of results. JC performed immunohistochemical analysis of mouse tissues. KR, RS, and PD synthesized hippuristanol that was used in this study. JAP synthesized and provided CR-131b. SWL designed the CAGs-RIK mice and revised the manuscript. JP generated the CAGs-RIK mice, designed the study, drafted the manuscript, and revised the manuscript. All authors read and approved the final manuscript.

Acknowledgements

This work was supported by grants from the Canadian Institutes of Health Research (CIHR) (MOP-106530) to J.P and from the National Cancer Institute (NCI) (1U01 CA168409) and a Program Project Grant (P01 CA 87497) to S.L.

Author details

[1]Departments of Biochemistry, McGill University, Montreal, Quebec H3G 1Y6, Canada. [2]Memorial Sloan-Kettering Cancer Center, New York, USA. [3]Département de Pathologie et de Microbiologie, Faculté de Médecine Vétérinaire, Université de Montréal, Saint-Hyacinthe, Québec J2S 2 M2, Canada. [4]Howard Hughes Medical Institute, New York, NY 10065, USA.
[5]Département de Chimie, Université Laval, Ste-Foy, Quebec G1V 0A6, Canada. [6]Center for Methodology and Library Development, Boston University, 590 Commonwealth Ave., Boston, MA 02215, USA. [7]Department of Oncology, McGill University, Montreal, Quebec H3G 1Y6, Canada. [8]The Rosalind and Morris Goodman Cancer Research Center, McGill University, Montreal, Quebec H3G 1Y6, Canada.

References

1.   de Boer-Dennert M, De Wit R, Schmitz PI, Djontono J, V Beurden V, Stoter G, Verweij J: **Patient perceptions of the side-effects of chemotherapy: the influence of 5HT3 antagonists.** Br J Cancer 1997, **76**(8):1055–1061.
2.   Paus R, Haslam IS, Sharov AA, Botchkarev VA: **Pathobiology of chemotherapy-induced hair loss.** Lancet Oncol 2013, **14**(2):e50–59.
3.   Cheok CF, Verma CS, Baselga J, Lane DP: **Translating p53 into the clinic.** Nat Rev Clin Oncol 2011, **8**(1):25–37.
4.   van Leeuwen IM: **Cyclotherapy: opening a therapeutic window in cancer treatment.** Oncotarget 2012, **3**(6):596–600.
5.   Cheok CF, Kua N, Kaldis P, Lane DP: **Combination of nutlin-3 and VX-680 selectively targets p53 mutant cells with reversible effects on cells expressing wild-type p53.** Cell Death Differ 2010, **17**(9):1486–1500.
6.   Carvajal D, Tovar C, Yang H, Vu BT, Heimbrook DC, Vassilev LT: **Activation of p53 by MDM2 antagonists can protect proliferating cells from mitotic inhibitors.** Cancer Res 2005, **65**(5):1918–1924.
7.   Kranz D, Dobbelstein M: **Nongenotoxic p53 activation protects cells against S-phase-specific chemotherapy.** Cancer Res 2006, **66**(21):10274–10280.
8.   Tokalov SV, Abolmaali ND: **Protection of p53 wild type cells from taxol by nutlin-3 in the combined lung cancer treatment.** BMC Cancer 2010, **10**:57.
9.   Sur S, Pagliarini R, Bunz F, Rago C, Diaz LA Jr, Kinzler KW, Vogelstein B, Papadopoulos N: **A panel of isogenic human cancer cells suggests a therapeutic approach for cancers with inactivated p53.** Proc Natl Acad Sci USA 2009, **106**(10):3964–3969.
10. Vassilev LT, Vu BT, Graves B, Carvajal D, Podlaski F, Filipovic Z, Kong N, Kammlott U, Lukacs C, Klein C, et al: **In vivo activation of the p53 pathway by small-molecule antagonists of MDM2.** Science 2004, **303**(5659):844–848.
11. Verma R, Rigatti MJ, Belinsky GS, Godman CA, Giardina C: **DNA damage response to the Mdm2 inhibitor nutlin-3.** Biochem Pharmacol 2010, **79**(4):565–574.
12. Valentine JM, Kumar S, Moumen A: **A p53-independent role for the MDM2 antagonist Nutlin-3 in DNA damage response initiation.** BMC Cancer 2011, **11**:79.
13. Brenner C, Nakayama N, Goebl M, Tanaka K, Toh-e A, Matsumoto K: **CDC33 encodes mRNA cap-binding protein eIF-4E of Saccharomyces cerevisiae.** Mol Cell Biol 1988, **8**(8):3556–3559.
14. Lin CJ, Nasr Z, Premsrirut PK, Porco JA Jr, Hippo Y, Lowe SW, Pelletier J: **Targeting Synthetic Lethal Interactions between Myc and the eIF4F Complex Impedes Tumorigenesis.** Cell Rep 2012, **1**(4):325–333.
15. Lynch M, Fitzgerald C, Johnston KA, Wang S, Schmidt EV: **Activated eIF4E-binding protein slows G1 progression and blocks transformation by c-myc without inhibiting cell growth.** J Biol Chem 2004, **279**(5):3327–3339.
16. Hinnebusch AG, Lorsch JR: **The mechanism of eukaryotic translation initiation: new insights and challenges.** In Protein Synthesis and Translational Control. Edited by John WB, Hershey, Nahum S, Michael B. Mathews: Cold Spring Harbor Laboratory Press; 2012:29–53.
17. Malina A, Mills JR, Pelletier J: **Emerging therapeutics targeting mRNA translation.** In Protein Synthesis and Translational Control. Edited by John WB, Hershey, Nahum S, Michael B. Mathews: Cold Spring Harbor Laboratory Press; 2012:327–343.
18. Premsrirut PK, Dow LE, Kim SY, Camiolo M, Malone CD, Miething C, Scuoppo C, Zuber J, Dickins RA, Kogan SC, et al: **A rapid and scalable system for studying gene function in mice using conditional RNA interference.** Cell 2011, **145**(1):145–158.
19. Cencic R, Carrier M, Galicia-Vazquez G, Bordeleau ME, Sukarieh R, Bourdeau A, Brem B, Teodoro JG, Greger H, Tremblay ML, et al: **Antitumor activity and mechanism of action of the cyclopenta[b]benzofuran, silvestrol.** PLoS ONE 2009, **4**(4):e5223.
20. Paus R, Handjiski B, Eichmuller S, Czarnetzki BM: **Chemotherapy-induced alopecia in mice. Induction by cyclophosphamide, inhibition by**

cyclosporine A, and modulation by dexamethasone. *Am J Pathol* 1994, **144**(4):719–734.

21. Lin CJ, Cencic R, Mills JR, Robert F, Pelletier J: c-Myc and eIF4F are components of a feedforward loop that links transcription and translation. *Cancer Res* 2008, **68**(13):5326–5334.

22. Rousseau D, Kaspar R, Rosenwald I, Gehrke L, Sonenberg N: Translation initiation of ornithine decarboxylase and nucleocytoplasmic transport of cyclin D1 mRNA are increased in cells overexpressing eukaryotic initiation factor 4E. *Proc Natl Acad Sci USA* 1996, **93**(3):1065–1070.

23. Hendrix S, Handjiski B, Peters EM, Paus R: A guide to assessing damage response pathways of the hair follicle: lessons from cyclophosphamide-induced alopecia in mice. *J Invest Dermatol* 2005, **125**(1):42–51.

24. Rodrigo CM, Cencic R, Roche SP, Pelletier J, Porco JA: Synthesis of rocaglamide hydroxamates and related compounds as eukaryotic translation inhibitors: synthetic and biological studies. *J Med Chem* 2012, **55**(1):558–562.

25. Bordeleau ME, Robert F, Gerard B, Lindqvist L, Chen SM, Wendel HG, Brem B, Greger H, Lowe SW, Porco JA Jr, *et al*: Therapeutic suppression of translation initiation modulates chemosensitivity in a mouse lymphoma model. *J Clin Invest* 2008, **118**(7):2651–2660.

26. Bordeleau M-E, Mori A, Oberer M, Lindqvist L, Chard LS, Higa T, Belsham GJ, Wagner G, Tanaka J, Pelletier J: Functional Characterization of IRESes by an inhibitor of the RNA helicase eIF4A. *Nat Chem Biol* 2006, **2**:213–220.

27. Cencic R, Hall DR, Robert F, Du Y, Min J, Li L, Qui M, Lewis I, Kurtkaya S, Dingledine R, *et al*: Reversing chemoresistance by small molecule inhibition of the translation initiation complex eIF4F. *Proc Natl Acad Sci USA* 2011, **108**(3):1046–1051.

28. Wang J, Lu Z, Au JL: Protection against chemotherapy-induced alopecia. *Pharm Res* 2006, **23**(11):2505–2514.

29. Jimenez JJ, Yunis AA: Protection from chemotherapy-induced alopecia by 1,25-dihydroxyvitamin D3. *Cancer Res* 1992, **52**(18):5123–5125.

30. Paus R, Schilli MB, Handjiski B, Menrad A, Henz BM, Plonka P: Topical calcitriol enhances normal hair regrowth but does not prevent chemotherapy-induced alopecia in mice. *Cancer Res* 1996, **56**(19):4438–4443.

31. Schilli MB, Paus R, Menrad A: Reduction of intrafollicular apoptosis in chemotherapy-induced alopecia by topical calcitriol-analogs. *J Invest Dermatol* 1998, **111**(4):598–604.

32. Nasr Z, Robert F, Porco JA Jr, Muller WJ, Pelletier J: eIF4F suppression in breast cancer affects maintenance and progression. *Oncogene* 2013, **32**(7):861–871.

33. Zhou FF, Yan M, Guo GF, Wang F, Qiu HJ, Zheng FM, Zhang Y, Liu Q, Zhu XF, Xia LP: Knockdown of eIF4E suppresses cell growth and migration, enhances chemosensitivity and correlates with increase in Bax/Bcl-2 ratio in triple-negative breast cancer cells. *Med Oncol* 2011, **28**(4):1302–1307.

34. Soni A, Akcakanat A, Singh G, Luyimbazi D, Zheng Y, Kim D, Gonzalez-Angulo A, Meric-Bernstam F: eIF4E knockdown decreases breast cancer cell growth without activating Akt signaling. *Mol Cancer Ther* 2008, **7**(7):1782–1788.

35. Rosenwald IB, Kaspar R, Rousseau D, Gehrke L, Leboulch P, Chen JJ, Schmidt EV, Sonenberg N, London IM: Eukaryotic translation initiation factor 4E regulates expression of cyclin D1 at transcriptional and post-transcriptional levels. *J Biol Chem* 1995, **270**(36):21176–21180.

36. Rosenwald IB, Lazaris-Karatzas A, Sonenberg N, Schmidt EV: Elevated levels of cyclin D1 protein in response to increased expression of eukaryotic initiation factor 4E. *Mol Cell Biol* 1993, **13**(12):7358–7363.

37. Blagosklonny MV, Darzynkiewicz Z: Cyclotherapy: protection of normal cells and unshielding of cancer cells. *Cell Cycle* 2002, **1**(6):375–382.

38. Keyomarsi K, Pardee AB: Selective protection of normal proliferating cells against the toxic effects of chemotherapeutic agents. *Prog Cell Cycle Res* 2003, **5**:527–532.

39. Wendel HG, De Stanchina E, Fridman JS, Malina A, Ray S, Kogan S, Cordon-Cardo C, Pelletier J, Lowe SW: Survival signalling by Akt and eIF4E in oncogenesis and cancer therapy. *Nature* 2004, **428**(6980):332–337.

40. Cencic R, Robert F, Galicia-Vazquez G, Malina A, Ravindar K, Somaiah R, Pierre P, Tanaka J, Deslongchamps P, Pelletier J: Modifying chemotherapy response by targeted inhibition of eukaryotic initiation factor 4A. *Blood Cancer J* 2013, **3**:e128.

41. Robert F, Carrier M, Rawe S, Chen S, Lowe S, Pelletier J: Altering chemosensitivity by modulating translation elongation. *PLoS ONE* 2009, **4**(5):e5428.

3

Antihypertensive drug treatment changes in the general population: the colaus study

Vanessa Christe[1], Gérard Waeber[2], Peter Vollenweider[2] and Pedro Marques-vidal[1*]

Abstract

Background: Changes in antihypertensive drug treatment are paramount in the adequate management of patients with hypertension, still, there is little information regarding changes in antihypertensive drug treatment in Switzerland. Our aim was to assess those changes and associated factors in a population-based, prospective study.

Methods: Data from the population-based, CoLaus study, conducted among subjects initially aged 35–75 years and living in Lausanne, Switzerland. 772 hypertensive subjects (371 women) were followed for a median of 5.4 years. Data Subjects were defined as continuers (no change), switchers (one antihypertensive class replaced by another), combiners (one antihypertensive class added) and discontinuers (stopped treatment). The distribution and the factors associated with changes in antihypertensive drug treatment were assessed.

Results: During the study period, the prescription of diuretics decreased and of ARBs increased: at baseline, diuretics were taken by 46.9% of patients; angiotensin receptor blockers (ARB) by 44.7%, angiotensin converting enzyme inhibitors (ACEI) by 28.8%, beta-blockers (BB) by 28.0%, calcium channel blockers (CCB) by 18.9% and other antihypertensive drugs by 0.3%. At follow-up (approximately 5 years later), their corresponding percentages were 42.8%, 51.7%, 25.5%, 33.0% 20.7% and 1.0%. Among all participants, 54.4% (95% confidence interval: 50.8-58.0) were continuers, 26.9% (23.8-30.2) combiners, 12.7% (10.4-15.3) switchers and 6.0% (4.4-7.9) discontinuers. Combiners had higher systolic blood pressure values at baseline than the other groups (p < 0.05). Almost one third (30.6%) of switchers and 29.3% of combiners improved their blood pressure status at follow-up, versus 18.8% of continuers and 8.7% of discontinuers (p < 0.001). Conversely, almost one third (28.3%) of discontinuers became hypertensive (systolic ≥140 mm Hg or diastolic ≥90 mm Hg), vs. 22.1% of continuers, 16.3% of switchers and 11.5% of combiners (p < 0.001). Multivariate analysis showed baseline uncontrolled hypertension, ARBs, drug regimen (monotherapy/polytherapy) and overweight/obesity to be associated with changes in antihypertensive therapy.

Conclusion: In Switzerland, ARBs have replaced diuretics as the most commonly prescribed antihypertensive drug. Uncontrolled hypertension, ARBs, drug regimen (monotherapy or polytherapy) and overweight/obesity are associated with changes in antihypertensive treatment.

Keywords: Antihypertensive drug therapy, Prospective study, Switzerland, Switching, Persistence, Blood pressure, Combination, Discontinuation

* Correspondence: Pedro-Manuel.Marques-Vidal@chuv.ch
[1]Institute of Social and Preventive Medicine (IUMSP), Lausanne University Hospital, Bâtiment Biopôle 2, Route de la Corniche 10, 1010 Lausanne, Switzerland
Full list of author information is available at the end of the article

Background

Hypertension is an important manageable risk factor of Cardiovascular Diseases (CVD), a major cause of morbidity and mortality worldwide [1], and its prevalence has been estimated at 36% in Switzerland [2]. Hypertension has considerable humanistic and economic consequence [3] and an effective and appropriate treatment must be provided to achieve blood pressure (BP) levels < 140/90 mmHg [4].

In many cases, a lifetime antihypertensive drug treatment is recommended [3] and combination therapy is often necessary to achieve BP control [5]. However, poor adherence to antihypertensive drug treatment has repeatedly been showed: in a Canadian study, 55% of participants on diuretics discontinued treatment after 1 year [6], and a similar discontinuation rate (53%) was found in Italy [7]. The absence of clinical symptoms of hypertension identifiable by the patient along with a low tolerability of certain antihypertensive drugs are the most common explanations why patients stop their treatment or take their medication at inappropriate intervals or wrong doses [3].

In a previous study [2], we assessed the prevalence and management of hypertension in Switzerland. Still, there is little if no information regarding changes in or discontinuation of antihypertensive drug treatment in this country. The aim of this study was thus to assess the therapeutic changes in hypertensive participants treated over a period of approximately five years using data from a population-based, prospective study and to identify the factors associated with those changes.

Methods

The CoLaus study

The sampling procedure of the Cohorte Lausannoise (CoLaus) study has been described previously [8]. The CoLaus study has been accepted by the Ethics Committee of the Canton Vaud and aims at assessing the genetic determinants of cardiovascular disease in the Caucasian population of Lausanne. The non-genetic part of the CoLaus study included all participants, irrespective of their ethnicity. Hence, only Caucasians were included in the main study to avoid population stratification and to increase genetic homogeneity for association studies. Still, non Caucasian subjects were also examined (but not included in the main study). The following inclusion criteria were applied: (i) written informed consent; (ii) age 35–75 years; (iii) willingness to take part in the examination and to have a blood sample drawn. Recruitment began in June 2003 and ended in May 2006. Quickly, the complete list of the Lausanne inhabitants aged 35–75 years (n = 56,694) was provided by the population registry of the city and a simple, nonstratified random sample of 35% was drawn. An invitation letter with a quick description of the study was sent to all randomized participants. Interested individuals were contacted telephonically within 14 days by one of the staff members who provided more information about the study and arranged for an appointment. Participation rate was 41% and 6,733 participants (3,544 women and 3,189 men) were recruited. In this study, all participants, irrespective of their ethnicity, were included.

Baseline risk factor assessment

All participants attended the outpatient clinic of the University Hospital of Lausanne in the morning after an overnight fast (minimum fasting time 8 hours). Data were collected by trained field interviewers in a single visit lasting about 60 min.

Participants received a questionnaire to record information about their status and lifestyle factors. Educational level was stratified into basic, apprenticeship, secondary school and university. Smoking status was classified as never, current or former smoker. Physical activity was defined as the practice of leisure time physical activity at least twice per week. During a face-to-face meeting, family history (mother and father) of myocardial infarction, stroke, hypertension, dyslipidemia or diabetes was collected. No data was available for other first degree relatives such as parents and siblings . Participants were also asked if they had previously experienced myocardial infarction, stroke or any other type of cardiovascular disease such as angina or peripheral artery disease. Personal history of and current treatment for hypercholesterolemia or diabetes were also determined. Information on the use of prescription and over the counter drugs was collected, together with their main indications. Collection was done by asking the participant to bring the drugs to the visit and the number of non-antihypertensive drugs prescribed was assessed.

Body weight and height were measured in light indoor clothes with shoes off. Body weight was measured in kilograms to the nearest 100 g using a Seca® scale, which was calibrated regularly. Height was measured to the nearest 5 mm using a Seca® height gauge. Body Mass Index (BMI) was calculated as weight (kg) divided by the square of the height (m). Overweight was defined by a BMI ≥ 25 kg/m^2 and <30 kg/m^2, and obesity by a BMI ≥ 30 kg/m^2. A similar procedure was performed at follow-up. Waist was measured with a non-stretchable tape over the unclothed abdomen at the narrowest point between the lowest rib and the iliac crest. Two measures were made and the mean (expressed in centimeters) used for analyses. Abdominal obesity was considered for a waist ≥ 102 cm for men and ≥ 88 cm for women [9].

After a median follow-up time of 5.4 years (interquartile range: 5.3–5.6 years), participants were invited to attend a second examination, which included the same assessments as for baseline.

Antihypertensive drug treatment and blood pressure status

The names of all antihypertensive drugs were collected and coded using the Anatomical Therapeutic Chemical (ATC) classification system [10]. In both baseline and follow-up, antihypertensive drugs were classified into six different categories: 1) Diuretics (isolated or associated with other drugs); 2) Calcium channel blockers (CCBs); 3) Beta-blockers (BBs); 4) Angiotensin-converting enzyme inhibitors (ACEIs); 5) Angiotensin receptor blockers (ARB) and 6) Other (reserpine). Combinations were split into the drug classes they contained; for example ATC code C08GA01, corresponding to nifedipine and diuretics, was split into "diuretics associated with other drugs" and "calcium channel blockers". As a single medicine can be a combination of up to three antihypertensive drug classes, two further classifications were used according to the number of antihypertensive drug classes or of antihypertensive pills: monotherapy (i.e. taking a single drug class)/combination therapy and single medicated (i.e. taking a single pill, which can eventually be a combination of drugs)/polymedicated.

According to the evolution of their antihypertensive treatment, participants were assigned into 4 different groups determined by drugs brought to visit at baseline and approximately 5 years later as suggested in a previous study [7]: 1) *Continuers*: participants continuing the initial treatment (including combinations) without changes; 2) *Switchers*: treatment from one class to another class of antihypertensive therapy (for example a CCB for an ARB); 3) *Combiners*: participants treated with an additional type of antihypertensive class but continuing the initial medication (for example adding a diuretic to an ARB) and 4) *Discontinuers*: participants stopping the therapy without having another antihypertensive drug prescription added.

On baseline and follow-up, BP was measured on the left arm, with an appropriately sized cuff. The reading was taken following at least 10 minute rest in the seated position, using an Omron® HEM-907 automated oscillometric sphygmomanometer. Three readings were taken and the average of the last two was used to compute systolic (SBP) and diastolic (DBP) blood pressure. A participant was considered as adequately controlled if her/his SBP was <140 mm Hg and her/his DBP was <90 mm Hg in the absence of diabetes, and if her/his SBP was <130 mm Hg and her/his DBP was <80 mm Hg in the presence of diabetes [11].

Statistical analysis

Statistical analyses were completed using Stata v.12.0 (Stata Corp, College Station, TX, USA). Results were expressed as number of participants (percentage) or as mean ± standard deviation. Between-group comparisons were performed using Chi-square for qualitative variables or Student's t-test or one-way analysis of variance (ANOVA) for quantitative variables. Post-hoc analyses after ANOVA were conducted using the Scheffe method. Multivariate analysis was conducted using Multinomial (polytomous) logistic regression and the results were expressed as relative risk ratio and (95% confidence interval). Statistical significance was considered for $p < 0.05$.

Results

Sample's characteristics

Among the 6,733 participants initially assessed, 4,973 (73.9%) had follow-up data at the present time, of which 772 (15.5%, 371 women) were treated for hypertension at baseline. Their clinical characteristics at baseline are summarized in Additional file 1: Table S1.

Distribution of antihypertensive drug classes

Distribution of antihypertensive drug classes at baseline and follow-up are summarized in Table 1. At baseline, the main antihypertensive classes were diuretics (mainly in association with other antihypertensive drugs) and ARBs, followed by ACE inhibitors and BBs. At follow-up, the percentage of participants on ARBs and BBs increased while the percentage of participants on diuretics and ACE inhibitors decreased. At baseline, almost half of the patients were treated with a single antihypertensive class, and less than one sixth with 3 or more antihypertensive classes. At follow-up, the percentage of participants treated with a single antihypertensive class decreased, while the percentage

Table 1 Antihypertensive drug treatment at baseline and follow-up, CoLaus study

	Baseline	Follow-up
Diuretics (%)	392 (46.9)	330 (42.8)
As main treatment (%)	93 (12.1)	108 (14.0)
Associated with other drugs (%)	293 (38.0)	240 (31.1)
Angiotensin receptor blockers (%)	345 (44.7)	399 (51.7)
Angiotensin converting enzyme inhibitors (%)	222 (28.8)	197 (25.5)
Beta-blockers (%)	216 (28.0)	255 (33.0)
Calcium channel blockers (%)	146 (18.9)	160 (20.7)
Other (%)	2 (0.3)	8 (1.0)
Number of antihypertensive classes (%)		
0	-	46 (6.0)
1	368 (47.7)	293 (38.0)
2	296 (38.3)	270 (35.0)
3+	108 (14.0)	163 (21.0)

Results are expressed as number of participants and (percentage). The total number of participants (772) was used as denominator to calculate percentages.

of patients treated with three or more antihypertensive classes increased to one fifth (Table 1).

Changes in antihypertensive drug treatment

Among all (mono or combination therapy) participants, 54.4% (95% confidence interval: 50.8-58.0) were continuers, 26.9% (23.8-30.2) combiners, 12.7% (10.4-15.3) switchers and 6.0% (4.4-7.9) discontinuers (Table 2). Among participants on monotherapy, the results were 42.1% (37.0-47.3), 35.9% (31.0-41.0), 13.3% (10.0-17.2) and 8.7% (6.0-12.1).

The distribution of continuers, combiners, switchers and discontinuers according to the pharmacological class of the antihypertensive drug is summarized in Figure 1 for participants on monotherapy only. The need for an additional antihypertensive class (combination) were higher in participants treated with CCBs (46.9%), ARBs (39.6%) and diuretics (37.5%). Participants treated with ARBs, ACEIs

Table 2 Baseline individual factors associated with antihypertensive drug changes, CoLaus study

	Continuers	Combiners	Switchers	Discontinuers	p-value
N	420 (54.4)	208 (26.9)	98 (12.7)	46 (6.0)	
Women (%)	213 (50.7)	93 (44.7)	50 (51.0)	15 (32.6)	0.08
Age (years)	60.2 ± 9.0	61.2 ± 8.9	59.2 ± 10.1	57.7 ± 8.2	0.06
Educational status (%)					
Basic	94 (22.4)	46 (22.1)	22 (22.5)	10 (21.7)	
Apprenticeship	186 (44.3)	90 (43.3)	37 (37.8)	18 (39.1)	0.90
High school/college	91 (21.7)	47 (22.6)	26 (26.5)	9 (19.6)	
University	49 (11.7)	25 (12.0)	13 (13.3)	9 (19.6)	
Smoking status (%)					
Never	169 (40.2)	75 (36.1)	43 (43.9)	19 (41.3)	
Former	160 (38.1)	94 (45.2)	35 (35.7)	18 (39.1)	0.67
Current	91 (21.7)	39 (18.8)	20 (20.4)	9 (19.6)	
Physically active (%)	205 (48.8)	100 (48.1)	56 (57.1)	26 (56.5)	0.34
BMI (kg/m^2)	28.4 ± 4.9	29 ± 4.4	27.9 ± 4.9	27.7 ± 4.2	0.15
BMI categories (%)					
Normal	105 (25.0)	36 (17.3)	29 (29.6)	12 (26.1)	
Overweight	181 (43.1)	92 (44.2)	41 (41.8)	26 (56.5)	<0.05
Obese	134 (31.9)	80 (38.5)	28 (28.6)	8 (17.4)	
Waist (cm)	97 ± 14	99 ± 14	95 ± 13	96 ± 12	0.13
Abdominal obesity (%)	219 (52.1)	121 (58.2)	48 (49.0)	16 (34.8)	<0.05
Alcohol drinker (%)	301 (71.7)	160 (76.9)	74 (75.5)	31 (67.4)	0.39
Personal history of (%)					
Myocardial infarction	27 (6.4)	16 (7.7)	2 (2.0)	1 (2.2)	NA
Stroke	11 (2.6)	8 (3.9)	5 (5.1)	1 (2.2)	NA
CVD	52 (12.4)	35 (16.8)	11 (11.2)	6 (13.0)	0.41
Dyslipidemia	182 (43.3)	105 (50.5)	39 (39.8)	19 (41.3)	0.23
Diabetes	64 (15.2)	31 (14.9)	10 (10.2)	4 (8.7)	0.41
Family history of (%)					
Myocardial infarction	110 (26.2)	44 (21.2)	26 (26.5)	14 (30.4)	0.43
Stroke	88 (21.0)	35 (16.8)	23 (23.5)	10 (21.7)	0.51
Hypertension	200 (47.6)	106 (51.0)	49 (50.0)	27 (58.7)	0.51
Dyslipidemia	72 (17.1)	41 (19.7)	19 (19.4)	12 (26.1)	0.48
Diabetes	85 (20.2)	44 (21.2)	20 (20.4)	12 (26.1)	0.83
Number of other drugs [§§]	2.9 ± 2.4	3.1 ± 2.5	3.0 ± 2.2	2.7 ± 2.7	0.80

Results are expressed as mean ± standard deviation or as number of participants and (percentage). [§]defined as the practice of leisure time physical activity at least twice per week; [§§]non-antihypertensive drugs prescribed. BMI, body mass index;. Statistical analysis comparing all groups by Chi-square or one-way analysis of variance: NA, not assessable.

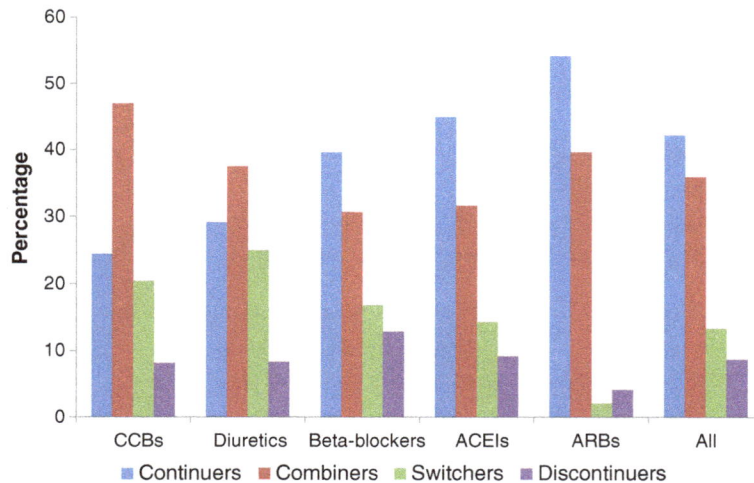

Figure 1 Distribution of continuers, combiners, switchers and discontinuers, according to the pharmacological category of the antihypertensive drug, CoLaus study. ACEIs, angiotensin converting enzyme inhibitors; ARBs, angiotensin receptor blockers; BBs, beta-blockers; CCBs, calcium channel blockers.

and BBs had a better continuation's rate, with a percentage of 54.2%, 44.9% and 33.6% respectively. Finally, treatment switching was more common among participant using diuretics (25.0%), CCBs (20.4%) and BBs (16.8%).

Factors associated with changes in antihypertensive drug treatment

The associations between changes in antihypertensive drug treatment and several personal, family and clinical characteristics at baseline are summarized in Tables 2 and 3. Prevalence of overweight/obesity and abdominal obesity differed between groups, but no differences were found regarding BMI or waist levels. Conversely, no differences were found between groups for personal and family history, number of other prescribed drugs and other clinical and biological variables (Table 2). SBP and DBP differed significantly between groups: combiners presented higher SBP values at baseline than the other

Table 3 Baseline blood pressure factors associated with antihypertensive drug changes, CoLaus study

	Continuers	Combiners	Switchers	Discontinuers	p-value
N	420 (54.4)	208 (26.9)	98 (12.7)	46 (6.0)	
BP status baseline					
SBP (mm Hg)	137 ± 17	146 ± 19	138 ± 16	137 ± 15	<0.001
DBP (mm Hg)	83 ± 11	86 ± 12	83 ± 11	83 ± 9	<0.05
Hypertension§	220 (52.4)	138 (66.4)	54 (55.1)	20 (43.5)	<0.001
Antihypertensive drug					
Diuretics (%)	236 (56.2)	64 (30.8)	47 (48.0)	15 (32.6)	<0.001
Beta-blockers (%)	120 (28.6)	50 (24.0)	30 (30.6)	16 (34.8)	0.38
CCB (%)	76 (18.1)	42 (20.2)	23 (23.5)	5 (10.9)	0.30
ACE inhibitors (%)	119 (28.3)	58 (27.9)	32 (32.7)	13 (28.3)	0.84
ARBs (%)	224 (53.3)	82 (39.4)	26 (26.5)	13 (28.3)	<0.001
Treatment regimen (%)					
One pill, single drug	155 (36.9)	132 (63.5)	49 (50.0)	32 (69.6)	
One pill, combination	119 (28.3)	34 (16.4)	26 (26.5)	7 (15.2)	<0.001
Several pills	146 (34.8)	42 (20.2)	23 (23.5)	7 (15.2)	

Results are expressed as mean ± standard deviation or as number of participants and (percentage). §defined as a systolic blood pressure ≥140 mm Hg or diastolic blood pressure ≥90 mm Hg if absence of diabetes, or as a systolic blood pressure ≥130 mm Hg or diastolic blood pressure ≥80 mm Hg if presence of diabetes. CCB, calcium channel blockers; ACE, angiotensin converting enzyme; ARB, angiotensin receptor blockers. Statistical analysis comparing all groups by Chi-square or one-way analysis of variance.

groups (Scheffe's $p < 0.05$), while for DBP only the difference between combiners and continuers was statistically significant. Combiners and discontinuers took diuretics less frequently, while switchers took ARBs less frequently. Combiners and discontinuers also had the highest prevalence of a one pill, single drug treatment (Table 3).

The results of the multivariate analysis of the factors associated with changes in antihypertensive drug treatment relative to continuers group are summarized in Table 4. Compared to continuers, discontinuers were less likely to be women, to take ARBs and more likely to be on a single pill, single drug regimen. Combiners were more likely to present with uncontrolled blood pressure at baseline, to be on a single pill, single drug regimen and to be overweight or obese. Switchers were less likely to take ARBs (Table 4). No association was found between antihypertensive drug changes and being on a single pill, combination regimen (Table 4). Similarly, in an extended model, no association was found between changes in antihypertensive drug treatment and marital status, educational level, smoking status, being physically active, personal history of CVD, age or number of other non-antihypertensive drugs prescribed (not shown).

Impact of changes in antihypertensive drug treatment on blood pressure status
Compared to continuers, combiners and switchers improved their blood pressure status at follow-up ($p < 0.001$, Table 5). Among continuers, 18.6% improved their blood pressure while 20.7% worsened (net result: 2.1% worsening); the corresponding values for combiners were 28.9% and 13.0% (net result: 15.9% improvement) and for switchers 30.6% and 14.3% (net result: 16.3% improvement). Finally, 8.7% of discontinuers improved their

blood pressure while 26.1% worsened (net result: 17.6% worsening, Table 5).

Continuers with uncontrolled BP at follow-up were more frequently men (54.1% vs. 44.6, $p = 0.05$), were more frequently uncontrolled (55.5% vs. 37.4%, $p < 0.001$) and on diuretics at baseline (15.8% vs. 8.5%, $p < 0.05$), while no differences were found for the other variables (not shown).

Discussion
Distribution of antihypertensive drug classes
The most commonly prescribed antihypertensive drug classes were ARBs and diuretics, a finding in agreement with another Swiss study [4]. The prescription rate for ARBs at follow-up was considerably higher than reported in other countries (51.7% vs. 18-36%) [12] but in accordance with the guidelines of the Swiss Society of Hypertension [13] and others [12]. Indeed, the Swiss guidelines recommend that ACEIs, ARBs, CCBs and diuretics be first line antihypertensives, BBs being considered second line drugs. A possible reason could be the choice of practitioners to prescribe an antihypertensive class with the lowest side effects but just as effective as the others [4]; further, the fact that antihypertensive medication is reimbursed by the Swiss health system might also induce practitioners to choose better tolerated, albeit more expensive antihypertensive drugs. Conversely, the low rate of ACE inhibitor prescriptions was not strictly in keeping with the guideline recommendations at baseline [11,12], which consider ACEIs as first-line antihypertensive drugs. This can be explained by the fact that the guidelines recommend not to combine ACE inhibitors with ARBs for the treatment of hypertension [12]. As ARBs are the most commonly prescribed

Table 4 Multivariate analysis of the baseline factors associated with changes in antihypertensive drug treatment, CoLaus study

	Combiners	Switchers	Discontinuers
Women vs. men	0.79 (0.55 - 1.12)	0.94 (0.60 - 1.48)	0.42 (0.21 - 0.81)
ARB (yes vs. no)	0.77 (0.53 - 1.13)	0.31 (0.18 - 0.52)	0.48 (0.23 - 0.98)
Hypertension (yes vs. no)	1.69 (1.18 - 2.42)	1.09 (0.69 - 1.72)	0.66 (0.35 - 1.23)
Treatment regimen			
Several pills	1 (ref)	1 (ref)	1 (ref)
One pill, combination	1.06 (0.63 - 1.79)	1.78 (0.94 - 3.38)	1.48 (0.49 - 4.47)
One pill, single drug	3.21 (2.06 - 5.00)	1.55 (0.88 - 2.74)	4.06 (1.68 - 9.83)
BMI status			
Normal	1 (ref)	1 (ref)	1 (ref)
Overweight	1.83 (1.13 - 2.95)	0.95 (0.55 - 1.66)	1.52 (0.71 - 3.24)
Obese	2.35 (1.42 - 3.88)	0.96 (0.53 - 1.76)	0.76 (0.29 - 1.98)

ARB, angiotensin receptor blocker; BMI, body mass index. Statistical analysis by multinomial (polytomous) logistic regression, using continuers as the reference group. Hypertension was defined as a systolic blood pressure ≥140 mm Hg or a diastolic blood pressure ≥90 mm Hg. Results are expressed as relative risk ratio and (95% confidence interval).

Table 5 Evolution of blood pressure status according to changes in antihypertensive drug treatment, CoLaus study

	Continuers	Combiners	Switchers	Discontinuers
N	420	208	98	46
C to HT	87 (20.7)	27 (13.0)	14 (14.3)	12 (26.1)
HT to HT	142 (33.8)	78 (37.5)	24 (24.5)	16 (34.8)
C to C	113 (26.9)	43 (20.7)	30 (30.6)	14 (30.4)
HT to C	78 (18.6)	60 (28.9)	30 (30.6)	4 (8.7)

Results are expressed as number of participants and (percentage). C, controlled blood pressure (systolic <140 mm Hg and diastolic <90 mm Hg); HT, hypertension (systolic ≥140 mm Hg or diastolic ≥90 mm Hg). Statistical analysis by Chi-square comparing all BP evolutions between groups: p < 0.001.

drug in our study, this might have led to a decrease in the number of ACE inhibitor prescriptions.

The recent 2013 ESH/ESC guidelines on management of arterial hypertension indicate that diuretics, beta-blockers, calcium antagonists, ACEI and ARBs are all suitable for the initiation and maintenance of antihypertensive treatment [13]. Still, after an approximate follow-up of five years, our results show that diuretics were more frequently replaced and ARBs were more frequently prescribed. Thus, our results suggest that practitioners on everyday's practice tend to switch from diuretics to ARB treatment.

Changes in antihypertensive drug treatment

Almost four out of ten participants (39.6%) changed their antihypertensive drug regimen during an approximately 5.4 year follow-up (26.9% combination and 12.7% switching), a value higher than reported previously (18%) [4]. Conversely, the rate of discontinuers was very low compared to other studies (Additional file 1: Table S2). Possible reasons include more motivated, health-conscious participants, the prescription of better tolerated antihypertensive drugs, and the reimbursement of any type of antihypertensive drug by the Swiss health insurances. Further, it has been shown that a high proportion of patients discontinuing treatment are returning on therapy within 1 year [6]. Hence, it is possible that the high discontinuation rates reported in other studies [7,14] might be overestimated due to a short follow-up time. Overall, our results suggest that, contrary to other countries, antihypertensive drug treatment maintenance is very high in Switzerland when assessed over a period of years.

Discontinuation of diuretics was higher than all other antihypertensive drugs. This is likely to be associated with the well described side effects such as hypotension and/or sodium or potassium abnormalities and/or metabolic disturbance. All side effects known to be associated with ARBs, ACEI, CCB or BB were not specifically recorded for this large population-based study but the discontinuation rate is strictly in agreement with other

studies [15,16] (Additional file 1: Table S3; for a review, see [3]) and in accordance with adverse effects well established in several studies [3,7-19].

Factors associated with changes in antihypertensive drug treatment

Presence of uncontrolled hypertension was positively associated with antihypertensive drug combination, a finding also reported elsewhere [7]. These findings are in agreement with the guidelines of the Swiss Society of Hypertension [13] and others [20] which indicate that combination therapy should be prescribed if monotherapy fails to control blood pressure levels.

Being treated by ARBs was negatively associated with switching or discontinuing antihypertensive drug treatment, a finding in agreement with the literature [7]. The most likely explanation is the lower rate of adverse effects of ARBs relative to the other antihypertensive drugs [19].

Being on a one pill, single drug regimen was positively associated with combining or discontinuing treatment. Indeed, the single drug regimen might favor discontinuation because of fewer co-morbidities and the fact that most patients are symptom-free and might experience more side effects from the treatment than the disease itself [7].

Women had a lower risk of discontinuing antihypertensive drug treatment, a finding in agreement with some studies [21,22] but not with others [23]. Contrary to previous studies [14,24], no association was found between antihypertensive drug changes and smoking, physical activity, marital status, educational level, personal history of cardiovascular diseases. These findings suggest that changes in anti-hypertensive drug treatment are mainly due to factors related to blood pressure and/or to possible side effects of antihypertensive drug treatment rather than to the socio-economic status of the patients.

Impact of changes in antihypertensive drug treatment on blood pressure status

Unlike larger studies [7,14,25], our study was able to assess the impact of antihypertensive drug treatment on blood pressure control. Overall, our results confirm that adjusting the antihypertensive drug regimen leads to favorable changes in blood pressure status. Conversely, discontinuing treatment leads to a deleterious increase in blood pressure levels, which could partly explain the greater incidence of CVD events among discontinuers [25].

Continuers with uncontrolled blood pressure at follow-up were more frequently men, with uncontrolled blood pressure and on diuretics at baseline. These findings suggest that diuretics might be less effective in controlling blood pressure than the other antihypertensive drugs, or that their side effects might lead to a lower compliance and thus worse BP control. Indeed, diuretics have been shown to have the lowest persistence rate of all antihypertensive drugs (Additional file 1: Table S3). They also indicate that practitioners should be more aggressive towards uncontrolled hypertension, as continuing the same treatment will not improve blood pressure control.

Strengths and limitations

The main strength of this study is that it is population-based and used a representative sample of subjects with hypertension. Hence, the conclusions are applicable to the general population and to daily clinical practice compared to those from randomized controlled trials. This study also allowed the analysis of a considerable number of factors associated with antihypertensive drug changes. Further, several studies that assessed changes in antihypertensive drug treatment used only two [1,26,27] or three categories such as "continuers", "switchers" and "discontinuers" [14]. In this study, we opted for a four-category classification as suggested by Mazzaglia and colleagues [7] because it reflected more accurately the behavior of a practitioner when managing a patient with hypertension. Indeed, our results suggest that the factors associated with combining antihypertensive drugs are different from those associated with maintenance of the antihypertensive drug regimen.

This study has also some limitations. Generalization might be limited by the modest participation rate (41%), but this rate is comparable to other epidemiological studies as reported by Wolff and colleagues [28]. It is also possible that the CoLaus participants are more health-conscious than the general population, thus biasing the observed prevalence of discontinuers and data on past medical history and clinical features. Unlike other studies [29], no record of adverse effects was available; hence, the impact of adverse effects of antihypertensive drugs could not be assessed. Further, it was not possible to objectively assess adherence to treatment. Compared to other studies [14,25], our sample size was rather small but blood pressure data was available while in the other studies it was not. Hence, the effect of antihypertensive drug changes could be objectively assessed, while the other studies lacked such information or relied on administrative data only. Participants might present with outdated prescription boxes or may forget to bring a box with them. This may have led to misclassification of the patient's baseline drug therapy status. No information was available regarding dosage of antihypertensive drugs at baseline; thus, no analysis of possible dosage escalation could be performed. Similarly, for logistic and economic reasons no yearly follow-up of the cohort could be performed, so it is possible that therapy adjustments and interventions may have been missed. Although incidence of CVD events was available, it was not possible to establish whether the changes in antihypertensive drug treatment occurred before or after the occurrence of the CVD event. The next follow-up of the cohort will start in April 2014 and will allow evaluating the impact of antihypertensive drug treatment changes in preventing CVD events Finally, we do not know the precise reason(s) for discontinuation, namely if it was a patient or practitioner decision.

Conclusion

In Switzerland, ARBs have replaced diuretics as the most commonly prescribed antihypertensive drug. The percentage of patients with hypertension who discontinue their treatment is considerably lower than in other countries. Uncontrolled hypertension, ARBs, drug regimen (monotherapy or polytherapy) and overweight/obesity are associated with changes in antihypertensive drug treatment.

Additional file

> **Additional file 1: Table S1.** Baseline characteristics of CoLaus participants treated for hypertension (n=772). **Table S2.** Comparison of the proportion of continuers, combiners, switchers, and discontinuers in several studies. **Table S3.** Persistence with initial treatment in different studies.

Competing interests
PV and GW received a research grant from GlaxoSmithKline to conduct the CoLaus baseline Study. The other authors (VC and PMV) indicate no conflict of interest.

Authors' contributions
VC completed part of the statistical analyses and wrote most of the article; PMV collected data, completed part of the statistical analysis and wrote part of the article; PV and GW revised the article for important intellectual content. PMV had full access to the data and is the guarantor of the study. All authors read and approved the final manuscript.

Acknowledgements
The authors also express their gratitude to the participants in the Lausanne CoLaus study and to the investigators who have contributed to the recruitment, in particular Yolande Barreau, Anne-Lise Bastian, Binasa Ramic, Martine Moranville, Martine Baumer, Marcy Sagette, Jeanne Ecoffey, Sylvie Mermoud, Nicole Bonvin, Laure Bovy, Nathalie Maurer, Vanessa Jaquet and Nattawan Laverrière.

Funding
The CoLaus/PsyCoLaus study was and is supported by research grants from GlaxoSmithKline, the Faculty of Biology and Medicine of Lausanne, Switzerland and three grants of the Swiss National Science Foundation (grants #3200B0–105993, #3200B0-118308, #33CSCO-122661 and FN 33CSC0-139468).

Author details
[1]Institute of Social and Preventive Medicine (IUMSP), Lausanne University Hospital, Bâtiment Biopôle 2, Route de la Corniche 10, 1010 Lausanne, Switzerland. [2]Department of Medicine, Internal Medicine, Lausanne University Hospital (CHUV) and Faculty of biology and medicine, Lausanne, Switzerland.

References
1. Elliott WJ, Plauschinat CA, Skrepnek GH, Gause D: **Persistence, adherence, and risk of discontinuation associated with commonly prescribed**

antihypertensive drug monotherapies. *J Am Board Fam Med* 2007, **20**(1):72–80.

2. Danon-Hersch N, Marques-Vidal P, Bovet P, Chiolero A, Paccaud F, Pecoud A, Hayoz D, Mooser V, Waeber G, Vollenweider P: **Prevalence, awareness, treatment and control of high blood pressure in a Swiss city general population: the CoLaus study.** *Eur J Cardiovasc Prev Rehabil* 2009, **16**(1):66–72.

3. Bramlage P, Hasford J: **Blood pressure reduction, persistence and costs in the evaluation of antihypertensive drug treatment–a review.** *Cardiovasc Diabetol* 2009, **8**:18.

4. Brenner R, Waeber B, Allemann Y: **Medical treatment of hypertension in Switzerland. The 2009 Swiss Hypertension Survey (SWISSHYPE).** *Swiss Med Wkly* 2011, **141**:w13169.

5. Brixner DI, Jackson KC 2nd, Sheng X, Nelson RE, Keskinaslan A: **Assessment of adherence, persistence, and costs among valsartan and hydrochlorothiazide retrospective cohorts in free-and fixed-dose combinations.** *Curr Med Res Opin* 2008, **24**(9):2597–2607.

6. Bourgault C, Senecal M, Brisson M, Marentette MA, Gregoire JP: **Persistence and discontinuation patterns of antihypertensive therapy among newly treated patients: a population-based study.** *J Hum Hypertens* 2005, **19**(8):607–613.

7. Mazzaglia G, Mantovani LG, Sturkenboom MC, Filippi A, Trifiro G, Cricelli C, Brignoli O, Caputi AP: **Patterns of persistence with antihypertensive medications in newly diagnosed hypertensive patients in Italy: a retrospective cohort study in primary care.** *J Hypertens* 2005, **23**(11):2093–2100.

8. Firmann M, Mayor V, Vidal PM, Bochud M, Pecoud A, Hayoz D, Paccaud F, Preisig M, Song KS, Yuan X, Danoff TM, Stirnadel HA, Waterworth D, Mooser V, Waeber G, Vollenweider P: **The CoLaus study: a population-based study to investigate the epidemiology and genetic determinants of cardiovascular risk factors and metabolic syndrome.** *BMC Cardiovasc Disord* 2008, **8**:6.

9. Lean ME, Han TS, Morrison CE: **Waist circumference as a measure for indicating need for weight management.** *BMJ* 1995, **311**(6998):158–161.

10. **Anatomical Therapeutic Chemical (ATC) classification system.** http://www.whocc.no/atc/structure_and_principles/.

11. **2009 Swiss Society of Hypertension Guidelines.** http://swisshypertension. ch/guidelines.htm.

12. **Hypertension: Clinical Management of Primary Hypertension in Adults.** http://publications.nice.org.uk/hypertension-cg127/guidance#choosing-antihypertensive-drug-treatment-2.

13. Mancia G, Fagard R, Narkiewicz K, Redon J, Zanchetti A, Böhm M, Christiaens T, Cifkova R, De Backer G, Dominiczak A, Galderisi M, Grobbee DE, Jaarsma T, Kirchhof P, Kjeldsen SE, Laurent S, Manolis AJ, Nilsson PM, Ruilope LM, Schmieder RE, Sirnes PA, Sleight P, Viigimaa M, Waeber B, Zannad F, Dominiczak A, Narkeiwicz K, Nilsson PM, Burnier M, Viigimaa M, et al: **2013 ESH/ESC guidelines for the management of arterial hypertension: the task force for the management of arterial hypertension of the European Society of Hypertension (ESH) and of the European Society of Cardiology (ESC).** *Eur Heart J* 2013, **34**(28):2159–219.

14. Degli Esposti L, Degli Esposti E, Valpiani G, Di Martino M, Saragoni S, Buda S, Baio G, Capone A, Sturani A: **A retrospective, population-based analysis of persistence with antihypertensive drug therapy in primary care practice in Italy.** *Clin Ther* 2002, **24**(8):1347–1357. discussion 1346.

15. Veronesi M, Cicero AF, Prandin MG, Dormi A, Cosentino E, Strocchi E, Borghi C: **A prospective evaluation of persistence on antihypertensive treatment with different antihypertensive drugs in clinical practice.** *Vasc Health Risk Manag* 2007, **3**(6):999–1005.

16. Lachaine J, Petrella RJ, Merikle E, Ali F: **Choices, persistence and adherence to antihypertensive agents: evidence from RAMQ data.** *Can J Cardiol* 2008, **24**(4):269–273.

17. Aellig WH: **Adverse reactions to antihypertensive therapy.** *Cardiovasc Drugs Ther* 1998, **12**(2):189–196.

18. Gregoire JP, Moisan J, Guibert R, Ciampi A, Milot A, Cote I, Gaudet M: **Tolerability of antihypertensive drugs in a community-based setting.** *Clin Ther* 2001, **23**(5):715–726.

19. Chen K, Chiou CF, Plauschinat CA, Frech F, Harper A, Dubois R: **Patient satisfaction with antihypertensive therapy.** *J Hum Hypertens* 2005, **19**(10):793–799.

20. Sever PS, Messerli FH: **Hypertension management 2011: optimal combination therapy.** *Eur Heart J* 2011, **32**(20):2499–2506.

21. Friedman O, McAlister FA, Yun L, Campbell NR, Tu K, Canadian Hypertension Education Program Outcomes Research T: **Antihypertensive drug persistence and compliance among newly treated elderly hypertensives in ontario.** *Am J Med* 2010, **123**(2):173–181.

22. Bautista LE: **Predictors of persistence with antihypertensive therapy: results from the NHANES.** *Am J Hypertens* 2008, **21**(2):183–188.

23. Erkens JA, Panneman MM, Klungel OH, van den Boom G, Prescott MF, Herings RM: **Differences in antihypertensive drug persistence associated with drug class and gender: a PHARMO study.** *Pharmacoepidemiol Drug Saf* 2005, **14**(11):795–803.

24. Ho PM, Spertus JA, Masoudi FA, Reid KJ, Peterson ED, Magid DJ, Krumholz HM, Rumsfeld JS: **Impact of medication therapy discontinuation on mortality after myocardial infarction.** *Arch Intern Med* 2006, **166**(17):1842–1847.

25. Corrao G, Zambon A, Parodi A, Merlino L, Mancia G: **Incidence of cardiovascular events in Italian patients with early discontinuations of antihypertensive, lipid-lowering, and antidiabetic treatments.** *Am J Hypertens* 2012, **25**(5):549–555.

26. Weiss R, Buckley K, Clifford T: **Changing patterns of initial drug therapy for the treatment of hypertension in a Medicaid population, 2001–2005.** *J Clin Hypertens (Greenwich)* 2006, **8**(10):706–712.

27. Wong MC, Jiang JY, Griffiths SM: **Switching of antihypertensive drugs among 93,286 Chinese patients: a cohort study.** *J Hum Hypertens* 2010, **24**(10):669–677.

28. Wolf HK KK, Tolonen H, Ruokokoski E: **Participation Rates, Quality of Sampling Frames and Sampling Fractions in the MONICA Surveys.** In *WHO MONICA*; 1998. Available at www.thl.fi/publications/monica/nonres/ nonres.htm assessed May 2013.

29. Engel-Nitz NM, Darkow T, Lau H: **Antihypertensive medication changes and blood pressure goal achievement in a managed care population.** *J Hum Hypertens* 2010, **24**(10):659–668.

The association between statin therapy during intensive care unit stay and the incidence of venous thromboembolism: a propensity score-adjusted analysis

Shmeylan A Al Harbi[1], Mohammad Khedr[2], Hasan M Al-Dorzi[2], Haytham M Tlayjeh[3], Asgar H Rishu[3] and Yaseen M Arabi[2]*

Abstract

Background: Studies have shown that statins have pleiotropic effects on inflammation and coagulation; which may affect the risk of developing venous thromboembolism (VTE). The objective of this study was to evaluate the association between statin therapy during intensive care unit (ICU) stay and the incidence of VTE in critically ill patients.

Methods: This was a post-hoc analysis of a prospective observational cohort study of patients admitted to the intensive care unit between July 2006 and January 2008 at a tertiary care medical center. The primary endpoint was the incidence of VTE during ICU stay up to 30 days. Secondary endpoint was overall 30-day hospital mortality. Propensity score was used to adjust for clinically and statistically relevant variables.

Results: Of the 798 patients included in the original study, 123 patients (15.4%) received statins during their ICU stay. Survival analysis for VTE risk showed that statin therapy was not associated with a reduction of VTE incidence (crude hazard ratio (HR) 0.66, 95% confidence interval (CI) 0.28-1.54, P = 0.33 and adjusted HR 0.63, 95% CI 0.25-1.57, P = 0.33). Furthermore, survival analysis for hospital mortality showed that statin therapy was not associated with a reduction in hospital mortality (crude HR 1.26, 95% CI 0.95-1.68, P = 0.10 and adjusted HR 0.98, 95% CI 0.72-1.36, P = 0.94).

Conclusion: Our study showed no statistically significant association between statin therapy and VTE risk in critically ill patients. This question needs to be further studied in randomized control trials.

Keywords: Venous thromboembolism, Outcome assessment, Intensive care, Hospital mortality, Propensity scores, Statins

Background

Venous thromboembolism (VTE), encompassing deep vein thrombosis (DVT) and pulmonary embolism (PE), is a common complication of critical illness and is associated with significant morbidity and mortality [1,2]. In general, the incidence of VTE is 1–2 per 1,000 individuals per year [3] and reaches 1% per year in those aged over 70 years [4]. In critically ill patients, the incidence has been reported up to 10% despite thromboprophylaxis [2]. Statins (Hydroxy-3- methylglutaryl conenzyme A reductase inhibitors) have demonstrated efficacy in reducing cholesterol levels and improving cardiovascular outcomes when administered for both primary and secondary indications. Additionally, through their effects on inflammation and coagulation [5], statins may have antithrombotic properties that can affect not only arterial but also venous thrombosis. Although, venous and arterial thrombosis have largely been considered separate diseases [6-8], multiple studies have suggested that they

* Correspondence: yaseenarabi@yahoo.com
[2]College of Medicine, King Saud bin Abdulaziz University for Health Sciences, King Abdulaziz Medical City, MC 1425, PO Box 22490, Riyadh 1426, Saudi Arabia
Full list of author information is available at the end of the article

both share certain risk factors, pathogenesis and possibly statin effects [9-11]. The antithrombotic properties of statins may be related to decreasing platelet aggregation, inhibition of tissue factor and plasminogen activator-inhibitor 1 expression, increasing expression of tissue plasminogen activator activity, and increasing expression of thrombomodulin that activates protein C and prevent thrombin-induced platelet and factor V activation and fibrinogen clotting [12,13]. Clinical studies have yielded variable estimates of the statin effect on VTE [14-19]. Observational studies in outpatient population as well as one randomized controlled trial in healthy older adults have suggested a protective effect of statin therapy [14-17]. In critically ill medical-surgical patients, there are limited studies examining this association. Therefore, we sought to assess the association between statins and VTE incidence in a cohort of critically ill patients.

Methods

Setting

The study was conducted in the adult medical-surgical intensive care unit (ICU) of King Abdulaziz Medical City, a tertiary care academic referral center in Riyadh, Saudi Arabia. The ICU admits medical, surgical, and trauma patients, and operates as a closed unit with 24-hr, 7-day onsite coverage by critical care board certified intensivists [20]. The nurse-to-patient ratio in the unit is approximately 1:1.2.

Study design

This is a post-hoc analysis of a recently published cohort study of the effect of mechanical thromboprophylaxis, intermittent pneumatic compression (IPC) or graduated compression stocking (GCS) on the incidence of VTE in patients admitted to the ICU between July 2006 and January 2008 [21]. The original study included 798 patients. Inclusion criteria were age ≥18 years and expected ICU length of stay of more than 48 hours. Patients were excluded if they were on therapeutic anticoagulation with warfarin or heparin, admitted to the ICU with acute PE, DVT, or had do-not-resuscitate or brain death status on or within first 24 hours of ICU admission. The patients were followed for a total of 30 days from admission to ICU. The study was approved by institutional review board of the hospital. The analysis included all patients who were in the original cohort study. Informed consent was not required.

Statin therapy

Data about statin therapy in the ICU were collected from the ICU pharmacy database and were matched and combined to the original clinical study database [21]. Statins were continued if they had been prescribed in the pre-ICU period or could have been initiated in the

ICU for patients admitted with stroke or acute coronary syndrome. Dosage was at the discretion of the treating physician.

Data collection

We used the following data for the analysis: age, Acute Physiology and Chronic Health Evaluation (APACHE II) score [22], admission Glasgow coma scale (GCS) score, creatinine, international normalized ratio (INR), activated partial thromboplastin time (aPTT), diagnosis of trauma, femur fracture, presence of central line, bedridden status for more than 3 days whether this was at home or in the hospital, malignancy, recent surgery, previous VTE, presence of hemodialysis catheter, the use of graduated compression stocking, the use of intermittent pneumatic compression device, the use of unfractionated heparin or enoxaparin, packed red blood cells (PRBC) and platelet transfusion. The use of aspirin was tested later in a separate analysis.

Outcomes

The primary outcome was the effect of statin therapy on VTE incidence (lower extremities DVT, PE, or both) during the ICU stay and up to 5 days after ICU discharge. Overall 30-day hospital mortality was secondary outcome. In this study, VTE was clinically ascertained and confirmed either by Doppler ultrasound for DVT or by helical chest tomography for PE.

Statistical analysis

Due to the non-random allocation of study groups, propensity scores were used to balance baseline characteristics (Table 1). The scores were derived from a logistic regression model using "pscore" program in Stata/SE version 11 for Windows (StatCorp LP, College Station, TX, USA). The model satisfied Hosmer-Lemeshow goodness-of-fit test ($P = 0.41$) and showed excellent discrimination ability (the area under ROC = 84%). The derived propensity scores were then divided into 6 blocks and used later in analysis as stratification factor or as an adjusting covariate. Variables included in the propensity score generation model were selected according to their relationship to the outcome (VTE) rather than the exposure (statin therapy). However, some of these variables were also related to the exposure. This approach is one of three possible ways (related to exposure and outcome, related to outcome alone, and related to exposure alone) for variable selection. It has been shown to reduce bias and variance of estimated exposure effect [23,24]. Those variables were: age, APACHE II score, GCS, diagnosis of trauma, presence of femur fracture, creatinine level, INR, aPTT level, central venous line presence, history of malignancy, recent surgery, history of previous VTE, PRBC and platelet transfusion, hemodialysis catheter

Table 1 Baseline characteristics of the statins and non-statin therapy groups

	Statin (n =123)	Non-Statin (n = 675)	P-value	PS Adjusted P-Value
Age, mean ± SD, years	67.1 ± 11.3	47.1 ± 21.1	<0.001	0.59
APACHE II, mean ± SD	26.7 ± 8.1	23.5 ± 9.1	0.0002	0.90
GCS, mean ± SD,	9.0 ± 4.6	8.5 ± 4.0	0.20	0.96
Creatinine, mean ± SD, µmol/L*	228.0 ± 179.3	146.4 ± 133.8	<0.001	0.81
INR, mean ± SD	1.3 ± 0.5	1.4 ± 0.7	0.03	0.93
aPTT, mean ± SD,	43.4 ± 57.1	42.2 ± 60.8	0.83	1.00
Trauma, No%	3 (2.4)	223 (33.0)	<0.001	0.007
Femur fracture, No.%	2 (1.6)	50 (7.4)	0.02	0.45
Any central line present, No. (%)	91(74.0)	504 (74.7)	0.87	0.78
Bedridden for > 3 days, No. (%)	84 (68.3)	310 (45.9)	<0.001	0.44
Malignancy, No. (%)	8 (6.5)	86 (12.7)	0.05	0.77
Recent surgery, No. (%)	22 (17.9)	221(32.7)	0.001	0.65
Previous VTE, No. (%)	4 (3.3)	8 (1.2)	0.08	0.98
Hemodialysis catheter, No. (%)	33 (26.8)	125 (18.5)	0.03	0.71
Compression stocking, No. (%)	26 (21.1)	172 (25.5)	0.31	0.79
Sequential compression device, No. (%)	29 (23.6)	227 (33.6)	0.03	0.75
Unfractionated heparin, No. (%)	97 (78.9)	405 (60.0)	<0.001	0.58
Enoxaparin, No. (%)	16 (13.0)	212 (31.4)	<0.001	0.21
Platelet transfusion, No. (%)	12 (9.8)	132 (19.6)	0.009	0.97

P-values are provided for the differences between the two groups significant before and after propensity score adjustment.
APACHE: Acute physiology and chronic health evaluation, GCS: Glasgow coma scale, INR: International normalized ratio.
aPTT: activated partial thromboplastin time, VTE: Venous thromboembolism, PS: propensity score.
*To convert to conventional units in mg/dL, divide by 88.4.

use, use of graduated compression stocking, use of intermittent pneumatic compression device, and unfractionated heparin or enoxaparin.

For hospital mortality analysis, follow-up time was censored at 30 days or at the time of hospital discharge if less than 30 days. Cox-proportional hazard regression was used to evaluate the effect of statins on the incidence of VTE. In addition to crude model, propensity score stratified, propensity score-adjusted and multivariate-adjusted models were assembled for verification. The potential cofounder effect of aspirin use was tested with multivariate models for both VTE and hospital mortality. Hazard ratios (HR) were derived and presented with their 95% confidence intervals (CI). All tests were considered significant at 0.05 alpha level.

Results

Patient's characteristics

Baseline characteristics are shown in Table 1. Of the 798 patients enrolled in the study, 123 (15.4%) received statins during their ICU stay and 57 (7.1%) patients developed VTE (Table 2). Patients who received statins were more likely to be bedridden and had higher BMI. In contrast, non-statin therapy group were more likely to be admitted with the diagnosis of trauma. Atorvastatin was

used in 100 patients (81%) at doses 10 to 40 mg/day and simvastatin was used in 23 patients (19%) at 20 mg/day.

VTE occurred in 6 (7.6%) patients in the statin therapy group and 51 (4.9%) patients in the non-statin therapy group (Table 2). The median follow-up time for statin-therapy and non statin-therapy groups were 17 days (IQR 7–30) and 14 days (IQR 7–26), respectively.

Statins were not associated with reduced VTE incidence on univariate analysis (HR 0.66, 95% CI 0.28-1.54, P = 0.33) and on propensity score stratified analysis (HR 0.63, 95% CI 0.25-1.57, P = 0.33) (Table 3 and Figure 1). The analyses using propensity score as an adjustment variable and multivariate analysis revealed similar findings. Adding aspirin as covariate to the multivariate model did not alter the results.

Table 2 Distribution of hospital mortality and VTE cumulative incidence according to statin use

Statin use*	Hospital mortality**	Incident VTE**
(n,%)	n (%)	n (%)
Yes (123, 15.4%)	58(47.2%)	6 (7.6%)
No (675, 84.6%)	256 (38%)	51 (4.9%)
Total (798)	314 (39.4%)	57 (7.1%)

*Numbers between parentheses reflect counts and percentages, respectively.
**Numbers between parentheses reflect percentage within statin category.

Table 3 Crude and PS stratified analysis of VTE risk and Hospital Mortality in statin and non-statin groups

Type of analysis	HR	SE	95% CI	P-value
VTE risk				
Crude analysis	0.66	0.29	(0.28-1.54)	0.33
PS stratified analysis*	0.63	0.29	(0.25-1.57)	0.33
Hospital Mortality				
Crude analysis	1.26	0.18	(0.95-1.68)	0.10
PS stratified analysis*	0.98	0.16	(0.72-1.36)	0.94

*Adjusted for age, APACHE II score, GCS, creatinine, INR, aPTT, Trauma, femoral fracture, central line presence, malignancy, recent surgery, previous VTE, hemodialysis catheter use, use of graduated compression stocking, use of sequential compression device, DVT prophylaxis with unfractionated heparin or enoxaparin, and platelet transfusion.

Hospital mortality

During the study, there were 58 (47.2%) deaths in statin-therapy group and 256 (38%) deaths in no-statin therapy group (Table 2). Statin therapy was not associated with reduction of hospital mortality on crude analysis (HR 1.26, 95% CI 0.95-1.68, P = 0.10) (Table 3 and Figure 2) or on stratified propensity score analysis (HR 0.98, 95% CI 0.72-1.36, P = 0.94). The analyses using propensity score as an adjustment variable and multivariate analysis revealed similar findings. Adding aspirin to the multivariate model did not alter the result.

Discussion

Our data failed to show a statistically significant reduction in VTE incidence and hospital mortality by continuing statin therapy during patients stay in ICU.

Several other studies have shown that statin therapy reduces VTE incidence but in outpatient settings. The Heart and Estrogens/Progestin Replacement Study of postmenopausal women with heart disease was the first to indicate a relationship between statin therapy and the

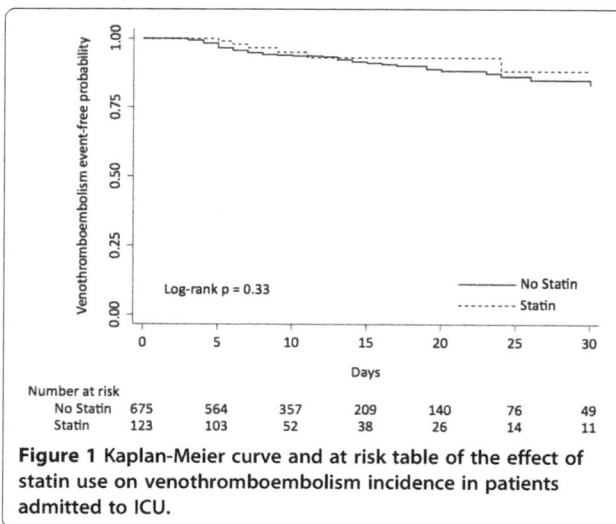

Figure 2 Kaplan-Meier curve and risk table of the effect of statin use on hospital mortality in patients admitted to ICU.

reduction in VTE risk, showing >50% decrease in VTE events among statin users compared with non-users (HR 0.45, 95% CI 0.23-0.88) [14]. Likewise, Doggen et al. found that statin therapy, among postmenopausal women, was associated with reduction in VTE risk (odds ratio [OR] 0.64, 95% CI 0.39-1.07) [15]. The association was observed in patients on simvastatin (OR 0.51, 95% CI 0.29-0.91) but not in patients on pravastatin (OR1.85, 95% CI 0.65-5.26) [15]. In a retrospective cohort study (N = 125, 862) over 8 years, Ray et al. found that statins were associated with significant DVT risk reduction (HR 0.78, 95% CI 0.69-0.87) among outpatient individuals aged ≥ 65 years [16]. In an age and sex-matched case–control study of hospitalized patients, Lacut et al. found that statin therapy was associated with a significant reduction in the risk of VTE (OR 0.42, 95% CI 0.23-0.76) [25]. In another population-based case–control study, Sorensen et al. found reduction in VTE risk (relative risk of 0.74, 95% CI (0.63-0.85)) in current statin therapy, which was observed whether simvastatin, pravastatin or atorvastatin was used [26]. Further, Ramcharan et al. found, in another population-based case–control study, that the current statin therapy was associated with lower risk of VTE in patients aged 18–70 years (adjusted OR 0.45, 95% CI 0.36-0.56) and this association was observed in all statins, including simvastatin, pravastatin, atorvastatin, fluvastatin, and rosuvastatin [27].

In contrast, two retrospective studies failed to demonstrate a benefit of statin therapy on VTE risk reduction. Yang et al. found no association between current, recent, or past statin therapy and the risk of VTE (OR 1.1, 95% CI 0.3-4.3) [18]. In a large population-based cohort study with a median follow-up period of 4.4 years using a propensity score-based adjustment, Smeeth et al. showed no VTE protective effect with statin therapy (adjusted HR 1.02, 95% CI 0.88-1.18) [19].

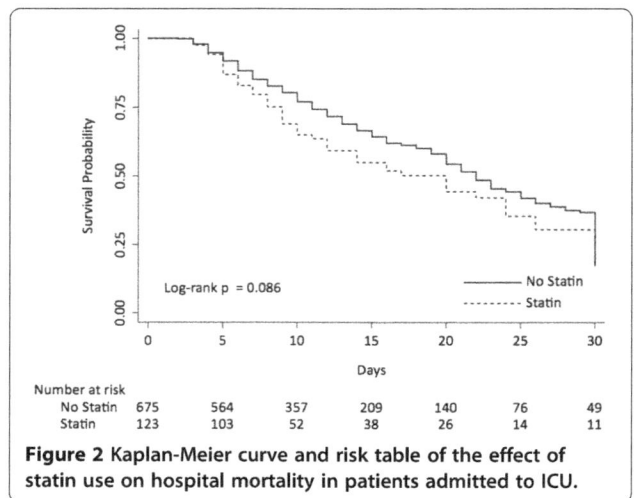

Figure 1 Kaplan-Meier curve and at risk table of the effect of statin use on venothromboembolism incidence in patients admitted to ICU.

Recently, JUPITER trial (Justification for the Use of statins in Prevention: an Intervention Trial Evaluating Rosuvastatin) showed that rosuvastatin (20 mg/day) was associated with lower VTE incidence compared to placebo (HR 0.57, 95% CI, 0.37-0.86) [17].

Three meta-analyses were published on the association of statin therapy in prevention of VTE. Agarwal et al. included one randomized controlled study (JUPITER) and nine observational studies (N = 971patients) and showed that statin therapy was associated with significant reduction in VTE risk (OR 0.68, 95% CI 0.54-0.86), DVT (OR 0.59, 95% CI 0.43-0.82), and PE (OR 0.70, 95% CI 0.53-0.94) [28]. Squizzato et al. included three randomized controlled trials, three cohort and eight case–control studies (N = 836 patients) [29] and demonstrated that statin therapy was associated with lower VTE risk (OR 0.81, 95% CI 0.66-0.99) [29]. Pia et al. included four cohort studies and four case–control studies found that statins were associated with lower risk for VTE (OR 0.67, 95% CI 0.53-0.84) and for DVT (OR 0.53, 95% CI 0.22-1.29) [30].

These studies, which showed benefit of statin therapy in reducing VTE risk, share long-term intervention in a low VTE risk outpatient population, and therefore are not applicable to ICU patients. Our study differs as it evaluates the effect of statin therapy on the short-term occurrence of VTE in a high-risk population.

In contrast to our study, a secondary analysis of the PROTECT (Prophylaxis of Thromboembolism in Critical Care) trial, published as an abstract, found a reduced risk for proximal leg DVT for any statin exposure in the week preceding enrolment (HR 0.46, 95% CI 0.27-0.77) [31]. Our study showed an adjusted HR for the association between statin therapy and VTE of 0.63, (95% CI of 0.25-1.57, P = 0.33). The direction of the point estimate towards protective effect of statins and the magnitude of the association are similar to previous studies in non-critically ill patients. Accordingly, one cannot dismiss beneficial effect of statin therapy on VTE risk during ICU stay, and therefore, further studies are required.

Among the limitations of our study are its monocenter nature, post-hoc design, and the lack of data on the duration of statin therapy prior to ICU admission, and statin side effects. Due the observational nature of the study, the presence of unobserved confounders and competing risks cannot also be entirely excluded. In our pragmatic approach for case ascertainment, we did not include surveillance ultrasounds to detect DVT. Our approach was based on clinical suspension and confirmation with Doppler ultrasound. Therefore, it is likely that some non-clinically evident DVTs were missed. This approach, currently, represents the standard of care and it has been shown to be more cost effective than surveillance approach [32].

We believe that these finding should trigger a larger well-designed randomized-controlled trial in critically ill patients. Such trial should evaluate the dose-effect relationship, the effect of duration of statin therapy on VTE risk, the mechanism of action whether related to the pleiotropic or lipid-lowering effect of statins and whether statins have an additive effect to anticoagulants. We hope that the ongoing clinical trials answer some of these questions [33-35] although trials in critically ill patients are still needed.

Conclusions

Our study failed to show a statically significant effect of continuing statin therapy during ICU stay on VTE risk and 30-day hospital mortality in critically ill patients. We suggest examining this important question in a randomized, control trial.

Abbreviations
VTE: Venous thromboembolism; DVT: Deep vein thrombosis; PE: Pulmonary embolism; INR: International normalized ratio; aPPT: Activated partial thromboplastin time; APACHE II: Acute Physiology and Chronic Health Evaluation.

Competing interests
The authors have no financial or non-financial competing interests to declare.

Authors' contribution
SAA: Conception and design, analysis and interpretation of data, drafting of the manuscript, critical revision of the manuscript for important intellectual content, supervision and final approval of the version to be published. MKH: Analysis and interpretation of data, drafting of the manuscript, critical revision of the manuscript for important intellectual content and final approval of the version to be published. HMD: Analysis and interpretation of data, drafting of the manuscript, critical revision of the manuscript for important intellectual content and final approval of the version to be published. HMT: Analysis and interpretation of data, critical revision of the manuscript for important intellectual content and final approval of the version to be published. AHR: Acquisition of data, critical revision of the manuscript for important intellectual content, and final approval of the version to be published. YMA: Conception and design, statistical analysis, critical revision of the manuscript and overall supervision. All authors read and approved the final manuscript.

Funding
The study was sponsored in part by an unrestricted grant from Sanofi-Aventis. However, the sponsors had no influence on data generation, analysis of the results or writing of the manuscript.

Author details
[1]College of Pharmacy, King Saud bin Abdulaziz University for Health Sciences, King Abdulaziz Medical City, Riyadh, Saudi Arabia. [2]College of Medicine, King Saud bin Abdulaziz University for Health Sciences, King Abdulaziz Medical City, MC 1425, PO Box 22490, Riyadh 1426, Saudi Arabia. [3]King Abdulaziz Medical City, Riyadh, Saudi Arabia.

References
1. Cook DJ, Crowther MA: Thromboprophylaxis in the intensive care unit: focus on medical-surgical patients. *Crit Care Med* 2010, 38(2 Suppl):S76–S82.
2. Cook D, Crowther M, Meade M, Rabbat C, Griffith L, Schiff D, Geerts W, Guyatt G: Deep venous thrombosis in medical-surgical critically ill

patients: prevalence, incidence, and risk factors. *Crit Care Med* 2005, **33**(7):1565–1571.

3.   Naess IA, Christiansen SC, Romundstad P, Cannegieter SC, Rosendaal FR, Hammerstrom J: **Incidence and mortality of venous thrombosis: a population-based study.** *J Thromb Haemost* 2007, **5**(4):692–699.

4.   Rosendaal FR, Vanhv A, Doggen CJ: **Venous thrombosis in the elderly.** *J Thromb Haemost* 2007, **5**(Suppl 1):310–317.

5.   Undas A, Brummel-Ziedins KE, Mann KG: **Statins and blood coagulation.** *Arterioscler Thromb Vasc Biol* 2005, **25**(2):287–294.

6.   Reich LM, Folsom AR, Key NS, Boland LL, Heckbert SR, Rosamond WD, Cushman M: **Prospective study of subclinical atherosclerosis as a risk factor for venous thromboembolism.** *J Thromb Haemost* 2006, **4**(9):1909–1913.

7.   Huerta C, Johansson S, Wallander MA, Rodriguez LA: **Risk of myocardial infarction and overall mortality in survivors of venous thromboembolism.** *Thromb J* 2008, **6**:10.

8.   Linnemann B, Schindewolf M, Zgouras D, Erbe M, Jarosch-Preusche M, Lindhoff-Last E: **Are patients with thrombophilia and previous venous thromboembolism at higher risk to arterial thrombosis?** *Thromb Res* 2008, **121**(6):743–750.

9.   Braekkan SK, Mathiesen EB, Njolstad I, Wilsgaard T, Stormer J, Hansen JB: **Family history of myocardial infarction is an independent risk factor for venous thromboembolism: the Tromso study.** *J Thromb Haemost* 2008, **6**(11):1851–1857.

10. Tsai AW, Cushman M, Rosamond WD, Heckbert SR, Polak JF, Folsom AR: **Cardiovascular risk factors and venous thromboembolism incidence: the longitudinal investigation of thromboembolism etiology.** *Arch Intern Med* 2002, **162**(10):1182–1189.

11. Prandoni P, Ghirarduzzi A, Prins MH, Pengo V, Davidson BL, Sorensen H, Pesavento R, Iotti M, Casiglia E, Iliceto S, *et al*: **Venous thromboembolism and the risk of subsequent symptomatic atherosclerosis.** *J Thromb Haemost* 2006, **4**(9):1891–1896.

12. Arslan F, Pasterkamp G, de Kleijn DP: **Unraveling pleiotropic effects of statins: bit by bit, a slow case with perspective.** *Circ Res* 2008, **103**(4):334–336.

13. Perez A, Bartholomew JR: **Interpreting the JUPITER trial: statins can prevent VTE, but more study is needed.** *Cleve Clin J Med* 2010, **77**(3):191–194.

14. Herrington DM, Vittinghoff E, Lin F, Fong J, Harris F, Hunninghake D, Bittner V, Schrott HG, Blumenthal RS, Levy R: **Statin therapy, cardiovascular events, and total mortality in the Heart and Estrogen/Progestin Replacement Study (HERS).** *Circulation* 2002, **105**(25):2962–2967.

15. Doggen CJ, Lemaitre RN, Smith NL, Heckbert SR, Psaty BM: **HMG CoA reductase inhibitors and the risk of venous thrombosis among postmenopausal women.** *J Thromb Haemost* 2004, **2**(5):700–701.

16. Ray JG, Mamdani M, Tsuyuki RT, Anderson DR, Yeo EL, Laupacis A: **Use of statins and the subsequent development of deep vein thrombosis.** *Arch Intern Med* 2001, **161**(11):1405–1410.

17. Glynn RJ, Danielson E, Fonseca FA, Genest J, Gotto AM Jr, Kastelein JJ, Koenig W, Libby P, Lorenzatti AJ, MacFadyen JG, *et al*: **A randomized trial of rosuvastatin in the prevention of venous thromboembolism.** *N Engl J Med* 2009, **360**(18):1851–1861.

18. Yang CC, Jick SS, Jick H: **Statins and the risk of idiopathic venous thromboembolism.** *Br J Clin Pharmacol* 2002, **53**(1):101–105.

19. Smeeth L, Douglas I, Hall AJ, Hubbard R, Evans S: **Effect of statins on a wide range of health outcomes: a cohort study validated by comparison with randomized trials.** *Br J Clin Pharmacol* 2009, **67**(1):99–109.

20. Arabi Y, Alshimemeri A, Taher S: **Weekend and weeknight admissions have the same outcome of weekday admissions to an intensive care unit with onsite intensivist coverage.** *Crit Care Med* 2006, **34**(3):605–611.

21. Arabi YM, Khedr M, Dara SI, Dhar GS, Bhat SA, Tamim HM, Afesh LY: **Intermittent pneumatic compression and not graduated compression stockings Are associated with lower incident venous thromboembolism in critically Ill patients: a multiple propensity scores adjusted analysis.** *Chest* 2013, **144**(1):152–159.

22. Knaus WA, Draper EA, Wagner DP, Zimmerman JE: **APACHE II: a severity of disease classification system.** *Crit Care Med* 1985, **13**(10):818–829.

23. Austin PC, Grootendorst P, Anderson GM: **A comparison of the ability of different propensity score models to balance measured variables between treated and untreated subjects: a Monte Carlo study.** *Stat Med* 2007, **26**(4):734–753.

24. Brookhart MA, Schneeweiss S, Rothman KJ, Glynn RJ, Avorn J, Sturmer T: **Variable selection for propensity score models.** *Am J Epidemiol* 2006, **163**(12):1149–1156.

25. Lacut K, Oger E, Le Gal G, Couturaud F, Louis S, Leroyer C, Mottier D: **Statins but not fibrates are associated with a reduced risk of venous thromboembolism: a hospital-based case–control study.** *Fundam Clin Pharmacol* 2004, **18**(4):477–482.

26. Sorensen HT, Horvath-Puho E, Sogaard KK, Christensen S, Johnsen SP, Thomsen RW, Prandoni P, Baron JA: **Arterial cardiovascular events, statins, low-dose aspirin and subsequent risk of venous thromboembolism: a population-based case–control study.** *J Thromb Haemost* 2009, **7**(4):521–528.

27. Ramcharan AS, Van Stralen KJ, Snoep JD, Mantel-Teeuwisse AK, Rosendaal FR, Doggen CJ: **HMG-CoA reductase inhibitors, other lipid-lowering medication, antiplatelet therapy, and the risk of venous thrombosis.** *J Thromb Haemost* 2009, **7**(4):514–520.

28. Agarwal V, Phung OJ, Tongbram V, Bhardwaj A, Coleman CI: **Statin use and the prevention of venous thromboembolism: a meta-analysis.** *Int J Clin Pract* 2010, **64**(10):1375–1383.

29. Squizzato A, Galli M, Romualdi E, Dentali F, Kamphuisen PW, Guasti L, Venco A, Ageno W: **Statins, fibrates, and venous thromboembolism: a meta-analysis.** *Eur Heart J* 2010, **31**(10):1248–1256.

30. Pai M, Evans NS, Shah SJ, Green D, Cook D, Crowther MA: **Statins in the prevention of venous thromboembolism: a meta-analysis of observational studies.** *Thromb Res* 2011, **128**(5):422–430.

31. Zarchanski R, Lim W, Rocha M, McIntyre L, Lamontagne F, Dodek P, Pai M, Cooper D, Alhashemi J, Zytaruk N: **112: DO Statins Influence Dvt Risk in the Critically Ill Patients?** *Crit Care Med* 2011, **39**(12):22.

32. Sud S, Mittmann N, Cook DJ, Geerts W, Chan B, Dodek P, Gould MK, Guyatt G, Arabi Y, Fowler RA: **Screening and prevention of venous thromboembolism in critically ill patients: a decision analysis and economic evaluation.** *Am J Respir Crit Care Med* 2011, **184**(11):1289–1298.

33. *Detecting the Impact of Statin Therapy on Lowering Risk of Venous Thrombo-Embolic Events (DISOLVE). NCT01524653.* http://clinicaltrials.gov/ct2/show/NCT01524653. Accessed on January 12, 2013.

34. *Re-STOP DVT: Reload of high dose atorvastatin for preventing deep vein thrombosis in statin user. NCT01063426.* http://clinicaltrials.gov/ct2/show/NCT01063426. Accessed January 12, 2013.

35. *Lowering the Risk of Operative Complications Using Atorvastatin Loading Dose (LOAD). NCT01543555.* http://clinicaltrials.gov/ct2/show/NCT01543555. Accessed on January 12, 2013.

5

Higher dose versus lower dose of antiviral therapy in the treatment of herpes zoster infection in the elderly: a matched retrospective population-based cohort study

Ngan N Lam[1,2,4*], Jamie L Fleet[1], Eric McArthur[3], Peter G Blake[1] and Amit X Garg[1,2,3]

Abstract

Background: Higher versus lower doses of antiviral drugs used to treat herpes zoster infection may lead to more adverse drug events in older adults, particularly those with chronic kidney disease.

Methods: We conducted a matched retrospective population-based cohort study of older adults (mean 77 years) in Ontario, Canada who initiated in the outpatient setting a higher (n = 23,256) or lower (n = 3,876) dose of one of three oral antivirals for the treatment of herpes zoster between 2002 and 2011. The primary outcome was hospitalization within 30 days with evidence of a computed tomography (CT) scan of the head (a proxy for acute neurotoxicity). The secondary outcome was 30-day all-cause mortality.

Results: A higher compared to lower dose of antiviral drug was not associated with an increased risk of hospitalization with an urgent CT scan of the head (247 [1.06%] events with higher dose versus 43 [1.11%] events with lower dose, relative risk 0.96, 95% confidence interval 0.69 to 1.33, p-value 0.79) and was not associated with a higher risk of all-cause mortality (63 [0.27%] events versus 15 [0.39%] events, relative risk 0.70, 95% confidence interval 0.40 to 1.23, p-value 0.21). Results were consistent in all subgroups, including those with and without chronic kidney disease.

Conclusions: Initiating a higher compared to a lower dose of an antiviral drug for the treatment of herpes zoster was not associated with an increased risk of adverse drug events. The findings support the safety of these drugs in older adults as currently prescribed in routine care.

Keywords: Administrative database, Epidemiology, Mortality, Neurotoxicity

Background

Acyclovir, valacyclovir (a pro-drug which is metabolized to acyclovir), and famciclovir are prescribed for the treatment of herpes zoster infection [1,2]. These drugs are commonly prescribed to older adults who are at risk of dose-related adverse drug reactions, particularly neurotoxicity with delirium [3,4]. In older patients with chronic kidney disease, the recommendation is to reduce the dose of these drugs to prevent systemic accumulation from reduced elimination (Table 1) [5-12]. There have been many case reports and case series of reversible acute neurological symptoms, such as delirium, resulting in hospitalization soon after the initiation of acyclovir, valacyclovir, or famciclovir [13-20]. Whether preferential use of a low dose of the antiviral drug minimizes this risk is unknown. Therefore, we conducted this study of older patients with herpes zoster infection to investigate whether initiation of a higher rather than lower dose of an oral antiviral drug in the outpatient setting is associated with more adverse drug events (neurotoxicity, death) within 30 days of prescription. We also considered whether any association between dose and adverse events differed in the presence of chronic kidney disease.

* Correspondence: nlam5@uwo.ca
[1]Department of Medicine, Division of Nephrology, Western University, London, ON N6A 3 K7, Canada
[2]Department of Epidemiology and Biostatistics, Western University, London, ON N6A 3 K7, Canada
Full list of author information is available at the end of the article

Table 1 Oral antiviral dosing for acute herpes zoster in popular drug prescribing references

	Higher dose (mg/day)[a]	Lower dose (mg/day)[a]	UpToDate recommendations (dose in mg/day) [7-9]	Compendium of pharmaceuticals and specialties (dose in mg/day) [10-12]
Acyclovir	4,000	3,200	4,000	4,000
		2,400	CrCl 10–25 mL/min/1.73 m²: 2,400	CrCl 10–25 mL/min/1.73 m²: 2,400
		1,600	CrCl <10 mL/min/1.73 m²: 1,600	CrCl <10 mL/min/1.73 m²: 1,600
		800		
Valacyclovir	3,000	2,000	3,000	3,000
		1,500	CrCl 15–30 mL/min: 2,000	CrCl 15–30 mL/min: 2,000
		1,000	CrCl <15 mL/min: 1,000	CrCl <15 mL/min: 1,000
		500		
Famciclovir	1,500	1,000	1,500	1,500
		500	CrCl 40–59 mL/min: 1,000	CrCl 40–59 mL/min/1.73 m²: 1,000
		350[b]	CrCl 20–39 mL/min: 500	CrCl 20–39 mL/min/1.73 m²: 500
			CrCl <20 mL/min: 250	CrCl <20 mL/min/1.73 m²: 250

[a]Dose categories as defined in this study include 50 mg dose above or below the cut-points.
[b]A dose of 350 mg/day was used instead of 250 mg/day because it was more commonly dispensed in our region with <20 patients being prescribed a dose of <300 mg/day.
Abbreviation: CrCl Creatinine Clearance.

Methods

Design and setting

We conducted this study at the Institute for Clinical Evaluative Sciences (ICES) according to a pre-specified protocol that was approved by the research ethics board at Sunnybrook Health Sciences Centre (Toronto, Canada). Participant informed consent was not required for this study. We conducted a retrospective, population-based, matched cohort study of older adults using linked healthcare databases in Ontario, Canada. Ontario has approximately 13 million residents, 2 million of whom are aged 65 years or older [21]. Residents have universal access to hospital care and physician services and those aged 65 or older have universal prescription drug coverage. The reporting of this study follows guidelines set out for observational studies (Additional file 1: Table S1) [22].

Data sources

We ascertained patient characteristics, drug use, covariate information, and outcome data using records from six databases. We obtained vital statistics from the Registered Persons Database (RPDB), which contains demographic information on all Ontario residents ever issued a health card. We used the Ontario Drug Benefit (ODB) database to identify prescription drug use, including dispensing date, quantity of pills, dose, and number of days supplied. This database contains highly accurate records of all outpatient prescriptions dispensed to patients aged 65 years or older, with an error rate of less than 1% [23]. We identified diagnostic and procedural information on all hospitalizations and emergency room visits from the Canadian Institute for Health Information Discharge Abstract Database (CIHI-DAD) and the National Ambulatory Care

Reporting System (NACRS), respectively. We obtained covariate information from the Ontario Health Insurance Plan (OHIP) database, which includes health claims for inpatient and outpatient physician services. We used the ICES Physician Database (IPDB) to ascertain antiviral drug prescriber information. Previously, we have used these databases to research health adverse drug events and health outcomes, including acyclovir-induced acute kidney injury [24-26]. With the exception of antiviral prescriber specialty and income quintile (missing in 14.5% and 0.4% of patients, respectively), the databases were complete for all variables used in this study. Given the ability of our databases to capture healthcare activity province-wide, the only loss to follow-up would be if patients emigrated from Ontario (a rate estimated to be less than 1% per year) [27]. The database codes used in the analysis are defined in Additional file 1: Table S2.

Patients

We established a cohort of residents aged ≥66 years in Ontario, Canada who filled a new outpatient prescription with ≥7-day supply for oral acyclovir, valacyclovir, or famciclovir from April 2002 to December 2011, a period spanning 9 years. We restricted our analysis to those who had evidence of a herpes zoster diagnosis in the 90 days prior to or 30 days following the time of the prescription (database diagnosis codes presented in Additional file 1: Table S2). The date of the first eligible prescription for a study antiviral served as the index date for that patient and marked the start date of follow-up. We excluded the following patients from the analysis: i) those in their first year of eligibility for prescription drug coverage (age 65) to avoid incomplete medication records,

ii) those living in long-term care facilities since residents may have frequent episodes of confusion or delirium for many reasons, iii) those with end-stage renal disease, iv) those who had a prescription for any antiviral in the prior 180 days in order to capture new usage, v) those who had a prescription for more than one type of antiviral on the index date in order to compare mutually exclusive groups, and vi) those who had a hospital admission or discharge on their index date or a hospital discharge in the prior two days to ensure these were new outpatient antiviral prescriptions (as patients continuing an antiviral treatment initiated in hospital would have their outpatient antiviral prescription dispensed on the same or next day of hospital discharge).

To select two groups of antiviral users that were well-balanced on the baseline characteristics we measured in this study, we matched each low-dose user with a high-dose user on a 1:6 basis using the following variables: age (within two years), sex, presence of chronic kidney disease, and type of antiviral prescribed (acyclovir, valacyclovir, or famciclovir). In Ontario, the validated algorithm for chronic kidney disease identifies older adults with a median estimated glomerular filtration rate (eGFR) of 38 mL/min per 1.73 m^2 (interquartile range 27 to 52), whereas its absence identifies those with a median eGFR of 69 mL/min per 1.73 m^2 (interquartile range 56 to 82) [28].

Antiviral dose

To align with recommendations in drug prescribing references, a higher dose of antiviral therapy was defined as at least 4,000 mg/day for acyclovir, 3,000 mg/day for valacyclovir, and 1,500 mg/day for famciclovir. A lower dose of antiviral therapy was defined as 3,200 mg/day, 2,400 mg/day, 1,600 mg/day or 800 mg/day for acyclovir, 2,000 mg/day, 1,500 mg/day, 1,000 mg/day, or 500 mg/day for valacyclovir, and 1,000 mg/day, 500 mg/day, or 350 mg/day for famciclovir (Table 1).

Outcomes

We followed all patients for 30 days after the index date for the assessment of two pre-specified outcomes. The primary outcome was hospital admission with evidence of an urgent computed tomography (CT) scan of the head within the first five days of admission (inclusive of any scans performed in the emergency room preceding an admission). Based on prospective studies of common clinical practice, neuroimaging is frequently used in the routine evaluation of patients who present to hospital acutely confused, even among those without focal neurological findings or head trauma [29-31]. Unlike diagnostic codes for acute delirium, the receipt of a CT scan of the head is well coded in our data sources (these codes have high sensitivity and specificity for receipt of

the imaging as they are associated with physician reimbursement) [32]. We also expected urgent CT scans of the head conducted for reasons unrelated to antiviral dosing to occur at a similar frequency in higher and lower dose groups; therefore, not impacting estimates of difference in risk. We have used this outcome of urgent CT scans of the head in other population-based drug safety studies to characterize the risk of drug-induced delirium [33]. Our secondary outcome was all-cause mortality. Death is accurately coded in our data sources (sensitivity 94%, positive predictive value 100%) [34].

Statistical analysis

We compared baseline characteristics between those prescribed a higher or lower antiviral dose using standardized differences [35]. This metric describes differences between group means relative to the pooled standard deviation and is considered a meaningful difference if greater than 10%. We estimated the odds ratio and 95% confidence intervals for inpatient CT scan of the head with higher antiviral dose compared to lower antiviral dose using conditional logistic regression analyses (accounting for matched sets). We interpreted odds ratios as relative risks which was appropriate given the low incidence of observed events. We examined the relative risk between higher dose and lower dose (referent dose) antiviral and each outcome first in the entire matched cohort and then in four pre-defined subgroups based on: age, sex, presence of chronic kidney disease, and antiviral type. We examined whether relative risks differed among subgroups using tests for interaction. We conducted all analysis with Statistical Analysis Software (SAS) version 9.2 (SAS Institute Incorporated, Cary, North Carolina, USA, 2008).

Results

We identified 77,381 eligible older adults who were prescribed outpatient oral antiviral drug for the treatment of herpes zoster infection (higher dose, n = 73,383 versus lower dose, n = 3,998). After the match, there were a total of 27,132 eligible patients of which 23,256 (85.7%) received a higher antiviral dose and 3,876 (14.3%) received lower antiviral dose (referent dose). A diagram of the cohort selection is represented in Additional file 1: Figure S1. The baseline characteristics of patients before and after the match are presented in Table 2. After the match, the baseline characteristics of the two dose groups were nearly identical (all standardized differences for 17 measured variables between the groups were ≤8%). The mean age was 77 years (standard deviation 7.1 years) and 63% were women. Three-quarters of the prescriptions were written by primary care physicians with 67% of prescriptions written for valacyclovir. Ophthalmologist prescribed <1% of the antivirals and <0.3% of patients had a diagnosis for herpes zoster involving the eye.

Table 2 Baseline characteristics

	Unmatched			Matched		
	Higher dose[a] (n = 73,383)	Lower dose[b] (n = 3,998)	Standardized difference[c]	Higher dose[a] (n = 23,256)	Lower dose[b] (n = 3,876)	Standardized difference[c]
Demographics						
Age, years	75.9 [6.8]	77.0 [7.3]	0.15	76.7 [7.1]	76.7 [7.1]	0
Women	45,613 (62.2)	2,541 (63.6)	0.03	14,682 (63.1)	2,447 (63.1)	0
Year of cohort entry						
2002 - 2003	11,318 (15.4)	514 (12.9)	0.07	3,083 (13.3)	505 (13.0)	0.01
2004 - 2005	14,016 (19.1)	595 (14.9)	0.11	4,096 (17.6)	572 (14.8)	0.08
2006 - 2007	14,930 (20.3)	807 (20.2)	0	4,641 (20.0)	779 (20.1)	0
2008 - 2009	15,783 (21.5)	993 (24.8)	0.08	5,320 (22.9)	964 (24.9)	0.05
2010 - 2011	17,336 (23.6)	1,089 (27.2)	0.08	6,116 (26.3)	1,056 (27.2)	0.02
Income quintile[d]						
First (lowest)	13,937 (19.0)	831 (20.8)	0.04	4,404 (18.9)	804 (20.7)	0.05
Second	15,526 (21.2)	802 (20.1)	0.03	4,886 (21.0)	777 (20.1)	0.02
Third (middle)	14,231 (19.4)	842 (21.1)	0.04	4,469 (19.2)	818 (21.1)	0.05
Fourth	14,521 (19.8)	751 (18.8)	0.03	4,620 (19.9)	730 (18.8)	0.03
Fifth (highest)	14,976 (20.4)	755 (18.9)	0.04	4,808 (20.7)	731 (18.9)	0.05
Missing	192 (0.26)	17 (0.43)	0.03	69 (0.3)	16 (0.4)	0.02
Rural location[e]	10,864 (14.8)	505 (12.6)	0.06	3,027 (13.0)	491 (12.7)	0.01
Modified Charlson score[f]						
0	53,431 (72.8)	2,731 (68.3)	0.10	16,623 (71.5)	2,684 (69.3)	0.05
1	8,024 (10.9)	445 (11.1)	0.01	2,560 (11.0)	428 (11.0)	0
2	6,350 (8.7)	400 (10.0)	0.05	2,086 (9.0)	383 (9.9)	0.03
≥3	5,578 (7.6)	422 (10.6)	0.10	1,987 (8.5)	381 (9.8)	0.04
Co-morbidities[g]						
CKD[h]	3,799 (5.2)	425 (10.6)	0.20	1,896 (8.2)	316 (8.2)	0
Chronic liver disease	2,420 (3.3)	138 (3.5)	0.01	735 (3.2)	135 (3.5)	0.02
COPD	2,994 (4.1)	212 (5.3)	0.06	1,010 (4.3)	198 (5.1)	0.04
CAD[i]	25,840 (35.2)	1,548 (38.7)	0.07	8,427 (36.2)	1,478 (38.1)	0.04
Diabetes mellitus[j]	11,016 (15.0)	699 (17.5)	0.07	3,636 (15.6)	671 (17.3)	0.05
Heart failure	8,469 (11.5)	611 (15.3)	0.11	2,985 (12.8)	571 (14.7)	0.06
Stroke/TIA	1,556 (2.1)	109 (2.7)	0.04	513 (2.2)	99 (2.6)	0.02
Herpes zoster (eye)	89 (0.12)	8 (0.20)	0.02	30 (0.13)	8 (0.21)	0.02
Antiviral type						
Acyclovir	4,095 (5.6)	297 (7.4)	0.08	1,692 (7.3)	282 (7.3)	0
Valacyclovir	29,482 (40.2)	2,694 (67.4)	0.57	15,528 (66.8)	2,588 (66.8)	0
Famciclovir	39,806 (54.2)	1,007 (25.2)	0.62	6,036 (26.0)	1,006 (26.0)	0
Medications[k]						
Anticonvulsants	3,079 (4.2)	178 (4.5)	0.01	988 (4.3)	167 (4.3)	0
Gabapentin	420 (0.57)	24 (0.60)	0	137 (0.59)	22 (0.57)	0
Antidepressants	11,201 (15.3)	663 (16.6)	0.04	3,756 (16.2)	636 (16.4)	0.01
Antipsychotics	1,431 (2.0)	88 (2.2)	0.02	503 (2.2)	86 (2.2)	0
Barbituates	115 (0.16)	7 (0.18)	0	45 (0.19)	7 (0.18)	0
Benzodiazepines	13,794 (18.8)	809 (20.2)	0.04	4,446 (19.1)	774 (20.0)	0.02

Table 2 Baseline characteristics (Continued)

Histamine2-receptor antagonists	6,191 (8.4)	337 (8.4)	0	1,911 (8.2)	325 (8.4)	0.01
Dopamine agonists	326 (0.44)	22 (0.55)	0.02	124 (0.53)	22 (0.57)	0
Muscle relaxants	399 (0.54)	25 (0.63)	0.01	132 (0.57)	25 (0.64)	0.01
Opioids	15,738 (21.5)	957 (23.9)	0.06	5,076 (21.8)	923 (23.8)	0.05
Overactive bladder medications	2,169 (3.0)	149 (3.7)	0.04	704 (3.0)	142 (3.7)	0.04
Prescribing physician						
General practitioner	55,723 (75.9)	3,015 (75.4)	0.01	17,671 (76.0)	2,925 (75.5)	0.01
Ophthalmologist	272 (0.37)	28 (0.70)	0.05	90 (0.39)	27 (0.70)	0.04
Neurologist[l]	41 (0.06)	≤5 (−)	(−)	12 (0.05)	≤5 (−)	(−)
Other	7,538 (10.3)	372 (9.3)	0.03	2,350 (10.1)	360 (9.3)	0.03
Missing	9,809 (13.4)	581 (14.5)	0.03	3,133 (13.5)	562 (14.5)	0.03

Data presented as number (percent) except for age which is presented as mean [standard deviation].
Abbreviations: CAD Coronary Artery Disease, *CKD* Chronic Kidney Disease, *COPD* Chronic Obstructive Pulmonary Disease, *TIA* Transient Ischemic Attack.
[a]Higher dose of antiviral defined as 4,000 mg/day for acyclovir, 3,000 mg/day for valacyclovir, and 1,500 mg/day for famciclovir.
[b]A lower dose of antiviral defined as 3,200 mg/day, 2,400 mg/day, 1,600 mg/day or 800 mg/day for acyclovir, 2,000 mg/day, 1,500 mg/day, 1,000 mg/day, or 500 mg/day for valacyclovir, and 1,000 mg/day, 500 mg/day, or 350 mg/day for famciclovir.
[c]Standardized differences are less sensitive to sample size than traditional hypothesis tests. They provide a measure of the difference between groups divided by the pooled standardized difference; a value >10% (0.1) is interpreted as a meaningful difference between the groups [35].
[d]Income was categorized into quintiles based on average neighbourhood income on the index date.
[e]Rural location indicates a population <10,000.
[f]Assessed with an algorithm using diagnosis codes from hospitalizations in the five years prior; patients with no hospitalizations during this period were given a value of zero.
[g]Co-morbid diagnoses were ascertained from administrative database codes in the five years preceding the index date.
[h]Identified individuals with chronic kidney disease using an algorithm of diagnosis codes validated in our region for older adults [28]. The algorithm identified patients with a median estimated glomerular filtration rate (eGFR) of 38 mL/min per 1.73 m^2 (interquartile range 27 to 52), whereas its absence identified patients with a median eGFR of 69 mL/min per 1.73 m^2 (interquartile range 56 to 82).
[i]Coronary artery disease includes receipt of coronary artery bypass graft surgery, percutaneous coronary intervention, and diagnoses of angina.
[j]Identified individuals with diabetes through medication use including oral hypoglycemic and insulin.
[k]Medication use was assessed in the 180 days prior to the index date.
[l]Due to privacy issues, values ≤5 are suppressed.

Compared to lower antiviral dose, the initiation of higher antiviral dose was not associated with a higher risk of hospitalization with urgent CT scan of the head (247 [1.06%] events with higher dose versus 43 [1.11%] events with lower dose, relative risk 0.96, 95% confidence interval 0.69 to 1.33, p-value 0.79) (Table 3). Figure 1 presents the association between antiviral dose and the primary outcome in four pre-defined subgroups: by age, sex, presence of chronic kidney disease, and antiviral type. There was no association between antiviral dose and hospital admission with urgent CT scan of the head in any of the subgroups, including those with and without chronic kidney disease (p-value for interaction 0.25). There was also no difference between the two dose groups in the incidence of all-cause mortality (63 [0.27%] events with higher dose versus 15 [0.39%] events with lower dose, relative risk 0.70, 95% confidence interval 0.40 to 1.23, p-value 0.21) (Table 3).

Discussion

In this population-based study of over 27,000 older patients, we found no association between initiating oral antiviral treatment for herpes zoster at a higher versus lower dose and the risk of hospital admission within 30 days with evidence of an urgent CT scan of the head. A similar association was observed in patients with and without chronic kidney disease, although given the smaller number of patients with chronic kidney disease, the estimates were less precise with wider confidence

Table 3 30-day outcomes of hospital admission with urgent CT scan of the head and all-cause mortality

	Number of events (Percent)		Relative risk	P-value
	Higher dose[a] (n = 23,256)	Lower dose[b] (Referent) (n = 3,876)	[95% confidence interval]	
Hospital admission with urgent CT scan of the head	247 (1.06%)	43 (1.11%)	0.96 [0.69 to 1.33]	0.79
All-cause mortality	63 (0.27%)	15 (0.39%)	0.70 [0.40 to 1.23]	0.21

Abbreviations: CT, Computed Tomography.
[a]Higher dose of antiviral defined as 4,000 mg/day for acyclovir, 3,000 mg/day for valacyclovir, and 1,500 mg/day for famciclovir.
[b]A lower dose of antiviral defined as 3,200 mg/day, 2,400 mg/day, 1,600 mg/day or 800 mg/day for acyclovir, 2,000 mg/day, 1,500 mg/day, 1,000 mg/day, or 500 mg/day for valacyclovir, and 1,000 mg/day, 500 mg/day, or 350 mg/day for famciclovir.

	No. events / No. at risk		Proportion with event		Adjusted odds ratio (95% CI)	Interaction test (p value)
	Low dose	High dose	Low dose	High dose		
Overall	43/3,876	247/23,256	1.11	1.06	0.96 (0.69 to 1.33)	
Age						
66-80	11/2,663	94/15,978	0.41	0.59	1.42 (0.76 to 2.66)	} 0.117
>80	32/1,213	153/7,278	2.64	2.10	0.79 (0.54 to 1.17)	
Sex						
Male	15/1,429	93/8,574	1.05	1.08	1.03 (0.60 to 1.79)	} 0.727
Female	28/2,447	154/14,682	1.14	1.05	0.92 (0.61 to 1.37)	
CKD						
Yes	8/316	30/1,896	2.53	1.58	0.63 (0.29 to 1.36)	} 0.251
No	35/3,560	217/21,360	0.98	1.02	1.03 (0.72 to 1.48)	
Antiviral type						
Acyclovir	≤5/282	12/1,692	≤1.77	0.71	0.65 (0.18 to 2.41)	0.969
Valacyclovir	23/2,588	166/15,528	0.89	1.07	1.21 (0.78 to 1.87)	0.097
Famciclovir	17/1,006	69/6,036	1.69	1.14	0.67 (0.39 to 1.15)	

```
   0   0.5   1   1.5   2
   ←———————————————————→
   risk higher          risk higher
   with lower dose      with higher dose
```

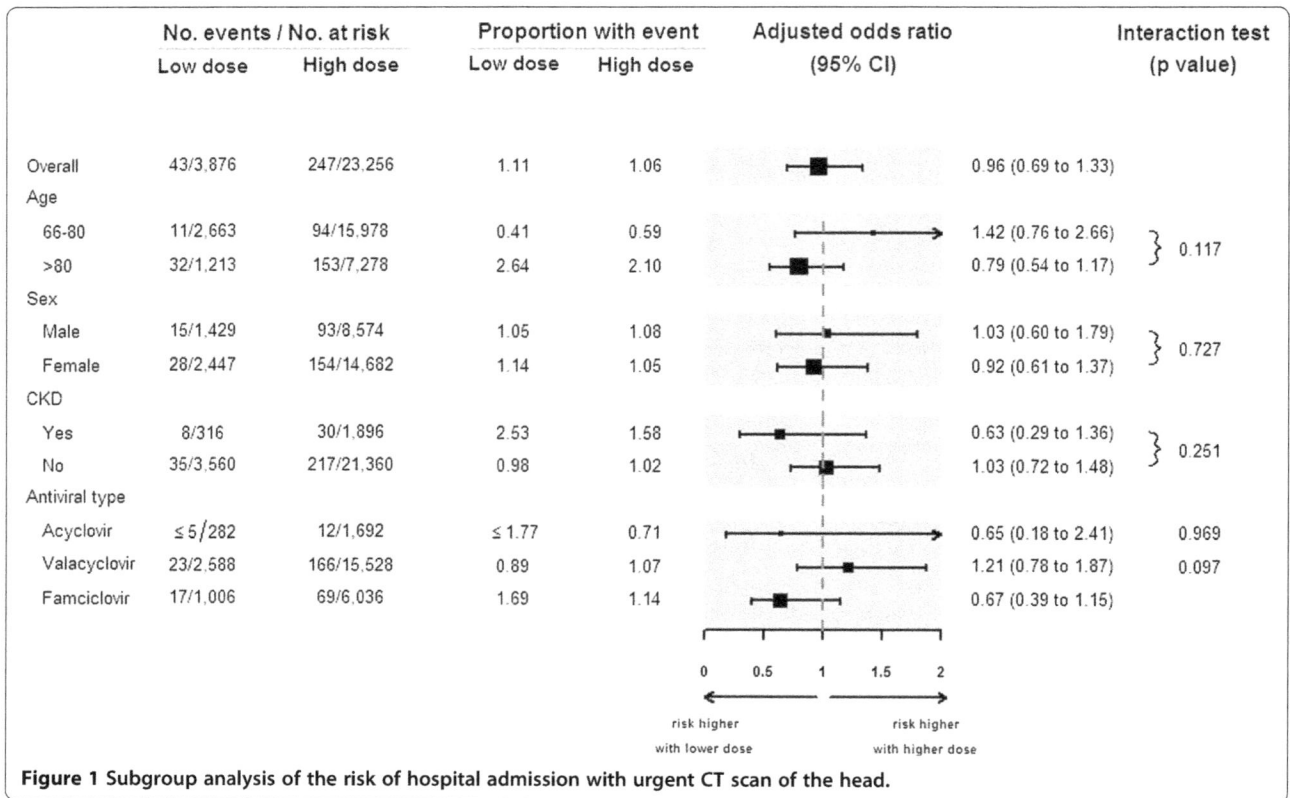

Figure 1 Subgroup analysis of the risk of hospital admission with urgent CT scan of the head.

intervals. The 30-day risk of mortality was also no different between the two dose groups.

Acyclovir, valacyclovir, and famciclovir are commonly prescribed antivirals used in routine outpatient care for the treatment of herpes zoster infection in the elderly. In randomized controlled trials, these drugs are similarly effective in reducing the duration and severity of painful lesions, preventing complications, and decreasing the frequency of recurrence [1,2]. A known adverse event of these oral antiviral drugs is neurotoxicity [13-20]. The symptoms of drug-induced neurotoxicity include tremor, confusion, hallucinations, and coma and can often be difficult to distinguish from herpes encephalitis. With these antivirals, symptoms typically occur within days of drug initiation and generally resolve with drug discontinuation. In one case series of 35 patients with neuropsychiatric symptoms during acyclovir treatment, risk factors included older age, the presence of chronic kidney disease, and co-administration of other potentially neurotoxic medications [13].

Given the results of these prior pharmacokinetic studies and case reports, we were concerned we would observe an increased risk of major adverse events when a higher rather than lower dose of an antiviral drug was initiated in older adults, particularly those with concomitant chronic kidney disease. The findings from this study are reassuring and support the safety of these drugs in older adults as currently prescribed in routine care.

Our study has a number of strengths. To our knowledge, it is the first population-based assessment of adverse outcomes from higher dose versus lower dose antiviral treatment. The study was made possible by our province's universal health care benefits, which provides information on all health care encounters for all Ontarians including accurate records of outpatient prescriptions to older patients. Consequently, there were a large number of patients who received antiviral prescriptions and this provided good precision for the estimates obtained for the primary outcome (there were over 200 events and the 95% confidence interval for the point estimate of the primary outcome was 0.69 to 1.33; confidently ruling out a 1.4 or higher risk).

Our study does have some limitations. For reasons of feasibility, in this retrospective study, we relied on urgent neuroimaging within the available data sources as a proxy for the diagnosis of acute altered mental status. A preferred methodology would be a prospective study with independent blinded outcome adjudication and detailed serial measures of cognitive function. In such an effort, kidney function values could also be recorded, rather than a validated algorithm for chronic kidney disease as used in our study. We were encouraged by the marked similarities in the baseline characteristics after matching and in the consistency of the observed association among various subgroups. However, in our study the antiviral dose was not randomly assigned, and with all observational studies, we may have failed to account for important unknown or unmeasured confounding variables. Our cohort consisted of patients over the age of 65 years. It is reassuring that 99% of elderly patients in routine care did not present to hospital with urgent CT scan of the head after use of either dose of oral antivirals. While we did not study younger patients in the present study, their incidence of adverse events would be expected to be even less.

Conclusions

In this study, initiating a higher compared to a lower dose of an antiviral drug for the treatment of herpes zoster was not associated with an increased risk of adverse drug events. The findings support the safety of these drugs in older adults as currently prescribed in routine care.

Additional file

> **Additional file 1: Table S1.** STROBE checklist. **Table S2.** Databases and coding definitions for baseline characteristics and study outcomes. **Figure S1.** Cohort selection.

Abbreviations

CIHI-DAD: Canadian Institute for Health Information Discharge Abstract Database; CT: Computed tomography; eGFR: Estimated Glomerular Filtration Rate; ICES: Institute for Clinical Evaluative Sciences; IPDB: ICES Physician Database; NACRS: National Ambulatory Care Reporting System; ODB: Ontario Drug Benefit; OHIP: Ontario Health Insurance Plan; RPDB: Registered Persons Database; SAS: Statistical Analysis Software.

Competing interests

The authors declare that they have no competing interests.

Authors' contributions

NNL, EM, and AXR conceived of the study, participated in its design, and drafted the manuscript. EM performed the statistical analysis. All authors read and approved the final manuscript.

Acknowledgements

We thank Ms. Lihua Li for her help with the graph and members of the provincial ICES Kidney Dialysis and Transplantation Program (www.ices.on.ca) for their support of this study. We thank Brogan Inc., Ottawa for use of its Drug Product and Therapeutic Class Database.

Author details

¹Department of Medicine, Division of Nephrology, Western University, London, ON N6A 3 K7, Canada. ²Department of Epidemiology and Biostatistics, Western University, London, ON N6A 3 K7, Canada. ³Institute for Clinical Evaluative Sciences (ICES), London, ON N6A 5 W9, Canada. ⁴Kidney Clinical Research Unit, Room ELL-111, London Health Sciences Centre, 800 Commissioners Road East, London, ON N6A 4G5, Canada.

References

1. Tyring SK, Beutner KR, Tucker BA, Anderson WC, Crooks RJ: **Antiviral therapy for herpes zoster: randomized, controlled clinical trial of valacyclovir and famciclovir therapy in immunocompetent patients 50 years and older.** *Arch Fam Med* 2000, **9:**863–869.
2. Beutner KR, Friedman DJ, Forszpaniak C, Andersen PL, Wood MJ: **Valaciclovir compared with acyclovir for improved therapy for herpes zoster in immunocompetent adults.** *Antimicrob Agents Chemother* 1995, **39:**1546–1553.
3. Moore AR, O'Keeffe ST: **Drug-induced cognitive impairment in the elderly.** *Drugs Aging* 1999, **15:**15–28.
4. Pretorius RW, Gataric G, Swedlund SK, Miller JR: **Reducing the risk of adverse drug events in older adults.** *Am Fam Physician* 2013, **87:**331–336.
5. Blum MR, Liao SH, de Miranda P: **Overview of acyclovir pharmacokinetic disposition in adults and children.** *Am J Med* 1982, **73:**186–192.
6. Smith JP, Weller S, Johnson B, Nicotera J, Luther JM, Haas DW: **Pharmacokinetics of acyclovir and its metabolites in cerebrospinal fluid and systemic circulation after administration of high-dose valacyclovir in subjects with normal and impaired renal function.** *Antimicrob Agents Chemother* 2010, **54:**1146–1151.
7. UpToDate: Acyclovir (systemic): *Drug Information.* [http://www-uptodate-com.proxy1.lib.uwo.ca/contents/acyclovir-systemic-drug-information?source=search_result&search=acyclovir&selectedTitle=1~148]
8. UpToDate: Valacyclovir: *Drug Information.* [http://www-uptodate-com.proxy1.lib.uwo.ca/contents/valacyclovir-drug-information?source=search_result&search=valacyclovir&selectedTitle=1~83]
9. UpToDate: Famciclovir: *Drug Information.* [http://www-uptodate-com.proxy1.lib.uwo.ca/contents/famciclovir-drug-information?source=search_result&search=famciclovir&selectedTitle=1~61]
10. Compendium of Pharmaceuticals and Specialties: *Zovirax Oral: Drug Monograph.* [https://www-e-therapeutics-ca.proxy1.lib.uwo.ca/cps.showMonograph.action?newSearch=true&simpleIndex=brand_generic&simpleQuery=zovirax&brandExactMatch=false]
11. Compendium of Pharmaceuticals and Specialties: *Valtrex: Drug Monograph.* [https://www-e-therapeutics-ca.proxy1.lib.uwo.ca/cps.select.preliminaryFilter.action?simplePreliminaryFilter=valacyclovir+HCl]
12. Compendium of Pharmaceuticals and Specialties: *Famvir: Drug Monograph.* [https://www-e-therapeutics-ca.proxy1.lib.uwo.ca/cps.select.preliminaryFilter.action?simplePreliminaryFilter=famciclovir]
13. Rashiq S, Briewa L, Mooney M, Giancarlo T, Khatib R, Wilson FM: **Distinguishing acyclovir neurotoxicity from encephalomyelitis.** *J Intern Med* 1993, **234:**507–511.
14. Johnson GL, Limon L, Trikha G, Wall H: **Acute renal failure and neurotoxicity following oral acyclovir.** *Ann Pharmacother* 1994, **28:**460–463.
15. Martinez-Diaz GJ, Hsia R: **Altered mental status from acyclovir.** *J Emerg Med* 2011, **41:**55–58.
16. Adair JC, Gold M, Bond RE: **Acyclovir neurotoxicity: clinical experience and review of the literature.** *South Med J* 1994, **87:**1227–1231.
17. Eck P, Silver SM, Clark EC: **Acute renal failure and coma after a high dose of oral acyclovir.** *N Engl J Med* 1991, **325:**1178–1179.
18. Swan SK, Bennett WM: **Oral acyclovir and neurotoxicity.** *Ann Intern Med* 1989, **111:**188.
19. Asahi T, Tsutsui M, Wakasugi M, Tange D, Takahashi C, Tokui K, Okazawa S, Okudera H: **Valacyclovir neurotoxicity: clinical experience and review of the literature.** *Eur J Neurol* 2009, **16:**457–460.
20. Gales BJ, Gales MA: **Confusion and bradykinesia associated with famciclovir therapy for herpes zoster.** *Am J Health Syst Pharm* 1996, **53:**1454–1456.
21. Statistics Canada: *Population by Sex and Age Group, by Province and Territory.* [http://www.statcan.gc.ca/tables-tableaux/sum-som/l01/cst01/demo31a-eng.htm]
22. von Elm E, Altman DG, Egger M, Pocock SJ, Gøtzsche PC, Vandenbroucke JP: **The strengthening the reporting of observational studies in epidemiology (STROBE) statement: guidelines for reporting observational studies.** *J Clin Epidemiol* 2008, **61:**344–349.
23. Levy AR, O'Brien BJ, Sellors C, Grootendorst P, Willison D: **Coding accuracy of administrative drug claims in the Ontario drug benefit database.** *Can J Clin Pharmacol* 2003, **10:**67–71.
24. Lam NN, Weir MA, Yao Z, Blake PG, Beyea MM, Gomes T, Gandhi S, Mamdani M, Wald R, Parikh CR, Hackam DG, Garg AX: **Risk of acute kidney injury from oral acyclovir: A population-based study.** *Am J Kidney Dis* 2013, **61:**723–729.

25. Zhao YY, Weir MA, Manno M, Cordy P, Gomes T, Hackam DG, Juurlink DN, Mamdani M, Moist L, Parikh CR, Paterson JM, Wald R, Yao Z, Garg AX: **New fibrate use and acute renal outcomes in elderly adults: a population-based study.** *Ann Intern Med* 2012, **156:**560–569.

26. Shih AW, Weir MA, Clemens KK, Yao Z, Gomes T, Mamdani MM, Juurlink DN, Hird A, Hodsman A, Parikh CR, Wald R, Cadarette SM, Garg AX: **Oral bisphosphonate use in the elderly is not associated with acute kidney injury.** *Kidney Int* 2012, **82:**903–908.

27. Ontario Ministry of Finance: *Ontario Population Projections Update.* [http://www.fin.gov.on.ca/en/economy/demographics/projections/#s4f]

28. Fleet JL, Dixon SN, Shariff SZ, Quinn RR, Nash DM, Harel Z, Garg AX: **Detecting chronic kidney disease in population-based administrative databases using an algorithm of hospital encounter and physician claim codes.** *BMC Nephrol* 2013, **14:**81.

29. Hardy JE, Brennan N: **Computerized tomography of the brain for elderly patients presenting to the emergency department with acute confusion.** *Emerg Med Australas* 2008, **20:**420–424.

30. Hirano LA, Bogardus ST Jr, Saluja S, Leo-Summers L, Inouye SK: **Clinical yield of computed tomography brain scans in older general medical patients.** *J Am Geriatr Soc* 2006, **54:**587–592.

31. Naughton BJ, Moran M, Ghaly Y, Michalakes C: **Computed tomography scanning and delirium in elder patients.** *Acad Emerg Med* 1997, **4:**1107–1110.

32. Williams J, Young W: *A Summary of Studies on the Quality of Health Care Administrative Databases in Canada.* Ottawa: Canadian Medical Association; 1996.

33. Weir MA, Fleet JL, Vinden C, Shariff SZ, Liu K, Song H, Jain AK, Gandhi S, Clark WF, Garg AX: **Hyponatremia and sodium picosulfate bowel preparations in older adults.** *Am J Gastroenterol* 2014, **109:**686–694.

34. Jha P, Deboer D, Sykora K, Naylor CD: **Characteristics and mortality outcomes of thrombolysis trial participants and nonparticipants: a population-based comparison.** *J Am Coll Cardiol* 1996, **27:**1335–1342.

35. Austin P: **Using the standardized difference to compare the prevalence of a binary variable between two groups in observational research.** *Commun Statistics Simulation Comput* 2009, **38:**1228–1234.

6

Palonosetron versus ondansetron as rescue medication for postoperative nausea and vomiting: a randomized, multicenter, open-label study

Keith A Candiotti[1*], Syed Raza Ahmed[2], David Cox[3] and Tong J Gan[4]

Abstract

Background: This study compared palonosetron and ondansetron as rescue medications for postoperative nausea and vomiting (PONV) in patients who received prophylactic ondansetron. Although guidelines recommend use of an agent from a different class when prophylaxis has failed, palonosetron has unique properties relative to other serotonin 5-HT$_3$ receptor antagonists. Prior trials assessing its use for rescue have had conflicting results. Although palonosetron has compared favorably with ondansetron for PONV prevention, the drugs have not been compared in the rescue setting of failure of 5-HT$_3$ receptor antagonist prophylaxis.

Methods: This was a randomized, open-label, multicenter trial comparing the efficacy and safety of intravenous palonosetron 0.075 mg and intravenous ondansetron 4 mg in patients experiencing PONV following laparoscopic abdominal or gynecological surgery despite prophylactic ondansetron.

Results: Of 239 patients screened, 220 were enrolled and 98 were treated for PONV: 48 and 50 in the palonosetron and ondansetron arms, respectively. Complete control during 72 hours after study drug administration was achieved in 25.0% of palonosetron recipients and 18.0% of ondansetron recipients (95% confidence interval [CI], −9.2, 23.3; p = 0.40). Corresponding incidences of vomiting were 29.2% for palonosetron and 48.0% for ondansetron (95% CI, −0.06, 37.7; p = 0.057), and 62.5% and 56.0% required additional rescue treatment, respectively (95% CI, −25.9, 12.9; p = 0.52). Other than a similar incidence of procedural pain in the 2 groups, the most common treatment-emergent adverse events, which were generally mild, were headache (14.6% vs 12.0%), constipation (8.3% vs 10.0%), and dizziness (6.3% vs 8.0%), for the palonosetron and ondansetron groups, respectively.

Conclusions: Palonosetron and ondansetron did not show differences in the primary efficacy endpoint of CC during the 72 hours after study drug administration. There was a trend toward less emesis in the 0–72 h time period favoring palonosetron. While larger studies are needed to fully assess any clinical benefits of palonosetron to rescue patients who have failed ondansetron prophylaxis for PONV, the benefit, if any, would be limited based on this study.

Trial registration: ClinicalTrials.gov, NCT00967499 (Registered August 27, 2009)

Keywords: Postoperative nausea and vomiting, Antiemetics, Palonosetron, Ondansetron

* Correspondence: KCandiot@med.miami.edu
[1]University of Miami–Jackson Memorial Hospital, 1611 NW 12th Avenue, Room 300, 33136 Miami, FL, USA
Full list of author information is available at the end of the article

Background

Postoperative nausea and vomiting (PONV) is a frequent complication of surgery, with considerable medical and economic impact, and is associated with high levels of patient discomfort and dissatisfaction [1]. PONV is an especially distressing adverse event to many patients, often feared more than postoperative pain [1,2]. The incidence of PONV is estimated at 25% to 30% in all patients and as high as 80% in patients with multiple high-risk factors [3,4].

PONV, alone or combined with pain, is one of the leading causes for delayed discharge or unplanned hospital admission following outpatient surgery [5-7]. PONV can occur during the day after a surgical procedure or beyond [8]. In the first 24 hours postoperatively, the highest incidence of emetic sequelae is observed in patients undergoing laparoscopic gynecologic surgery or receiving general anesthesia [9,10]. Abdominal surgery is also a risk factor for PONV, with an incidence in excess of 50% [1]. The overall incidence of PONV after general anesthesia in outpatients has been reported to be 37%, although several factors, including sex, age, history of PONV, and opiate administration, influence the risk [11].

The serotonin 5-HT$_3$ receptor antagonists (RAs) commonly are used for prophylaxis of PONV; however, there are fewer trials examining their use for treatment and rescue of PONV. Guidelines from the Society for Ambulatory Anesthesia (SAMBA) recommend that when PONV occurs after antiemetic prophylaxis, an agent from a different class should be used as rescue treatment [12]. Candiotti and colleagues investigated 88 women who developed PONV after ondansetron prophylaxis; these patients were randomly assigned to receive a repeat dose of ondansetron 4 mg, granisetron 1 mg, or granisetron 0.1 mg and were then followed for 24 hours [13]. The authors concluded that patients who failed ondansetron prophylaxis did not have a significant response to crossover administration of another 5-HT$_3$ RA (ie, granisetron). In contrast, de Wit et al. demonstrated a benefit to rescue administration using granisetron and dexamethasone in patients receiving highly emetogenic chemotherapy who had failed ondansetron and dexamethasone prophylaxis [14]. Note that the former study evaluated PONV, while the latter assessed cancer-induced nausea and vomiting; differences may exist between these 2 populations. Thus, this issue remains unsettled.

Palonosetron is a pharmacologically distinct 5-HT$_3$ RA with a greater binding affinity and longer half-life than older agents in this class [15]. Binding isotherms, equilibrium diagnostic tests, and kinetic diagnostic tests show that palonosetron is an allosteric antagonist with positive cooperativity, unlike ondansetron and granisetron. Differential effects on [^{3}H]-ligand binding indicate that palonosetron interacts at different or additional sites on the 5-HT$_3$ receptor compared with the binding profiles of granisetron or ondansetron. Unlike these agents, palonosetron also elicits 5-HT$_3$ receptor internalization and promotes extended inhibition of receptor activity [16].

Two studies have shown that, compared with placebo, a single intravenous dose of palonosetron 0.075 mg effectively reduced emesis, nausea intensity, and rescue medication use in patients, particularly within 24 hours after surgery [17,18]. When directly compared with ondansetron before laparoscopic surgery or thyroidectomy, palonosetron showed similar or superior efficacy for prevention of PONV [19-23]; however, to our knowledge use of palonosetron as rescue therapy after ondansetron failure has not been assessed. The pharmacological profile of palonosetron, combined with its efficacy and favorable comparisons with ondansetron for the prevention of PONV, prompted the hypothesis that palonosetron may be effective as rescue therapy in patients for whom preoperative prophylaxis with another 5-HT$_3$ RA had been unsuccessful, despite SAMBA recommendations to use an agent from another class [12]. The current phase II study evaluated the safety and efficacy of intravenous palonosetron 0.075 mg and intravenous ondansetron 4 mg (the currently approved doses) as rescue medications in patients experiencing PONV in the postanesthesia care unit (PACU) following unsuccessful prophylaxis with ondansetron.

Methods

This was a randomized, open-label, multicenter trial that compared palonosetron with ondansetron using a 1:1 ratio as rescue therapy in outpatients who developed PONV in the PACU after receiving prophylactic ondansetron. Study objectives were to assess efficacy and safety of palonosetron and ondansetron when used in outpatients as rescue therapy for PONV in the PACU. The study was registered with ClinicalTrials.gov on August 27, 2009 (NCT00967499). Approval of the research protocol was required by each study center's institutional review board/ethics committee prior to patient randomization, and the study complied with the Declaration of Helsinki and Good Clinical Practice guidelines (the International Conference on Harmonisation), with written informed consent obtained from all patients. This was an open-label study, and study drug preparation and dispensing were performed by the site pharmacist. A list of study sites and investigators is provided in Additional file 1.

Patient selection

Outpatients undergoing elective laparoscopic abdominal or gynecological surgery who required general endotracheal anesthesia for ≥30 minutes were eligible for randomization if they met these criteria: ≥18 years of age, American Society of Anesthesiologists (ASA) physical status I to III, and ≥2 of the following PONV risk factors: female, nonsmoker, and history of PONV and/or currently prone to motion sickness. Exclusion criteria included chemotherapy within 4 weeks or emetogenic radiotherapy within 8 weeks of study entry; body mass index >40 kg/m^2, use of investigational drugs within 30 days of study entry; use of drugs with potential antiemetic efficacy; or any nausea, vomiting, or retching within 24 hours prior to anesthesia.

Treatment regimen and study design

On the day of surgery, patients received preoperative intravenous ondansetron 4 mg before induction of anesthesia per dosing and timing approved by the Food and Drug Administration (FDA). All patients had intravenous induction of general anesthesia per the standard of care at each site, were intubated, and received neuromuscular blockade, with reversal at the end of surgery as indicated. Regional or total intravenous anesthesia was not allowed. Using a minimization random allocation ratio, patients were randomized to rescue treatment with either intravenous palonosetron 0.075 mg or intravenous ondansetron 4 mg, both provided by Eisai Inc. Patients with symptoms requiring a rescue antiemetic—nausea score ≥4 on an 11-point Numeric Rating Scale (NRS), retching or vomiting, or patient request—within 6 hours of PACU admission were given the randomized drug within 10 minutes of investigator determination of necessity. The NRS was an 11-point linear scale on which patients rated their nausea, with 0 meaning no nausea and 10 meaning the worst possible nausea. These doses were selected because they correspond with those approved by the FDA for prevention of PONV and were anticipated to provide maximal effect.

Patients were assessed for their overall response to the rescue medication, and discharge from the PACU was not affected by study participation. Baseline assessments occurred at a screening visit within 2 weeks before the surgery (day 1), and efficacy and safety were evaluated at 0.5, 1, 2, 6, 12, 24, 48, and 72 hours after dosing with the rescue medication. After discharge from the PACU, all patients received a follow-up telephone call to review the patient diary, in which they were instructed to record emetic episodes, nausea severity (subjectively rated by patient) and duration, use of additional rescue drugs, and functioning related to nausea/emesis. In addition to baseline, the NRS was completed at the previously mentioned evaluation time points, with patients asked to rate the most severe nausea they had experienced since the last assessment.

The primary efficacy endpoint was the proportion of patients who achieved complete control (CC), defined as no emetic episode, no rescue medication, and a nausea severity score of ≤3 on the NRS, from 0 to 72 hours after rescue dosing. The percentage of patients with CC 0 to 30, 30 to 60, and 60 to 120 minutes also was assessed. Secondary efficacy endpoints were complete response (CR), defined as no emetic episode and no rescue medication; the proportions of patients with no emesis and no additional rescue medication in the 72 hours following the rescue dose; and the change from baseline nausea score using the NRS. Treatment-emergent adverse events (TEAEs), regardless of suspected causal relationship to the study medication, were recorded throughout.

Statistical considerations

It was estimated that approximately 300 patients would need to be randomized to have 100 patients treated with either palonosetron or ondansetron; as this study was for proof of concept, no statistical justification of sample size was done. Patients were assigned to a treatment group using a minimization random allocation ratio. The primary efficacy parameter was analyzed using the full analysis set population, consisting of all patients who were randomized to and received study drug. Safety was evaluated for all randomized patients given rescue medication and who had ≥1 safety assessment after treatment.

Descriptive statistics were used for most primary and secondary efficacy parameters, as well as safety data. The Cochran-Mantel-Haenszel test was used to compare the CC rates between treatment groups, stratified to sex at a 2-sided significance level of 0.05. All secondary endpoints were analyzed using the same methods.

Results

Study disposition and baseline characteristics

Patients were recruited from July 2009 to December 2009. Of 239 patients screened, 220 patients were randomized from 10 centers. See Figure 1 for complete patient disposition. In all, 98 patients experienced PONV that required rescue medication within 6 hours of PACU admission and were included in the study assessment. The patient demographics and baseline characteristics were similar in the palonosetron and ondansetron groups (Table 1). All patients were female, and most were nonsmokers. Most patients had low ASA scores (I or II).

Complete control

As shown in Table 2, CC through 72 hours after dosing was achieved by 25.0% of palonosetron patients compared with 18.0% of ondansetron patients (95% confidence interval [CI], −9.2, 23.3; p = 0.40). Assessment of the initial 24 hours demonstrated a similar efficacy profile, while efficacy increased for both drugs during the 24- to 72-hour time period, with CC reached by a similar portion of patients in both groups.

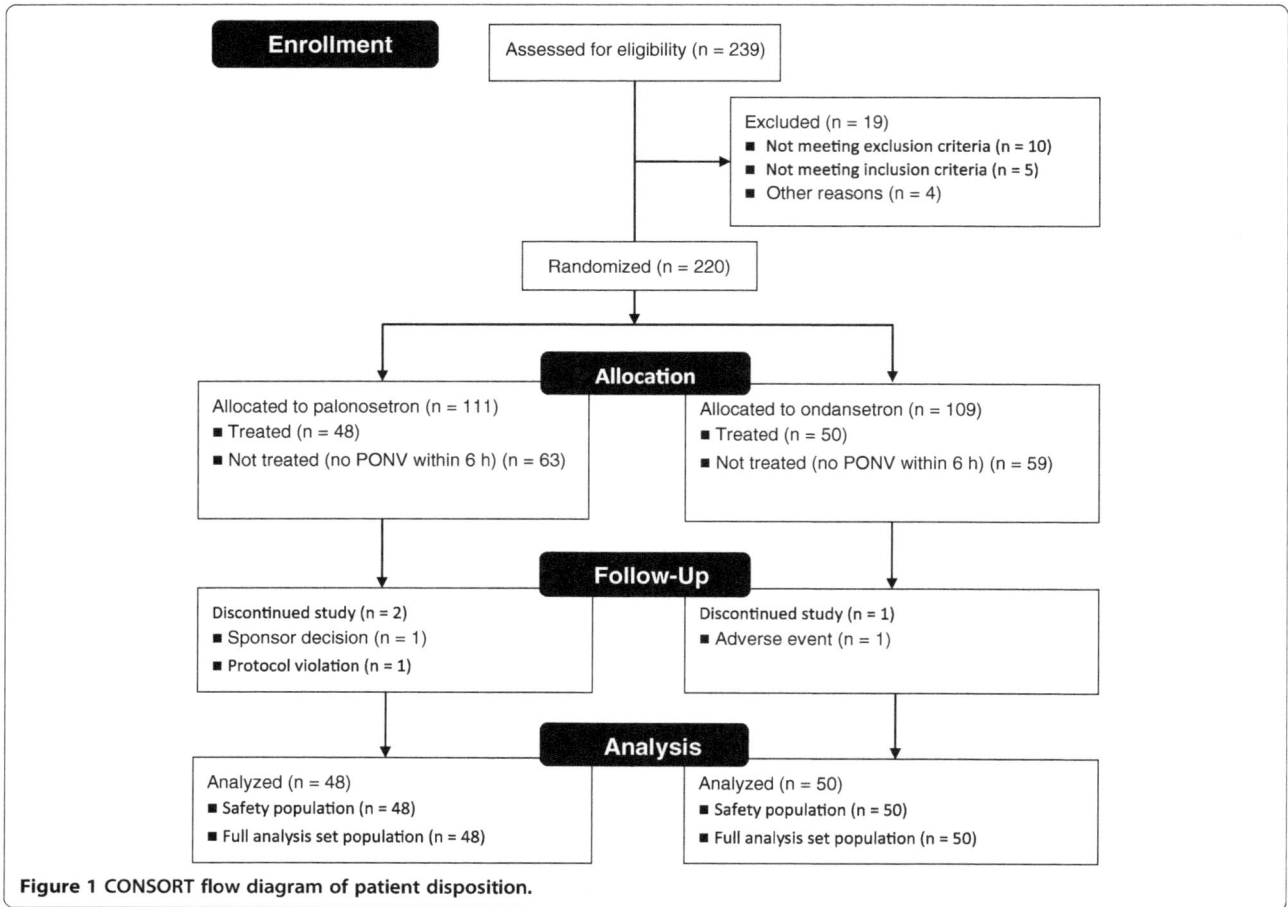

Figure 1 CONSORT flow diagram of patient disposition.

A total of 56.3% of palonosetron patients and 58.0% of ondansetron patients achieved CC within the first 30 minutes of dosing. Across the 3 time periods examined during the first 120 minutes, CC ranged from 50.0% to 66.7% in the palonosetron group and from 58.0% to 62.0% in the ondansetron group.

Secondary efficacy endpoints

The secondary endpoints of CR, no emesis, and no additional rescue medication are shown in Table 3 for the 0- to 72-, 0- to 24-, and 24- to 72-hour time periods. With the exception of a result that possibly favored palonosetron over ondansetron for no emesis over the entire 72-hour evaluation period (p = 0.057), none of the other comparisons approached statistical significance.

Prior to rescue medication administration, moderate nausea (as rated subjectively by patient) was experienced by 66.7% of patients in the palonosetron group and 62.0% of patients in the ondansetron group. After 24 hours no nausea was reported by 83.3% and 82.0% of patients treated with palonosetron and ondansetron, respectively, and at the end of 72 hours no nausea was recorded by 79.2% and 82.0% of palonosetron and ondansetron

patients, respectively. Baseline NRS severity scores were similar for the 2 groups (5.7 and 5.9 in the palonosetron and ondansetron arms, respectively). Changes were most substantial in the 24- to 72-hour time period, with similar decreases in NRS scores, ranging from –5.1 to –5.3 and –5.3 to –5.6 in the palonosetron and ondansetron arms, respectively.

Safety profile

The safety profiles for palonosetron and ondansetron were comparable, with a similar number of patients experiencing TEAEs during the 72-hour evaluation period (Table 4). Other than procedural pain, which was not substantially different between groups, the most common TEAEs in both groups were headache, constipation, and dizziness: 14.6%, 8.3%, and 6.3% and 12.0%, 10.0%, and 8.0% in the palonosetron and ondansetron groups, respectively. Most TEAEs were mild, but 6 palonosetron patients (12.5%) and 8 ondansetron patients (16.0%) experienced serious TEAEs, primarily gastrointestinal effects. No serious TEAEs were attributed to treatment with palonosetron, and 1 (2.0%) serious TEAE was thought to be related to ondansetron treatment.

Table 1 Baseline patient demographics and clinical characteristics

	Palonosetron (n = 48)	Ondansetron (n = 50)	Total (N = 98)
Age (y)			
Mean (SD)	41 (10.2)	43 (13.8)	42 (12.1)
Min, max	22, 62	21, 83	21, 83
Sex			
Female, n (%)	48 (100.0)	50 (100.0)	98 (100.0)
Race, n (%)			
White	36 (75.0)	36 (72.0)	72 (73.5)
Black or African American	7 (14.6)	9 (18.0)	16 (16.3)
Asian	1 (2.1)	3 (6.0)	4 (4.1)
Other	4 (8.3)	2 (4.0)	6 (6.1)
Nonsmoker*, n (%)	45 (93.8)	49 (98.0)	94 (95.9)
BMI (kg/m^2)			
Mean (SD)	27.2 (5.4)	27.8 (5.0)	27.5 (5.2)
Min, max	17, 38	20, 39	17, 39
Duration of laparoscopic surgery (min)			
Mean (SD)	113.3 (69.4)	102.0 (59.8)	107.6 (64.6)
Median	92.5	81.5	88.5
Min, max	26, 306	34, 282	26, 306
Baseline NRS for nausea severity			
n	47	48	95
Mean (SD)	5.7 (1.84)	5.9 (1.86)	5.8 (1.84)
Min, max	2, 10	3, 10	2, 10
History of PONV[†], n (%)	30 (62.5)	27 (54.0)	57 (58.2)
Type of laparoscopic surgery, n (%)			
Gynecological	37 (77.1)	31 (62.0)	68 (69.4)
Abdominal	11 (22.9)	19 (38.0)	30 (30.6)
ASA classification, n (%)			
I	20 (41.7)	20 (40.0)	40 (40.8)
II	25 (52.1)	24 (48.0)	49 (50.0)
III	3 (6.3)	6 (12.0)	9 (9.2)
Baseline opioid use, n (%)	47 (97.9)	50 (100.0)	97 (99.0)

Abbreviations: ASA American Society of Anesthesiologists, BMI body mass index, NRS Numeric Rating Scale, PONV postoperative nausea and vomiting, SD standard deviation.
*Never smoked or quit ≥12 months before participation in the study. [†]History of PONV and/or currently prone to motion sickness.

Table 2 Complete control achieved—primary efficacy endpoint

	Palonosetron (n = 48) n (%)	Ondansetron (n = 50) n (%)	Difference, % (95% CI)	p-value
0-72 h	12 (25.0)	9 (18.0)	7.0 (−9.2, 23.2)	0.40
0-24 h	12 (25.0)	10 (20.0)	5.0 (−11.5, 21.5)	0.56
24-72 h	40 (83.3)	40 (80.0)	3.3 (−12.0, 18.6)	0.67

Abbreviation: CI confidence interval.

Table 3 Secondary efficacy endpoints

	Palonosetron (n = 48)	Ondansetron (n = 50)	Difference, %	p-value
	n (%)	n (%)	(95% CI)	
Complete response				
0-72 h	15 (31.3)	13 (26.0)	5.3 (−12.6, 23.1)	0.57
0-24 h	15 (31.3)	15 (30.0)	1.3 (−17.0, 19.5)	0.89
24-72 h	43 (89.6)	41 (82.0)	7.6 (−6.1, 21.3)	0.29
No emesis				
0-72 h	34 (70.8)	26 (52.0)	18.8 (−0.06, 37.7)	0.057
0-24 h	34 (70.8)	29 (58.0)	12.8 (−5.9, 31.6)	0.19
24-72 h	45 (93.8)	44 (88.0)	5.8 (−5.6, 17.1)	0.33
No additional rescue medication				
0-72 h	18 (37.5)	22 (44.0)	−6.5 (−25.9, 12.9)	0.52
0-24 h	18 (37.5)	23 (46.0)	−8.5 (−28.0, 11.0)	0.40
24-72 h	44 (91.7)	43 (86.0)	5.7 (−6.7, 18.1)	0.38

Abbreviation: CI confidence interval.

Discussion

The use of prophylactic antiemetics is intended to prevent episodes of vomiting, eliminate or lessen the severity of nausea, and minimize or remove the need for PONV rescue medications. 5-HT$_3$ RAs have proven effective for the prevention and treatment of PONV, with minimal adverse effects [12]. As a class, 5-HT$_3$ RAs are generally safe at the usual doses used to prevent or treat PONV, with no dose-related sedation or extrapyramidal reactions and no significant effects on vital signs [24]. For prophylaxis of PONV, palonosetron has demonstrated efficacy similar to or superior to ondansetron [19-23]; however, they have not been compared for rescue after ondansetron failure. If patients who receive no antiemetic prophylaxis before surgery experience PONV, a 5-HT$_3$ RA may be of benefit [12]. According to the SAMBA guidelines, if patients experience PONV after prophylaxis was given, an agent should be chosen from a therapeutic class different from the one administered prophylactically [12]. Because the mechanism of action and pharmacokinetics for palonosetron differ substantially

from other 5-HT$_3$ RAs, its use seemed reasonable when ondansetron had failed. Ondansetron rescue of ondansetron prophylaxis served as an active drug comparator with previously known results.

The primary endpoint of the study, proportion of patients achieving CC over the 72-hour evaluation period, was achieved in 25.0% and 18.0% of patients receiving PONV rescue treatment with palonosetron and ondansetron, respectively, showing no statistical difference (p = 0.40). The lack of statistical significance affirms an earlier study assessing granisetron rescue therapy following failed ondansetron prophylaxis [13]. Contrary to our estimate that 100 patients per treatment group would be appropriate, a post hoc power analysis showed that approximately 540 patients actually would be needed per arm to demonstrate a statistically significant difference in the primary endpoint with the results seen here (25.0% vs 18.0%). However, at the time, the study was carried out assuming a much larger treatment difference between palonosetron and ondansetron arms.

The 95% CI for the difference ranged from −9.2% (favoring ondansetron) to 23.2% (favoring palonosetron). Because the pharmacology of palonosetron differs from other 5-HT$_3$ RAs, as described earlier, it seemed plausible that palonosetron might prove effective when another agent from the same class already has been used for PONV prophylaxis. If there is a difference, however, it would seem to be small based on this study. Differences in the 0- to 24-hour and 24- to 72-hour time periods also were not statistically significant.

Among the secondary outcomes of CR, no emesis, and no additional rescue medication, differences between the two arms showed a lack of statistical significance at all times. However, as with the primary endpoint, the 95%

Table 4 Treatment-emergent adverse events

	Palonosetron (n = 48)	Ondansetron (n = 50)	Total (N = 98)
TEAEs	43 (89.6)	49 (98.0)	92 (93.9)
Treatment-related AEs	5 (10.4)	4 (8.0)	9 (9.2)
Serious TEAEs	6 (12.5)	8 (16.0)	14 (14.3)
Treatment-related serious TEAEs	0 (0.0)	1 (2.0)	1 (1.0)
Deaths	0 (0.0)	0 (0.0)	0 (0.0)

Abbreviations: AEs adverse events, *TEAEs* treatment-emergent adverse events. All data reported as n (%).

CI had a wide overlap across zero, and clinically relevant differences between palonosetron and ondansetron cannot be ruled out. Over the entire 72-hour assessment period, a lack of emesis was reported by 70.8% and 52.0% (95% CI −0.06, 37.7; p = 0.057) of palonosetron and ondansetron patients, respectively, showing a trend toward statistical significance, possibly due to the much longer half-life of palonosetron. Patient self-reported nausea showed similar improvements with palonosetron and ondansetron. The safety analyses demonstrated that both palonosetron and ondansetron were well tolerated, with no notable differences in safety parameters between groups.

Limitations of the current study include the lack of blinding, the timing of ondansetron prophylaxis, and the dosing of drugs. Drug dosing and time of administration needed to be consistent with FDA-approved labeling, so alternative methods of administration recommended by others could not be evaluated here. The most recent SAMBA guidelines recommend giving prophylactic ondansetron at the end of surgery, while administering palonosetron prior to surgery [12]. In this study, ondansetron was given at the induction of anesthesia, as per product labeling; however, this is not likely to have influenced rescue therapy. In addition, SAMBA guidelines recommend use of a different class of agent from the one given for PONV prophylaxis for PONV rescue; however, palonosetron was evaluated in this trial because of its unique pharmacological properties compared with other 5-HT_3 RAs, as described earlier. The authors acknowledge that we could potentially learn more from a study designed with a different comparator than ondansetron (eg, an antiemetic with a different mechanism of action relative to the 5-HT_3 RAs). In addition, although the study was open to both males and females, male patients were unable to be recruited. The incidence of PONV is higher in females, but the results cannot necessarily be extrapolated to males.

Conclusions

Palonosetron and ondansetron did not show differences in the primary efficacy endpoint of CC during the 72 hours after study drug administration. At the earliest time points, there were no differences between palonosetron and ondansetron treatment, but in the full 0- to 72-hour period, there was a trend toward greater efficacy for palonosetron for patients experiencing no emesis after rescue, possibly because the longer half-life of palonosetron may make it more effective than ondansetron for delayed emesis. Outside of this trend toward less emesis overall, there does not appear to be a significant difference between palonosetron and ondansetron for rescue treatment of PONV after failure of ondansetron prophylaxis, supporting the SAMBA recommendations to use an antiemetic from another class.

Additional file

Additional file 1: Study site investigators.

Abbreviations

5-HT_3: Serotonin; ASA: American Society of Anesthesiologists; CC: Complete control; CI: Confidence interval; CR: Complete response; FDA: US Food and Drug Administration; PACU: Postanesthesia care unit; NRS: Numeric rating scale; PONV: Postoperative nausea and vomiting; RA: Receptor antagonist; SAMBA: Society for Ambulatory Anesthesia; SD: Standard deviation; TEAE: Treatment-emergent adverse event.

Competing interests
KAC receives grant/research support, serves as a consultant to, and serves on the speakers bureau of Helsinn; SRA was an employee of Eisai Inc. at the time of the study; DC is a current employee of Eisai Inc.; TJG receives research/grant support from Eisai Inc. and NIKOM, and serves on the speakers' bureaus of Baxter, Hospira, Pacira, and Fresenius.

Authors' contributions
KAC helped design and conduct the study, analyze the data, and write the manuscript. SRA helped design and coordinate the study. DC helped design and coordinate the study. TJG helped design the study. All authors reviewed drafts of the manuscript and provided final approval of the manuscript for submission.

Acknowledgements
The authors would like to thank all the patients who participated and the study site investigators who assisted in coordinating this trial (see Additional file 1). The authors acknowledge Christian Apfel, MD, for advising and commenting on the manuscript. The authors also acknowledge The Medicine Group for initial medical writing and editorial support of this manuscript, and Jeff Kuper, PharmD, of MedVal Scientific Information Services, LLC, for providing medical writing and editorial assistance. This manuscript was prepared according to the International Society for Medical Publication Professionals' "Good Publication Practice for Communicating Company-Sponsored Medical Research: the GPP2 Guidelines." Funding to support the study conduct and preparation of this manuscript was provided by Eisai Inc.

Author details
[1]University of Miami–Jackson Memorial Hospital, 1611 NW 12th Avenue, Room 300, 33136 Miami, FL, USA. [2]Becton, Dickinson and Company, 1 Becton Drive, 07417 Franklin Lakes, NJ, USA. [3]Eisai Inc., 100 Tice Boulevard, 07677 Woodcliff Lake, NJ, USA. [4]Duke University Medical Center, 2100 Erwin Road, 27710 Durham, NC, USA.

References
1. Apfel CC: Postoperative Nausea and Vomiting. In *Miller's Anesthesia*. 7th edition. Edited by Miller RD, Eriksson LI, Fleisher LA, *et al*. Philadelphia: Churchill Livingstone Elsevier; 2009:2729–2755.
2. Macario A, Weinger M, Carney S, Kim A: Which clinical anesthesia outcomes are important to avoid? The perspective of patients. *Anesth Analg* 1999, **89**:652–658.
3. Kovac AL: Prevention and treatment of postoperative nausea and vomiting. *Drugs* 2000, **59**:213–243.
4. Apfel CC, Laara E, Koivuranta M, Greim CA, Roewer N: A simplified risk score for predicting postoperative nausea and vomiting: conclusions from cross-validations between two centers. *Anesthesiology* 1999, **91**:693–700.
5. Carroll NV, Miederhoff P, Cox FM, Hirsch JD: Postoperative nausea and vomiting after discharge from outpatient surgery centers. *Anesth Analg* 1995, **80**:903–909.
6. Hedayati B, Fear S: Hospital admission after day-case gynaecological laparoscopy. *Br J Anaesth* 1999, **83**:776–779.

7. Junger A, Klasen J, Benson M, Sciuk G, Hartmann B, Sticher J, Hempelmann G: Factors determining length of stay of surgical day-case patients. *Eur J Anaesthesiol* 2001, **18**:314–321.

8. Odom-Forren J, Jalota L, Moser DK, Lennie TA, Hall LA, Holtman J, Hooper V, Apfel CC: Incidence and predictors of postdischarge nausea and vomiting in a 7-day population. *J Clin Anesth* 2013, **25**:551–559.

9. Sniadach MS, Alberts MS: A comparison of the prophylactic antiemetic effect of ondansetron and droperidol on patients undergoing gynecologic laparoscopy. *Anesth Analg* 1997, **85**:797–800.

10. Koivuranta M, Laara E, Snare L, Alahuhta S: A survey of postoperative nausea and vomiting. *Anaesthesia* 1997, **52**:443–449.

11. Apfel CC, Philip BK, Cakmakkaya OS, Shilling A, Shi YY, Leslie JB, Allard M, Turan A, Windle P, Odom-Forren J, Hooper VD, Radke OC, Ruiz J, Kovac A: Who is at risk for postdischarge nausea and vomiting after ambulatory surgery? *Anesthesiology* 2012, **117**:475–486.

12. Gan TJ, Diemunsch P, Habib AS, Kovac A, Kranke P, Meyer TA, Watcha M, Chung F, Angus S, Apfel CC, Bergese SD, Candiotti KA, Chan MT, Davis PJ, Hooper VD, Lagoo-Deenadayalan S, Myles P, Nezat G, Philip BK, Tramer MR: Consensus guidelines for the management of postoperative nausea and vomiting. *Anesth Analg* 2014, **118**:85–113.

13. Candiotti KA, Nhuch F, Kamat A, Deepika K, Arheart KL, Birnbach DJ, Lubarsky DA: Granisetron versus ondansetron treatment for breakthrough postoperative nausea and vomiting after prophylactic ondansetron failure: a pilot study. *Anesth Analg* 2007, **104**:1370–1373.

14. de Wit R, de Boer AC, vd Linden GHM, Stoter G, Sparreboom A, Verweij J: Effective cross-over to granisetron after failure to ondansetron, a randomized double blind study in patients failing ondansetron plus dexamethasone during the first 24 hours following highly emetogenic chemotherapy. *Br J Cancer* 2001, **85**:1099–1101.

15. Rojas C, Stathis M, Thomas AG, Massuda EB, Alt J, Zhang J, Rubenstein E, Sebastiani S, Cantoreggi S, Snyder SH, Slusher B: Palonosetron exhibits unique molecular interactions with the 5-HT3 receptor. *Anesth Analg* 2008, **107**:469–478.

16. Rojas C, Thomas AG, Alt J, Stathis M, Zhang J, Rubenstein EB, Sebastiani S, Cantoreggi S, Slusher BS: Palonosetron triggers 5-HT(3) receptor internalization and causes prolonged inhibition of receptor function. *Eur J Pharmacol* 2010, **626**:193–199.

17. Candiotti KA, Kovac AL, Melson TI, Clerici G, Joo GT: A randomized, double-blind study to evaluate the efficacy and safety of three different doses of palonosetron versus placebo for preventing postoperative nausea and vomiting. *Anesth Analg* 2008, **107**:445–451.

18. Kovac AL, Eberhart L, Kotarski J, Clerici G, Apfel C: A randomized, double-blind study to evaluate the efficacy and safety of three different doses of palonosetron versus placebo in preventing postoperative nausea and vomiting over a 72-hour period. *Anesth Analg* 2008, **107**:439–444.

19. Park SK, Cho EJ: A randomized, double-blind trial of palonosetron compared with ondansetron in preventing postoperative nausea and vomiting after gynaecological laparoscopic surgery. *J Int Med Res* 2011, **39**:399–407.

20. Moon YE, Joo J, Kim JE, Lee Y: Anti-emetic effect of ondansetron and palonosetron in thyroidectomy: a prospective, randomized, double-blind study. *Br J Anaesth* 2012, **108**:417–422.

21. Laha B, Hazra A, Mallick S: Evaluation of antiemetic effect of intravenous palonosetron versus intravenous ondansetron in laparoscopic cholecystectomy: a randomized controlled trial. *Indian J Pharmacol* 2013, **45**:24–29.

22. Kim SH, Hong JY, Kim WO, Kil HK, Karm MH, Hwang JH: Palonosetron has superior prophylactic antiemetic efficacy compared with ondansetron or ramosetron in high-risk patients undergoing laparoscopic surgery: a prospective, randomized, double-blinded study. *Korean J Anesthesiol* 2013, **64**:517–523.

23. Kim YY, Moon SY, Song DU, Lee KH, Song JW, Kwon YE: Comparison of palonosetron with ondansetron in prevention of postoperative nausea and vomiting in patients receiving intravenous patient-controlled analgesia after gynecological laparoscopic surgery. *Korean J Anesthesiol* 2013, **64**:122–126.

24. Kovac AL: Benefits and risks of newer treatments for chemotherapy-induced and postoperative nausea and vomiting. *Drug Saf* 2003, **26**:227–259.

7

Uridine prevents tamoxifen-induced liver lipid droplet accumulation

Thuc T Le[1,2,3*], Yasuyo Urasaki[1,2,3] and Giuseppe Pizzorno[1,2*]

Abstract

Background: Tamoxifen, an agonist of estrogen receptor, is widely prescribed for the prevention and long-term treatment of breast cancer. A side effect of tamoxifen is fatty liver, which increases the risk for non-alcoholic fatty liver disease. Prevention of tamoxifen-induced fatty liver has the potential to improve the safety of long-term tamoxifen usage.

Methods: Uridine, a pyrimidine nucleoside with reported protective effects against drug-induced fatty liver, was co-administered with tamoxifen in C57BL/6J mice. Liver lipid levels were evaluated with lipid visualization using coherent anti-Stokes Raman scatting (CARS) microscopy, biochemical assay measurement of triacylglyceride (TAG), and liquid chromatography coupled with mass spectrometry (LC-MS) measurement of membrane phospholipid. Blood TAG and cholesterol levels were measured. Mitochondrial respiration of primary hepatocytes in the presence of tamoxifen and/or uridine was evaluated by measuring oxygen consumption rate with an extracellular flux analyzer. Liver protein lysine acetylation profiles were evaluated with 1D and 2D Western blots. In addition, the relationship between endogenous uridine levels, fatty liver, and tamoxifen administration was evaluated in transgenic mice $UPase1^{-/-}$ and $UPase1$-TG.

Results: Uridine co-administration prevented tamoxifen-induced liver lipid droplet accumulation in mice. The most prominent effect of uridine co-administration with tamoxifen was the stimulation of liver membrane phospholipid biosynthesis. Uridine had no protective effect against tamoxifen-induced impairment to mitochondrial respiration of primary hepatocytes or liver TAG and cholesterol export. Uridine had no effect on tamoxifen-induced changes to liver protein acetylation profile. Transgenic mice $UPase1^{-/-}$ with increased pyrimidine salvage activity were protected against tamoxifen-induced liver lipid droplet accumulation. In contrast, $UPase1$-TG mice with increased pyrimidine catabolism activity had intrinsic liver lipid droplet accumulation, which was aggravated following tamoxifen administration.

Conclusion: Uridine co-administration was effective at preventing tamoxifen-induced liver lipid droplet accumulation. The ability of uridine to prevent tamoxifen-induced fatty liver appeared to depend on the pyrimidine salvage pathway, which promotes biosynthesis of membrane phospholipid.

Keywords: Coherent anti-Stokes Raman scattering microscopy, Drug-induced fatty liver, Lipidomics, Membrane phospholipid, Mitochondrial respiration, Protein lysine acetylation, Pyrimidine, Tamoxifen, Triacylglyceride, Uridine phosphorylase

* Correspondence: thuc@uchicago.edu; giuseppe.pizzorno@dri.edu
[1]Nevada Cancer Institute, One Breakthrough Way, Las Vegas, NV 89135, USA
[2]Desert Research Institute, 10530 Discovery Drive, Las Vegas, NV 89135, USA
Full list of author information is available at the end of the article

Background

Tamoxifen is an effective drug widely used for the treatment of estrogen receptor-positive breast cancer [1]. Women taking tamoxifen from 5 to 10 years exhibit reduced risks of breast cancer recurrence and mortality [2,3]. While generally well-tolerated, tamoxifen is known to induce fatty liver in 43% of women within the first 2 years of treatment [4-6]. Fatty liver is an established risk factor for non-alcoholic fatty liver disease (NAFLD) [7]. Prolonged tamoxifen treatment increases the risk of NAFLD, particularly in women with pre-existing metabolic condition [8].

The mechanism underlying tamoxifen-induced fatty liver is a topic of active investigation. Evidence from several independent research groups supports tamoxifen-induced impairment of mitochondrial fatty acid oxidation (FAO) as a primary cause of lipid accumulation in the liver [9-11]. Co-administration of tetradecylthioacetic acid, which improves mitochondrial and peroxisomal FAO, prevents tamoxifen-induced fatty liver [12]. Tamoxifen also inhibits hepatic triacylglyceride secretion leading to liver lipid accumulation [10,11]. Therapeutic intervention to prevent tamoxifen-induced fatty liver condition has the potential to improve the safety of long-term tamoxifen usage for breast cancer treatment.

Uridine, a pyrimidine nucleoside, has been shown to prevent fatty liver condition induced by several drugs with unrelated therapeutic usages and acting mechanisms [13,14]. Uridine could be salvaged into pyrimidine nucleotides or catabolized into uracil and subsequently β-alanine and acetyl-CoA (Figure 1) [15]. Homeostatic regulation of uridine is controlled by uridine phosphorylase, an enzyme that catalyzes the reversible phosphorylitic conversion of uridine to uracil [16]. Genetic knock-out of uridine phosphorylase in $UPase1^{-/-}$ mice elevates tissues and plasma levels of uridine [17]; whereas, transgenic overexpression of uridine phosphorylase in $UPase1$-TG mice depletes tissues and plasma levels of uridine [18]. The liver is actively regulating plasma uridine level by continuously degrading plasma uridine and replacing it with $de\ novo$ uridine synthesis [19]. The interaction between liver uridine homeostasis and lipid metabolism has been reported [18].

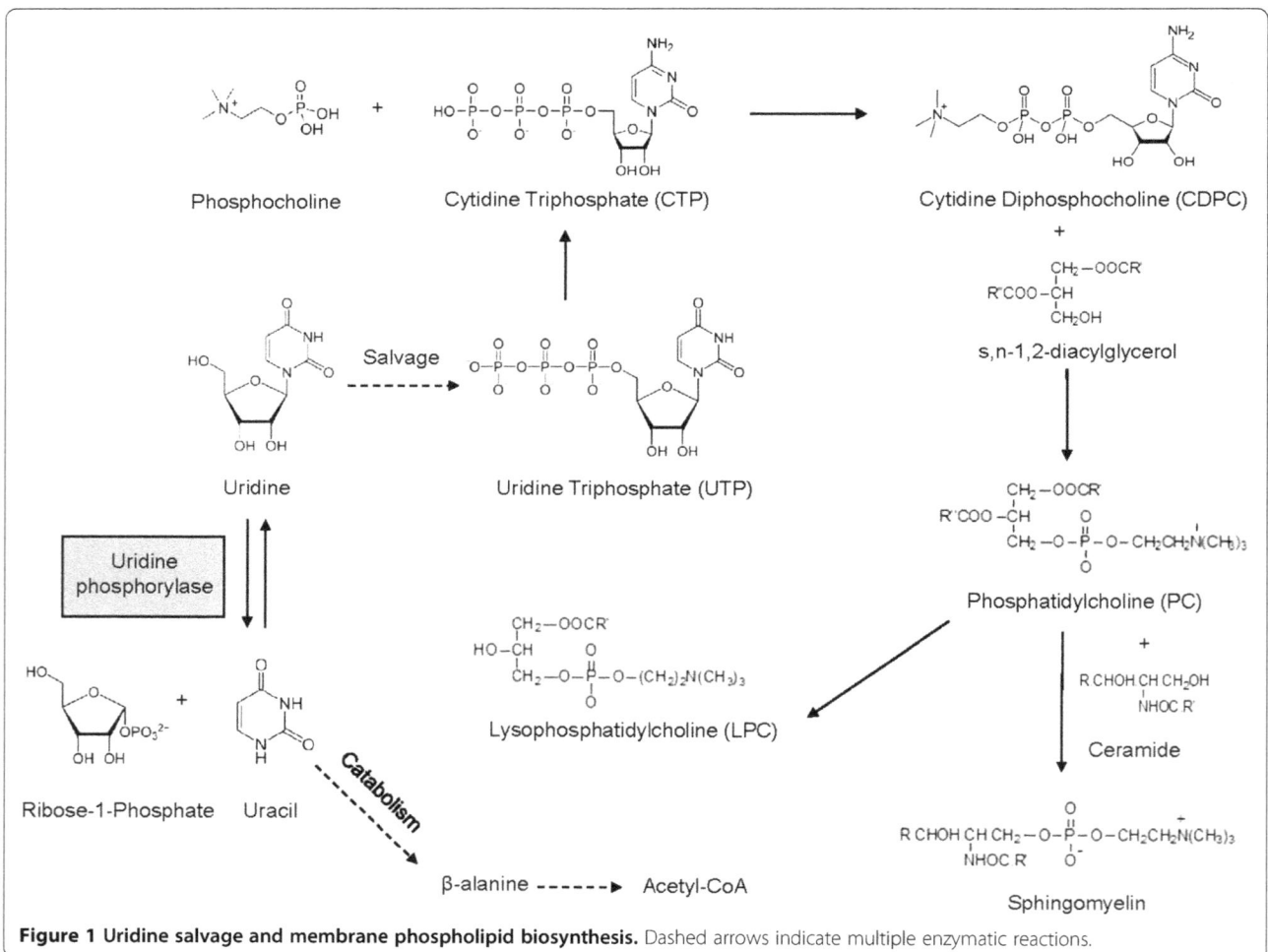

Figure 1 Uridine salvage and membrane phospholipid biosynthesis. Dashed arrows indicate multiple enzymatic reactions.

However, precise underlying mechanisms have not been determined. Consequently, therapeutic potential of uridine for treatment of fatty liver condition has not been realized.

In this study, we examine the effects of uridine coadministration with tamoxifen on liver lipid content in control C57BL/6J and transgenic $UPase1^{-/-}$ and $UPase1$-TG mice. Specifically, we examine the contribution of pyrimidine salvage and catabolism pathways to the biological activity of uridine. We aim to explore therapeutic potential of uridine for the prevention of drug-induced fatty liver and biological action of uridine on liver lipid metabolism.

Methods

Ethical statement
All animal studies were performed with the ethical approval of the Animal Care and Use Committees at Nevada Cancer Institute, Desert Research Institute, and Touro University Nevada. All experiments conducted on animals were in compliance with the guidelines of the U.S. Office of Laboratory Animal Welfare of the National Institutes of Health and the Public Health Service Policy on Humane Care and Use of Laboratory Animals.

Experimental animals
Three mice strains were used, C57BL/6J or wildtype mice (Jackson Laboratories, Bar Harbor, ME), $UPase1$-TG mice with ubiquitous genetic knock-in of uridine phosphorylase 1 [18], and $UPase1^{-/-}$ mice with ubiquitous genetic knock-out of uridine phosphorylase 1 [17]. Transgenic mice described in this study have been deposited into the Mutant Mouse Regional Resource Centers supported by the National Institutes of Health. The MMRRC strains are now known as B6;129-$Upp1^{tm1Gp}$/Mmucd (037119-UCD) for $UPase1^{-/-}$ mice and B6; FVB-Gt $(ROSA)$ $26Sor^{tm1.1(CAG-Upp1)Gp}$/Mmucd (037120-UCD) for $UPase1$-TG mice. All mice used were female at 10–12 weeks of age with average bodyweight of approximately 20 grams.

Study design
All mice were randomly divided into groups of 4 or 5 mice per cage and housed in a controlled environment with an average temperature of 22°C, a 12 hours of light and 12 hours of dark cycle, and with *ad libitum* access to food and water. For control C57BL/6J mice, 36 mice were randomly divided into 4 experimental groups of 9 mice per group: control diet (C57BL/6J), diet supplemented with uridine (C57BL/6J + U), diet supplemented with tamoxifen (C57BL/6J + Tmx), and diet supplemented with both tamoxifen and uridine (C57BL/6J + Tmx + U). For transgenic $UPase1^{-/-}$ and $UPase1$-TG mice, 18 mice per strain were randomly divided into the following 4 experimental groups of 9 mice per group: $UPase1^{-/-}$ mice

on control diet ($UPase1^{-/-}$), $UPase1^{-/-}$ mice on tamoxifen-supplemented diet, $UPase1$-TG mice on control diet ($UPase1$-TG), and $UPase1$-TG mice on tamoxifen-supplemented diet. In addition, 6 C57BL/6J mice were used for primary hepatocyte collection for bioenergetics experiments. The number of mice per experimental group was chosen to ensure that data obtained were statistically significant.

Experimental procedures
Control mice were fed with PicoLab Mouse Diet ground pellets (Cat. No. 5058, LabDiet, Brentwood, MO) that provide 4.6 kcal/g and consist of 22% protein and 9% fat. The lipid composition includes cholesterol (200 ppm), linoleic acid (2.32%), linolenic acid (0.21%), arachidonic acid (0.02%), and omega-3 fatty acid (0.32%). The total saturated and monounsaturated fatty acids are 2.72% and 2.88%, respectively. For mice receiving uridine supplementation alone, uridine was thoroughly mixed with ground pellets with a dosage of 400 mg/kg/day. For mice receiving tamoxifen treatment alone, tamoxifen was thoroughly mixed with ground pellets with a dosage of 200 mg/kg/day. For mice receiving both uridine and tamoxifen, uridine and tamoxifen were thoroughly mixed with ground pellets with a dosage of 400 mg/kg/day and 200 mg/kg/day, respectively. Mice were placed on control or supplemented diets for 5 days prior to terminal liver and blood samples collection. All samples were collected in early mornings. Blood samples were collected via the tail veins while mice were under anesthesia with isoflurane. Liver tissues were collected following cardiac perfusion under deep anesthesia with isoflurane. Cardiac perfusion was necessary to ensure collection of pure liver tissues devoid of blood and plasma contaminants. Mice were anaesthetized and incisions were made from the abdomen up to the torso. Diaphragms were severed and 22 gauge needles were inserted into the left ventricles. Phosphate buffered saline (PBS) was used as the perfusate. Approximately 50–100 ml of PBS was flushed through each mouse from the left ventricle and exited through the incision made to the right atrium. Following the perfusion procedure, liver tissues were collected for immediate usage or frozen in liquid nitrogen for future usage.

CARS imaging of liver tissues
A home-built CARS microscope was used to image lipid using CH_2 vibrational frequency at 2851 cm^{-1} as described previously [20]. Approximately 31 frames were taken along the vertical axis at 1-micron increment for volumetric evaluation of liver lipid content. Liver lipid level was the square root of resonant CARS signal intensity, which is the difference between total CARS signal intensity and CARS signal intensity arising from cellular membrane and non-resonant signal [21-23]. Liver lipid level was normalized to

1 for control wildtype mice and respectively for other mice strains or treatment conditions. Quantitative analysis of liver lipid level was performed using the NIH ImageJ software. Liver was perfused with PBS prior to collection. Liver tissues were sliced into 200-micron thick sections, transferred into glass-bottom chambered slides, overlaid with 200 microliter of 1% agarose, and imaged with CARS microscopy. On average, 9 imaging volumes were analyzed with CARS microscopy per liver sample. The xyz dimensions of each analysis volume were 167 μm × 167 μm × 30 μm. Nine liver samples from nine mice were used for CARS imaging analysis per animal group.

Biochemical measurement of liver triacylglyceride (TAG)

Liver samples of equal weight were used for chloroform/methanol total lipid extraction. TAG was determined using the commercial TAG quantitation kit (Cat. No. 10010303, Cayman Chemical, Ann Arbor, MI) according to manufacturer's protocol and normalized with liver tissue weight. Nine liver samples from nine mice were used for biochemical TAG measurement per animal group.

1D Western blots

Total liver protein extracts were separated on 10% SDS-PAGE gels, transferred to nitrocellulose membranes, incubated first with primary antibodies against proteins of interest and then with secondary antibodies conjugated with horseradish peroxidase (Cat. No. 31460, Thermo Scientific, Rockford, IL). Membrane was developed with enhanced chemiluminescence reagents (Cat. No. 34075, Thermo Scientific), stripped, and re-incubated with anti bodies against β-actin for evaluation of loading controls. Primary antibodies against acetylated lysine and β-actin were from Cell Signaling (Cat. No. 9441 & 4967, Danvers, MA).

2D Western blots

2D Western blots were performed by Kendrick Laboratories (Madison, WI). Approximately 500 μg of protein from each liver tissue was loaded per gel. Proteins were separated using isoelectric focusing (IEF) in the first dimension and SDS polyacrylamide gel electrophoresis (SDS-PAGE) in the second dimension. Primary and secondary antibodies were the same as in 1D Western blot. Molecular weight standards were: myosin (220,000), phosphorylase A (94,000), catalase (60,000), actin (43,000) carbonic anhydrase (29,000) and lysozyme (14,000) (Sigma Chemical Co., St. Louis, MO).

Bioenergetics of primary hepatocytes

Immediately after isolation, primary hepatocytes were plated into 24-well plates at a density of 1×10^5 cell per well. Plating media was consisted of DMEM with 25 mM glucose, 2 mM glutamine, 10% FBS, 0.1 mM sodium pyruvate, 1% Pen/Strep, and 1 mM HEPES at pH 7.4. At 4 hours after plating, primary hepatocytes were incubated for 24 hours with either uridine alone, tamoxifen alone, or a combination of tamoxifen and uridine depending on the treatment condition. The final concentration used for uridine was 100 μM and tamoxifen was 10 μM. At 90 minutes prior to assaying, plating media was replaced with Cellular Assay Solution consisting of DMEM, 25 mM glucose, 2 mM glutamine, 1 mM sodium pyruvate and adjusted to pH 7.2 with 25 mM of MOPS. Bioenergetics of primary hepatocytes were determined using the XF Cell Mito Stress Test Kit and a XF24-3 Analyzer (Seahorse Bioscience, North Billerica, MA) following manufacturer's suggested protocols and published protocols [24]. Bioenergetics experiments were performed at the UCLA's Cellular Bioenergetics Core Facilities. At least 24 repeated measurements were performed per experimental condition. Final concentrations of oligomycin, FCCP, rotenone, and myxothiazol were 1 μg/ml, 1 μM, 0.1 μM, and 2 μM, respectively. Oxygen consumption rates were reported as absolute values (pmol O_2 consumed per minute) on a per-unit of protein basis, where average protein concentration per well was normalized to 1.

Clinical blood lipid analysis

Analysis of blood lipid level (TAG, cholesterol, HDL, and LDL) were performed by Research Animal Diagnostic Laboratory (RADIL, Columbia, MO) on terminally collected blood samples of 6 mice per animal group. HDL and LDL were determined via direct measurement.

Measurement of phospholipid with LC-MS

Total liver lipid extracts of 6 mice per animal group were sent to Kansas Lipidomics Research Center (Kansas State University, Manhattan, KS) for LC-MS analysis of phospholipid species. Concentrations of phospholipid are expressed as nmol per mg of dried liver lipid weight.

Statistical analysis

Data were presented as average values ± standard deviations. Statistical analysis was performed using Excel's paired Student's t-test and analysis of variance (ANOVA) functions. Statistical significance was set at $p \leq 0.05$.

Results and discussion

The effects of tamoxifen treatment on liver lipid content were evaluated in C57BL/6J mice. Daily dosage of 200 milligrams tamoxifen per kilogram bodyweight was chosen for mice to reproduce equivalent dosage administered in humans after adjusting for differences in energy metabolism and pharmacokinetics between species [25]. Following 5 days of tamoxifen treatment, mice lost up to 5% of bodyweight. Traditional histopathology analysis does not have sufficient sensitivity to analyze mild hepatic microvesicular steatosis associated with tamoxifen treatment for 5 days [11,21]. Therefore, collected liver tissues were examined with CARS microscopy, a highly sensitive method for lipid visualization [22,23,26], to evaluate liver lipid content. Liver tissues of untreated control mice and mice treated with uridine did not exhibit any intracellular lipid accumulation (Figure 2A). In contrast, liver tissues of mice treated with tamoxifen had significant intracellular lipid droplet accumulation, which could be classified as microvesicular steatosis [27]. Quantitative analysis of liver lipid level using CARS signal intensity revealed that tamoxifen treatment increased intracellular liver lipid level by 76% (Figure 2B). Surprisingly, uridine co-administration completely prevented tamoxifen-induced hepatic steatosis (Figure 2A,B). Data obtained with CARS microscopy were corroborated with biochemical measurements of liver triacylglyceride content (Figure 2C). Oil Red O histology was also performed on all liver tissue samples. However, ORO histology was unable to detect mild hepatic microvesicular

steatosis associated with tamoxifen treatment (data not shown). The insensitivity of ORO histology to detect mild microvesicular steatosis had been described in the literature [21,28-30]. It is important to point out that while uridine co-administration completely suppressed tamoxifen-induced hepatic microvesicular steatosis, it had no impact on tamoxifen-induced weight loss in mice.

Uridine has the ability to modulate liver protein acetylation profile [14,18]. Uridine catabolism produces acetyl-CoA, which is a donor substrate for protein acetylation [18]. Uridine supplementation also elevates liver $NAD^+/NADH$ ratio, which alters the activity of NAD^+-dependent deacetylases [18]. Liver protein acetylation is highly correlated to energy metabolism [31,32]. To determine whether uridine prevented tamoxifen-induced fatty liver by modulating protein acetylation profile, 1D Western blots using antibodies against acetylated lysine residues were performed on total liver extracts (Figure 3A). Tamoxifen treatment increased acetylation of a protein band with molecular

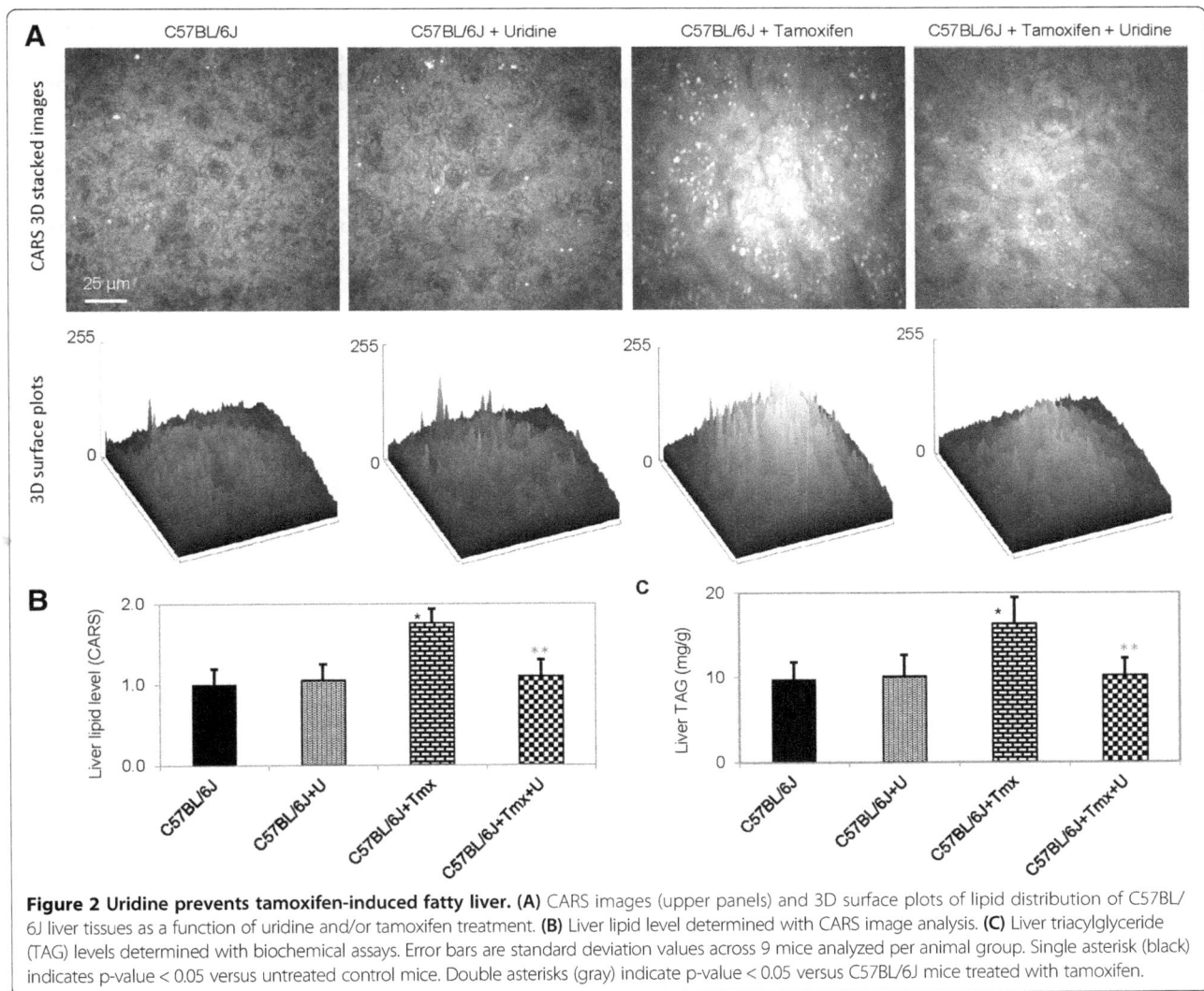

Figure 2 Uridine prevents tamoxifen-induced fatty liver. (A) CARS images (upper panels) and 3D surface plots of lipid distribution of C57BL/6J liver tissues as a function of uridine and/or tamoxifen treatment. **(B)** Liver lipid level determined with CARS image analysis. **(C)** Liver triacylglyceride (TAG) levels determined with biochemical assays. Error bars are standard deviation values across 9 mice analyzed per animal group. Single asterisk (black) indicates p-value < 0.05 versus untreated control mice. Double asterisks (gray) indicate p-value < 0.05 versus C57BL/6J mice treated with tamoxifen.

weight of ~80 kD. However, uridine co-administration with tamoxifen had no effect on the acetylation state of this protein band.

Next, 2D Western blots were employed for high resolution evaluation of liver protein acetylation profiles (Figure 3B). Consistent with 1D Western blots, 2D Western blots revealed that tamoxifen treatment induced acetylation of a protein spot with molecular weight of 80 kD (Figure 3B, box with dashed line). Also consistent with 1D Western blot, uridine co-administration with tamoxifen could not prevent the effect of tamoxifen-induced hyper-acetylation of this 80 kD protein spot. Overall, when uridine was co-administered with tamoxifen, it had no impact on liver protein acetylation profile. Therefore, it was unlikely that uridine prevented tamoxifen-induced fatty liver by modulating liver protein acetylation profiles.

Tamoxifen treatment is associated with impaired mitochondrial respiration [9,11]. To determine whether uridine co-administration could prevent the inhibitory effects of tamoxifen on mitochondrial respiration, primary hepatocyte cell cultures were employed. An Extracellular Flux Analyzer was employed to measure 5 key parameters of cellular bioenergetics: basal respiration, non-mitochondrial respiration, ATP production, proton leak, and maximal respiration using a previously described protocol [24]. Consistent with the literature, tamoxifen treatment severely reduced oxygen consumption rates in primary hepatocytes for all parameters evaluated (Figure 4A). Uridine administration by itself had no effect on mitochondrial respiration

of primary hepatocytes. Surprisingly, uridine co-administration could not prevent tamoxifen-induced impairment to mitochondrial respiration in primary hepatocytes. Thus, it was unlikely that uridine co-administration prevented fatty liver by restoring mitochondrial function impaired by tamoxifen.

Tamoxifen treatment is associated with reduced liver secretion of TAG and cholesterol [10,11]. To determine if uridine co-administration with tamoxifen could improve liver secretion of TAG and cholesterol, blood lipid profiles were evaluated (Figure 4B). Consistent with the literature, tamoxifen treatment caused reduction of blood TAG and cholesterol levels. Uridine treatment by itself had no effect on blood TAG and cholesterol levels. Neither could uridine co-administration prevent tamoxifen-induced reduction of blood TAG and cholesterol levels. Thus, there was no evidence to support a role of uridine in reversing tamoxifen-induced suppression of liver secretion of TAG and cholesterol.

Salvage of uridine to cytidine triphosphate promotes phospholipid biosynthesis in the presence of phosphocholine and diacylglycerol [15,33]. To determine if there was a role for uridine salvage in the prevention of tamoxifen-induced fatty liver, lipidomics profiling of liver phospholipid with LC-MS was carried out (Figure 4C, Table 1). When administered individually, both uridine and tamoxifen increased the levels of many liver phospholipid species. When administered together, uridine and tamoxifen further increased the levels of many

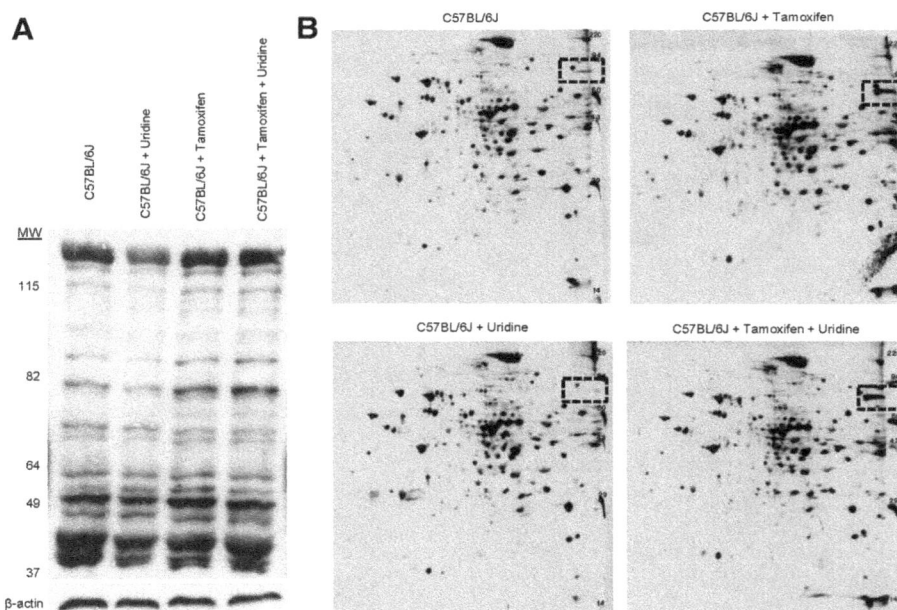

Figure 3 Effects of uridine and tamoxifen on liver protein acetylation profile. (A) 1D Western blot analysis of liver protein lysine acetylation profile. β-actin serves as a loading control. **(B)** 2D Western blot analysis of liver protein lysine acetylation profile. Box with dashed black lines highlights the locations of a protein band at 80 kD whose acetylation level increases with tamoxifen treatment.

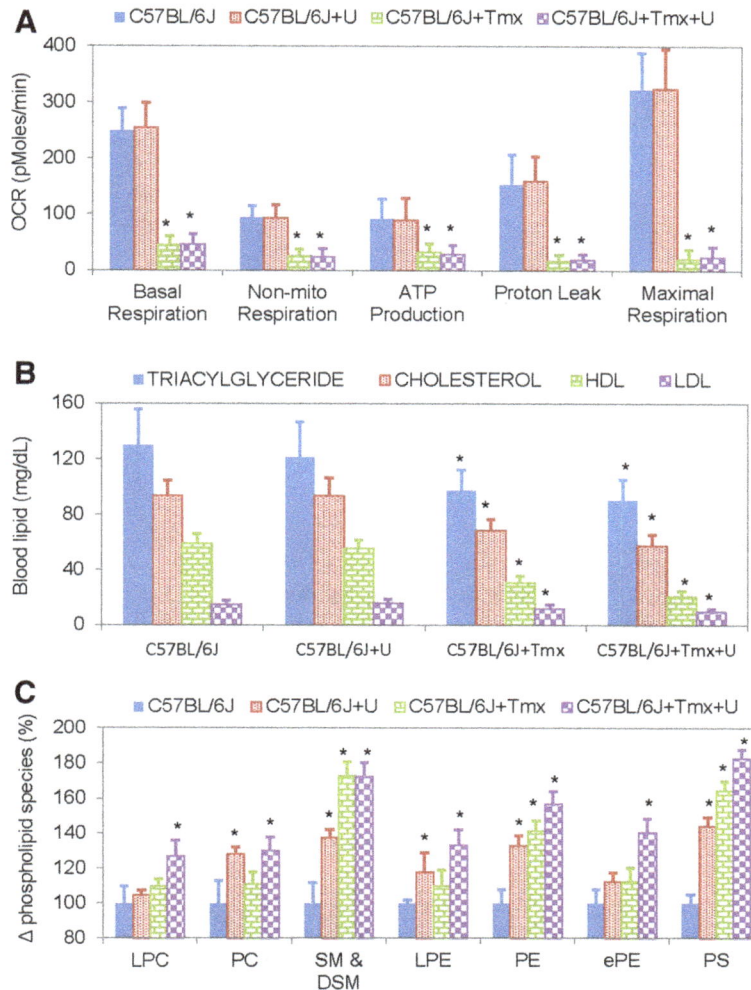

Figure 4 Effects of uridine and tamoxifen on hepatocyte mitochondrial respiration, blood lipid level, and liver phospholipid level.
(A) Oxygen consumption rate (OCR) of primary hepatocytes measured with an Extracellular Flux Analyzer. Error bars are standard deviation values across 24 repeated measurements per experimental condition. **(B)** Blood levels of triacylglyceride, cholesterol, high-density lipoprotein (HDL), and low-density lipoprotein (LDL) determined via direct measurements. **(C)** Changes in selective phospholipid species as a function of uridine and/or tamoxifen treatment. Lysophosphotidylcholine (LPC); phosphotidylcholine (PC); sphingomyelin (SM) & dihydrosphingomyelin (DSM); lysophosphoethanolamine (LPE); phosphoethanolamine (PE); ether-linked phosphoethanoamine (ePE); phosphatidylserine (PS). Error bars are standard deviation values across 6 mice analyzed per animal group. Asterisks indicate p-value < 0.05 versus untreated control mice.

liver phospholipid species. Among the most affected phospholipid species were sphingomyelin, phosphatidyl-serine, and phosphoethanolamine, where uridine co-administration with tamoxifen increased their levels by as much as 80%. The lipidomics data suggested that uridine could prevent tamoxifen-induced fatty liver by promoting membrane phospholipid biosynthesis.

To further evaluate the relationship between pyrimidine salvage pathway and the prevention of tamoxifen-induced fatty liver, $UPase1^{-/-}$ and $UPase1$-TG mice were employed. $UPase1^{-/-}$ mice have elevated liver and circulating uridine concentration due to genetic knock-out of a gene encoding for uridine phosphorylase 1, an enzyme that catalyzes uridine catabolism [17]. On average, $UPase1^{-/-}$ mice have

liver and plasma concentration of 42.8 μM and 7.2 μM, respectively; whereas, C57BL/6J mice have liver and plasma concentration of 6.8 μM and 1.5 μM, respectively [34]. For $UPase1^{-/-}$ strain, liver tissues of untreated control mice were devoid of intracellular lipid droplet (Figure 5A-C). Tamoxifen treatment of $UPase1^{-/-}$ mice did not lead to intracellular lipid droplet accumulation in the liver tissues. On the other hand, $UPase1$-TG mice have depleted liver and circulating uridine concentration due to genetic knock-in of a gene encoding for for uridine phosphorylase 1 [18]. On average, $UPase1$-TG mice have liver and plasma uridine concentration of 0.5 μM and 0.08 μM, respectively. For $UPase1$-TG strain, liver tissues of untreated control mice were already exhibiting microvesicular steatosis

Table 1 Liver phospholipid species quantified with LC-MS

Phospholipid species (nmol/mg)	C57BL/6J	C57BL/6J + U	C57BL/6J + Tmx	C57BL/6J + Tmx + U
Lysophosphotidylcholine	6.7 ± 0.7	7.1 ± 0.3	7.4 ± 0.4	8.6 ± 0.8*
Phosphotidylcholine	380.5 ± 51	486.8 ± 20*	421.9 ± 30.6	495.1 ± 39.6*
Sphingomyelin & dihydrosphingomyelin	29.1 ± 3.7	40.0 ± 2.8*	50.3 ± 3.9*	50.2 ± 3.7*
Ether-linked phosphotidylcholine	18.9 ± 2.2	18.5 ± 0.6	21.2 ± 1.4	22.5 ± 2.1
Lysophosphoethanolamine	1.9 ± 0.1	2.3 ± 0.26	2.1 ± 0.2	2.6 ± 2.1
Phosphoethanolamine	105.5 ± 8.9	140.1 ± 8.8*	149.2 ± 8.3*	165.6 ± 8.9*
Phosphoethanoamine-ceramide	0.01 ± 0.01	0.01 ± 0.01	0.016 ± 0.005	0.027 ± 0.013
Ether-linked Phosphoethanoamine	4.0 ± 0.4	4.5 ± 0.3	4.5 ± 0.3	5.6 ± 0.4*
Phosphatidylinositol	51.2 ± 6.9	60.0 ± 7.1	46.9 ± 3.7	58.4 ± 6.2
Phosphatidylserine	15.4 ± 0.8	22.3 ± 1.1*	25.4 ± 1.3*	28.2 ± 1.3*
Ether-linked phosphatidylserine	0.2 ± 0.03	0.3 ± 0.03*	0.36 ± 0.017*	0.4 ± 0.04*
Phosphatidic acid	19.9 ± 2.3	23.2 ± 2.4	15.2 ± 1.7	21.2 ± 1.4
Phosphatidylglycerol	27.2 ± 3.1	29.9 ± 2.7	33.0 ± 2.1	29.7 ± 2.2

Asterisks indicate p-value <0.05 versus untreated control.

(Figure 5A-C). Tamoxifen treatment of *UPase1*-TG mice increased liver lipid content by approximately 20% compared to untreated control *UPase1*-TG mice. Hence, *UPase1*$^{-/-}$ mice, which had increased pyrimidine salvage activity [17], were protected against tamoxifen-induced fatty liver. In contrast, *UPase1*-TG mice, which had increased uridine catabolism activity [18], were susceptible to further liver lipid accumulation following tamoxifen treatment.

Conclusions

In this study, we report that uridine co-administration is effective at completely preventing intracellular lipid droplet accumulation in the liver tissues of mice treated with tamoxifen. To examine the roles of uridine in the prevention of tamoxifen-induced fatty liver, several aspects of liver energy metabolism perturbed by tamoxifen were evaluated. Tamoxifen administration was associated with an increased in acetylation of a protein band at 80

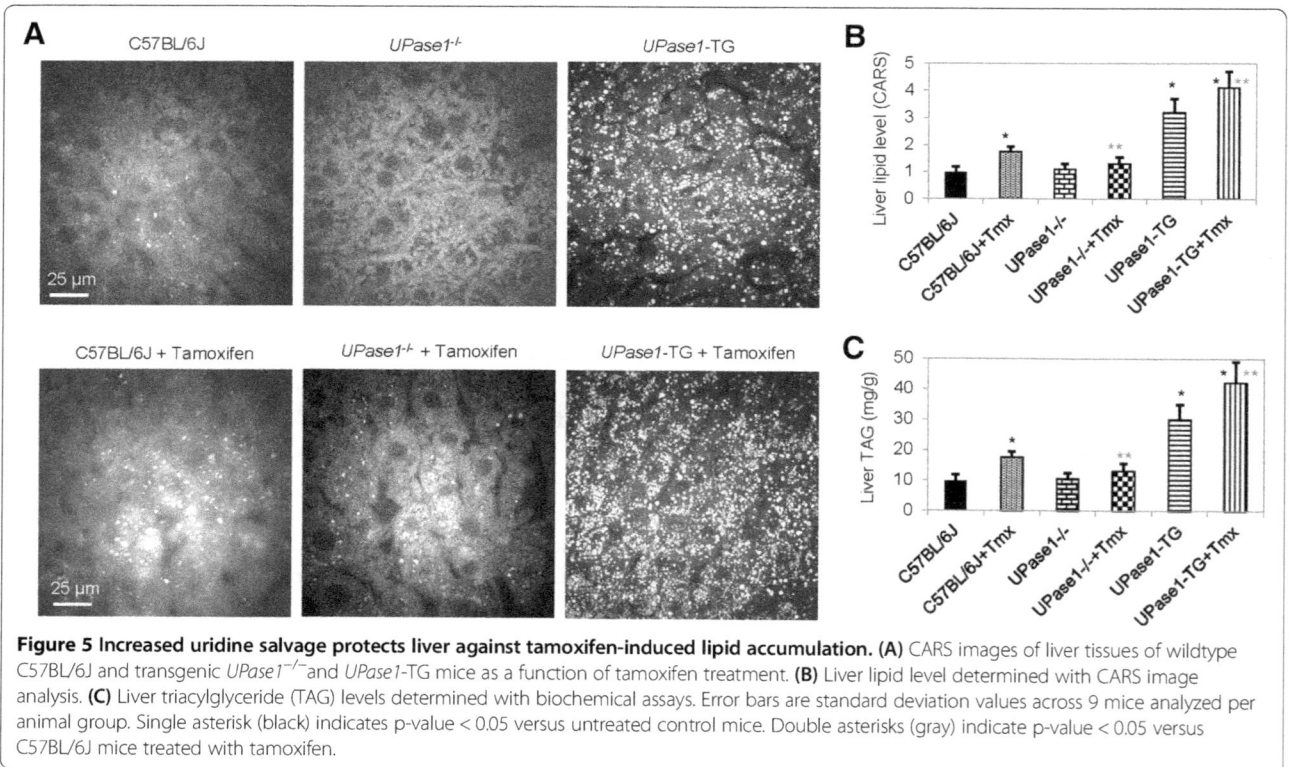

Figure 5 Increased uridine salvage protects liver against tamoxifen-induced lipid accumulation. (A) CARS images of liver tissues of wildtype C57BL/6J and transgenic *UPase1*$^{-/-}$ and *UPase1*-TG mice as a function of tamoxifen treatment. **(B)** Liver lipid level determined with CARS image analysis. **(C)** Liver triacylglyceride (TAG) levels determined with biochemical assays. Error bars are standard deviation values across 9 mice analyzed per animal group. Single asterisk (black) indicates p-value < 0.05 versus untreated control mice. Double asterisks (gray) indicate p-value < 0.05 versus C57BL/6J mice treated with tamoxifen.

kD and impaired mitochondrial respiration; however, both of these tamoxifen-induced effects could not be reversed by uridine co-administration. Neither could uridine prevent tamoxifen-induced reduction in blood TAG and cholesterol levels. Surprisingly, both uridine and tamoxifen when administered alone and together increased membrane phospholipid biosynthesis. The synthesis of phosphatidylcholine (PC), the key component of phospholipid, was dependent on the availability of diacylglycerol (DAG) and cytidine diphosphocholine (CDPC) (Figure 1) [33]. It is possible that tamoxifen-induced lipid accumulation in liver tissues made TAG and DAG to be readily available for PC synthesis. Uridine salvage into CTP promoted CDPC synthesis, which together with DAG availability stimulated PC synthesis. Transgenic mice $UPase1^{-/-}$ with increased uridine salvage into CTP were protected against tamoxifen-induced fatty liver. In contrast, $UPase1$-TG mice with overt catabolism of uridine had intrinsic fatty liver phenotype, which was aggravated following tamoxifen treatment. In summary, uridine co-administration was able to prevent tamoxifen-induced intracellular lipid droplet accumulation, but not able to prevent other side effects associated with tamoxifen treatment such as impaired mitochondrial respiration and reduced TAG and cholesterol export. A plausible means that uridine prevented tamoxifen-induced fatty liver was via the pyrimidine salvage pathway, which channeled neutral lipid into phospholipid biosynthesis and reduced cytoplasmic lipid accumulation.

A previous study on the anti-proliferative effect of tamoxifen in human MCF-7 breast cancer cells proposed that tamoxifen prevented DNA synthesis by blocking uridine transport, thus, inhibiting the pyrimidine salvage pathway [35]. In our study, C57BL/6J mice with dietary uridine supplementation or $UPase1^{-/-}$ mice with elevated endogenous uridine levels both had enhanced pyrimidine salvage activity [17]. Both mice strains were resistant to tamoxifen-induced fatty liver; however, they exhibited weight loss following tamoxifen treatment. In addition, uridine supplementation in primary hepatocyte cultures could not prevent tamoxifen-induced impairment to mitochondrial respiration. Our observation indicates that tamoxifen exert inhibitory effects beyond the pyrimidine salvage pathway. Indeed, tamoxifen has been shown to directly intercalate mitochondrial DNA (mtDNA) and impair mtDNA synthesis and mitochondrial respiration [11]. It is unlikely that uridine can prevent the interaction of cationic tamoxifen with mtDNA, hence, its inability to suppress the inhibitory effects of tamoxifen on mitochondrial function.

The balance between purine and pyrimidine nucleotides is critical for the maintenance of genomic stability and regulation. A surge in uridine concentration subsequently leads to a rise in pyrimidine nucleotides and perturbs the balance of the nucleotide pool [15]. Therefore, an adaptive mechanism must be in place to cope with excessive uridine concentration. In rodents, most tissues rely on the plasma for uridine supply [36]. The circulating uridine concentration is tightly regulated by the liver, where plasma uridine is cleared in a single pass and replaced with newly synthesized uridine [19]. Hence, the liver effectively serves as a regulator of uridine homeostasis. Rapid clearance of uridine in the liver involves both uridine salvage and catabolism, where uridine metabolites affect other cellular processes in a non-specific manner. Multi-targeted effects are evident by the ability of uridine to prevent fatty liver caused by different drugs with vastly different acting mechanisms [13,14]. Multi-targeted effects pose a challenge for precise therapeutic targeting using uridine. However, uridine homeostasis is regulated by uridine phosphorylase [16]. The enzymatic activity of uridine phosphorylase has been modulated by pharmaceutical compounds to prevent toxicity associated with 5-fluorouracil treatment of cancer [37]. Modulation of uridine phosphorylase enzymatic activity is a possible means to achieve precise therapeutic targeting of uridine for the prevention of drug-induced fatty liver.

Abbreviations
CARS: Coherent anti-Stokes Raman scattering; CDPC: Cytidine diphosphocholine; DAG: Diacylglycerol; HDL: High-density lipoprotein; LC-MS: Liquid chromatography coupled with mass spectrometry; LDL: Low-density lipoprotein; OCR: Oxygen consumption rate; PC: Phosphatidylcholine; TAG: Triacylglyceride.

Competing interests
The authors declare that they have no competing interest.

Authors' contribution
TTL and GP designed experiments. TTL and GP contributed reagents, samples, and analytical tools. TTL and YU performed experiments and analyzed data. TTL prepared the manuscript. All authors read and approved final manuscript.

Acknowledgements
This work was partially supported by the Nevada INBRE Program of the National Center for Research Resources (P20RR-016464, TTL), the Vons Breast Cancer Research Award (GP & TTL) and the American Cancer Society (IRG-08-062-04, TTL). The funders had no role in study design, data collection and analysis, decision to publish, or preparation of the manuscript. The authors thank Laurent Vergnes (UCLA) and Robert Kirsh (DRI) for help with some experiments.

Author details
[1]Nevada Cancer Institute, One Breakthrough Way, Las Vegas, NV 89135, USA. [2]Desert Research Institute, 10530 Discovery Drive, Las Vegas, NV 89135, USA. [3]Roseman University of Health Sciences, 11 Sunset Way, Henderson NV 89014, USA.

References
1.   Fisher B, Costantino JP, Wickerham DL, Redmond CK, Kavanah M, Cronin WM, Vogel V, Robidoux A, Dimitrov N, Atkins J, Daly M, Wieand S, Tan-Chiu E, Ford L, Wolmark N: **Tamoxifen for prevention of breast cancer: report of the national surgical adjuvant breast and bowel project P-1 study.** *J Natl Cancer Inst* 1998, **90**(18):1371–1388.

2.   Hackshaw A, Roughton M, Forsyth S, Monson K, Reczko K, Sainsbury R, Baum M: Long-term benefits of 5 years of tamoxifen: 10-year follow-up of a large randomized trial in women at least 50 years of age with early breast cancer. *J Clin Oncol* 2011, 29(13):1657–1663.

3.   Davies C, Pan H, Godwin J, Gray R, Arriagada R, Raina V, Abraham M, Alencar VH, Badran A, Bonfill X, Bradbury J, Clarke M, Collins R, Davis SR, Delmestri A, Forbes JF, Haddad P, Hou MF, Inbar M, Khaled H, Kielanowska J, Kwan WH, Matthew BS, Mittra I, Muller B, Nicolucci A, Peralta O, Pernas F, Petruzelka L, Pienkowski T, et al: Long-term effects of continuing adjuvant tamoxifen to 10 years versus stopping at 5 years after diagnosis of oestrogen receptor-positive breast cancer: ATLAS, a randomised trial. *Lancet* 2013, 381(9869):805–816.

4.   Nishino M, Hayakawa K, Nakamura Y, Morimoto T, Mukaihara S: Effects of tamoxifen on hepatic fat content and the development of hepatic steatosis in patients with breast cancer: high frequency of involvement and rapid reversal after completion of tamoxifen therapy. *AJR Am J Roentgenol* 2003, 180(1):129–134.

5.   Ogawa Y, Murata Y, Nishioka A, Inomata T, Yoshida S: Tamoxifen-induced fatty liver in patients with breast cancer. *Lancet* 1998, 351(9104):725.

6.   Nguyen MC, Stewart RB, Banerji MA, Gordon DH, Kral JG: Relationships between tamoxifen use, liver fat and body fat distribution in women with breast cancer. *Int J Obes Relat Metab Disord* 2001, 25(2):296–298.

7.   Cohen JC, Horton JD, Hobbs HH: Human fatty liver disease: old questions and new insights. *Science* 2011, 332(6037):1519–1523.

8.   Bruno S, Maisonneuve P, Castellana P, Rotmensz N, Rossi S, Maggioni M, Persico M, Colombo A, Monasterolo F, Casadei-Giunchi D, Desiderio F, Stroffolini T, Sacchini V, Decensi A, Veronesi U: Incidence and risk factors for non-alcoholic steatohepatitis: prospective study of 5408 women enrolled in Italian tamoxifen chemoprevention trial. *BMJ* 2005, 330(7497):932.

9.   Cardoso CM, Custodio JB, Almeida LM, Moreno AJ: Mechanisms of the deleterious effects of tamoxifen on mitochondrial respiration rate and phosphorylation efficiency. *Toxicol Appl Pharmacol* 2001, 176(3):145–152.

10. Lelliott CJ, Lopez M, Curtis RK, Parker N, Laudes M, Yeo G, Jimenez-Linan M, Grosse J, Saha AK, Wiggins D, Hauton D, Brand MD, O'Rahilly S, Griffin JL, Gibbons GF, Vidal-Puig A: Transcript and metabolite analysis of the effects of tamoxifen in rat liver reveals inhibition of fatty acid synthesis in the presence of hepatic steatosis. *FASEB J* 2005, 19(9):1108–1119.

11. Larosche I, Letteron P, Fromenty B, Vadrot N, Abbey-Toby A, Feldmann G, Pessayre D, Mansouri A: Tamoxifen inhibits topoisomerases, depletes mitochondrial DNA, and triggers steatosis in mouse liver. *J Pharmacol Exp Ther* 2007, 321(2):526–535.

12. Gudbrandsen OA, Rost TH, Berge RK: Causes and prevention of tamoxifen-induced accumulation of triacylglycerol in rat liver. *J Lipid Res* 2006, 47(10):2223–2232.

13. Lebrecht D, Vargas-Infante YA, Setzer B, Kirschner J, Walker UA: Uridine supplementation antagonizes zalcitabine-induced microvesicular steatohepatitis in mice. *Hepatology* 2007, 45(1):72–79.

14. Le TT, Urasaki Y, Pizzorno G: Uridine prevents fenofibrate-induced fatty liver. *PLoS One* 2014, 9(1):e87179.

15. Connolly GP, Duley JA: Uridine and its nucleotides: biological actions, therapeutic potentials. *Trends Pharmacol Sci* 1999, 20(5):218–225.

16. Pizzorno G, Cao D, Leffert JJ, Russell RL, Zhang D, Handschumacher RE: Homeostatic control of uridine and the role of uridine phosphorylase: a biological and clinical update. *Biochim Biophys Acta* 2002, 1587(2–3):133–144.

17. Cao D, Leffert JJ, McCabe J, Kim B, Pizzorno G: Abnormalities in uridine homeostatic regulation and pyrimidine nucleotide metabolism as a consequence of the deletion of the uridine phosphorylase gene. *J Biol Chem* 2005, 280(22):21169–21175.

18. Le TT, Ziemba A, Urasaki Y, Hayes E, Brotman S, Pizzorno G: Disruption of uridine homeostasis links liver pyrimidine metabolism to lipid accumulation. *J Lipid Res* 2013, 54(4):1044–1057.

19. Gasser T, Moyer JD, Handschumacher RE: Novel single-pass exchange of circulating uridine in rat liver. *Science* 1981, 213(4509):777–778.

20. Urasaki Y, Johlfs MG, Fiscus RR, Le TT: Imaging immune and metabolic cells of visceral adipose tissues with multimodal nonlinear optical microscopy. *PLoS One* 2012, 7(6):e38418.

21. Le TT, Ziemba A, Urasaki Y, Brotman S, Pizzorno G: Label-free evaluation of hepatic microvesicular steatosis with multimodal coherent anti-stokes Raman scattering microscopy. *PLoS One* 2012, 7(11):e51092.

22. Evans CL, Xie XS: Coherent anti-Stokes Raman scattering microscopy: chemically selective imaging for biology and medicine. *Annu Rev Anal Chem* 2008, 1(1):883–909.

23. Le TT, Yue S, Cheng JX: Shedding new light on lipid biology with coherent anti-Stokes Raman scattering microscopy. *J Lipid Res* 2010, 51(11):3091–3102.

24. Zhang J, Nuebel E, Wisidagama DR, Setoguchi K, Hong JS, Van Horn CM, Imam SS, Vergnes L, Malone CS, Koehler CM, Teitell MA: Measuring energy metabolism in cultured cells, including human pluripotent stem cells and differentiated cells. *Nat Protoc* 2012, 7(6):1068–1085.

25. Robinson SP, Langan-Fahey SM, Johnson DA, Jordan VC: Metabolites, pharmacodynamics, and pharmacokinetics of tamoxifen in rats and mice compared to the breast cancer patient. *Drug Metab Dispos* 1991, 19(1):36–43.

26. Pezacki JP, Blake JA, Danielson DC, Kennedy DC, Lyn RK, Singaravelu R: Chemical contrast for imaging living systems: molecular vibrations drive CARS microscopy. *Nat Chem Biol* 2011, 7(3):137–145.

27. Kleiner DE, Brunt EM, Van Natta M, Behling C, Contos MJ, Cummings OW, Ferrell LD, Liu YC, Torbenson MS, Unalp-Arida A, Yeh M, McCullough AJ, Sanyal AJ, Nonalcoholic Steatohepatitis Clinical Research Network: Design and validation of a histological scoring system for nonalcoholic fatty liver disease. *Hepatology* 2005, 41(6):1313–1321.

28. Garcia Urena MA, Colina Ruiz-Delgado F, Moreno Gonzalez E, Jimenez Romero C, Garcia Garcia I, Loinzaz Segurola C, Gonzalez P, Gomez Sanz R: Hepatic steatosis in liver transplant donors: common feature of donor population? *World J Surg* 1998, 22(8):837–844.

29. Markin RS, Wisecarver JL, Radio SJ, Stratta RJ, Langnas AN, Hirst K, Shaw BW Jr: Frozen section evaluation of donor livers before transplantation. *Transplantation* 1993, 56(6):1403–1409.

30. El-Badry AM, Breitenstein S, Jochum W, Washington K, Paradis V, Rubbia-Brandt L, Puhan MA, Slankamenac K, Graf R, Clavien PA: Assessment of hepatic steatosis by expert pathologists: the end of a gold standard. *Ann Surg* 2009, 250(5):691–697.

31. Kendrick AA, Choudhury M, Rahman SM, McCurdy CE, Friederich M, Van Hove JL, Watson PA, Birdsey N, Bao J, Gius D, Sack MN, Jing E, Kahn CR, Friedman JE, Jonscher KR: Fatty liver is associated with reduced SIRT3 activity and mitochondrial protein hyperacetylation. *Biochem J* 2011, 433(3):505–514.

32. Hirschey MD, Shimazu T, Jing E, Grueter CA, Collins AM, Aouizerat B, Stancakova A, Goetzman E, Lam MM, Schwer B, Stevens RD, Muehlbauer MJ, Kakar S, Bass NM, Kuusisto J, Laakso M, Alt FW, Newgard CB, Farese RV Jr, Kahn CR, Verdin E: SIRT3 deficiency and mitochondrial protein hyperacetylation accelerate the development of the metabolic syndrome. *Mol Cell* 2011, 44(2):177–190.

33. Kent C: Eukaryotic phospholipid biosynthesis. *Annu Rev Biochem* 1995, 64:315–343.

34. Cao D, Ziemba A, McCabe J, Yan R, Wan L, Kim B, Gach M, Flynn S, Pizzorno G: Differential expression of uridine phosphorylase in tumors contributes to an improved fluoropyrimidine therapeutic activity. *Mol Cancer Ther* 2011, 10(12):2330–2339.

35. Cai J, Lee CW: Tamoxifen inhibits nitrobenzylthioinosine-sensitive equilibrative uridine transport in human MCF-7 breast cancer cells. *Biochem J* 1996, 320(Pt 3):991–995.

36. Traut TW, Jones ME: Uracil metabolism–UMP synthesis from orotic acid or uridine and conversion of uracil to beta-alanine: enzymes and cDNAs. *Prog Nucleic Acid Res Mol Biol* 1996, 53:1–78.

37. Pizzorno G, Yee L, Burtness BA, Marsh JC, Darnowski JW, Chu MY, Chu SH, Chu E, Leffert JJ, Handschumacher RE, Calabresi P: Phase I clinical and pharmacological studies of benzylacyclouridine, a uridine phosphorylase inhibitor. *Clin Cancer Res* 1998, 4(5):1165–1175.

8

Prevalence of malaria and anaemia among HIV infected pregnant women receiving co-trimoxazole prophylaxis in Tanzania: a cross sectional study in Kinondoni Municipality

Vicent P Manyanga[1], Omary Minzi[1*] and Billy Ngasala[2]

Abstract

Background: HIV-infected pregnant women are particularly more susceptible to the deleterious effects of malaria infection particularly anaemia. In order to prevent opportunistic infections and malaria, a policy of daily co-trimoxazole prophylaxis without the standard Suphadoxine-Pyrimethamine intermittent preventive treatment (SP-IPT) was introduced to all HIV infected pregnant women in the year 2011. However, there is limited information about the effectiveness of this policy.

Methods: This was a cross sectional study conducted among HIV-infected pregnant women receiving co-trimoxazole prophylaxis in eight public health facilities in Kinondoni Municipality from February to April 2013. Blood was tested for malaria infection and anaemia (haemoglobin <11 g/dl). Data were collected on the adherence to co-trimoxazole prophylaxis and other risk factors for malaria infection and anaemia. Pearson chi-square test, Fischer's exact test and multivariate logistic regression were used in the statistical analysis.

Results: This study enrolled 420 HIV infected pregnant women. The prevalence of malaria infection was 4.5%, while that of anaemia was 54%. The proportion of subjects with poor adherence to co-trimoxazole was 50.5%. As compared to HIV infected pregnant women with good adherence to co-trimoxazole prophylaxis, the poor adherents were more likely to have a malaria infection (Adjusted Odds Ratio, AOR = 6.81, 95% CI = 1.35-34.43, P = 0.02) or anaemia (AOR = 1.75, 95% CI = 1.03-2.98, P = 0.039). Other risk factors associated with anaemia were advanced WHO clinical stages, current malaria infection and history of episodes of malaria illness during the index pregnancy.

Conclusion: The prevalence of malaria was low; however, a significant proportion of subjects had anaemia. Good adherence to co-trimoxazole prophylaxis was associated with reduction of both malaria infection and anaemia among HIV infected pregnant women.

Keywords: HIV, Malaria, Pregnancy, Anaemia, Co-trimoxazole prophylaxis

Background

Combined malaria and HIV infection during pregnancy increases the susceptibility of the pregnant women to the negative effects of malaria suggesting a synergistic interaction between HIV infection and malaria [1,2]. HIV-infected pregnant women have significant alterations in immunity to malaria, which render them more vulnerable to the negative effects related to malaria infection [3,4]. This population experiences consistently more peripheral and placental malaria, higher parasite densities, more febrile illnesses, severe anaemia, and adverse birth outcomes than HIV uninfected women regardless of the parity [2].

WHO has recommended a daily dose of co-trimoxazole among HIV-infected pregnant women during the whole pregnancy period in order to prevent opportunistic infections and malaria [5]. Concurrent administration of SP and co-trimoxazole is not advised to avoid adverse reactions [5]. Tanzania had adopted this policy since the year 2011 [6].

* Correspondence: minziobejayesu@gmail.com
[1]Unit of Pharmacology and Therapeutics, Muhimbili University of Health and Allied Sciences, Dar Es Salaam, Tanzania
Full list of author information is available at the end of the article

Unfortunately, there is limited information about the effectiveness of daily co-trimoxazole for preventing malaria and its deleterious effects particularly anaemia among HIV infected pregnant women.

This study was carried out in a malaria endemic area characterized by malaria transmission throughout the year [7]. In this area, peripheral parasitaemia among pregnant women can be absent or below the detection limit of the microscopic method [8,9]. To overcome this challenge, we used selected malaria rapid diagnostic tests (MRDT) targeting antigens called histidine rich protein 2 (HRP-2). These antigens are released by red blood cells infected by the malaria parasites; they can be detected in the peripheral circulation even when the parasites are sequestered within the placenta [9,10].

This cross sectional study reports the prevalence of malaria, anaemia and the associated risk factors among HIV infected pregnant women receiving co-trimoxazole prophylaxis in one district in Tanzania.

Methods

Study design and study area

The design of the study was a cross sectional. It was conducted between February and April 2013 in eight public health facilities in Kinondoni municipality, Dar Es Salaam. Kinondoni has a hot and humid tropical climate with two rainfall seasons: an intense one observed from the month of March to May, and a mild one in November and December. The average temperature ranges from a minimum of 18.1°C to a maximum of 32.1°C. The average annual rainfall is 1,115 mm. A theoretical model based on data for rainfall and temperature characterizes Kinondoni as an area with stable malaria transmission (holoendemic), with transmission occurring during the entire year [7]. Malaria is the leading cause of both the outpatient visits and inpatient admissions [11].

Study population

The targeted subjects were HIV infected pregnant women receiving co-trimoxazole prophylaxis for more than four weeks. Sample size for this study was calculated using the formula for cross-sectional study based on the study done in Uganda [12]. In that study; these prevalence of malaria infection among HIV infected pregnant women using co-trimoxazole prophylaxis (x) was found to be 19%. The formula used was:

$$n = \frac{z^2 x(100-x)}{\varepsilon^2}$$

n = Minimum sample size, z = point on standard normal distribution curve corresponding to significance level of 5% (its value is 1.96), x = previous prevalence of malaria infection among HIV infected pregnant women

receiving co-trimoxazole prophylaxis (19%), ε = margin of error on x (set at 4%). A total of 420 consented subjects on different trimesters and varied gravidities were enrolled into the study. Pregnant women with sickle cell disease, vaginal bleeding and severe medical conditions were excluded from the study.

Sampling procedure

Kinondoni municipality has a total of 33 public health facilities; among them two are hospitals, one is a health centre and thirty are dispensaries. Cluster sampling was used for selection of health facilities to be included in the study. The health facilities were divided into three clusters, namely hospitals, health centre and dispensaries. The two hospitals and the health centre were included in the study. Five out of the thirty dispensaries were selected using simple random sampling without replacement technique. Each name of the 30 dispensaries was written on a small piece of paper, and then the paper was folded to 'a ball like' figure and put in a mug. The mug was thoroughly shaken and five 'paper balls' were randomly picked to select the five dispensaries. Two hospitals involved in the study were Mwananyamala and Sinza. A Health Centre involved was Magomeni; and the five dispensaries were Kambangwa, Tandale, Mburahati, Kimara and Mbezi.

Due to the limited number of HIV infected pregnant women, all the subjects in the selected clusters who met the inclusion criteria were enrolled in the study.

Data collection methods

A structured interview schedule was used to obtain information on various characteristics of the subjects and supplemented by information from patients' files. These include age, weight, height, gravidity, marital status, education level, employment status, WHO clinical stage, use of insecticide treated nets (ITN), history of episodes of malaria illness, use of iron supplements, use of deworming drugs, anti-retroviral treatment category (prophylaxis or lifelong), duration of zidovudine use. The subjects were then tested for malaria and anaemia. The blood sample was collected for CD4 assay.

Adherence to co-trimoxazole prophylaxis

Adherence to co-trimoxazole prophylaxis was measured by using an interview schedule adapted from Morisky medication adherence scale (Table 1) [13,14].

Haemoglobin measurement

Haemoglobin was measured by *HemoCue Hb 201 +* ° machine manufactured by HemoCue AB Ängelholm, Sweden. The tip of the middle finger was cleaned by alcohol swab; then a blood sample was obtained by finger pricking procedure. The *Haemocue 201 +* ° cuvette was filled with blood, excess blood was cleaned from the cuvette and air

Table 1 A scale used to determine the adherence level for co-trimoxazole prophylaxis among HIV infected pregnant women

No.	Questions	Yes	No
i	Do you sometimes forget to take your co-trimoxazole tablets?	0	1
ii	People sometimes miss taking their medicines for reasons other than forgetting. Thinking over the past 2 weeks, were there any days when you did not take your co-trimoxazole tablets?	0	1
iii	Have you ever cut back or stopped taking co-trimoxazole without telling your doctor because you felt worse when you took it?	0	1
iv	When you travel or leave home, do you sometimes forget to bring along co-trimoxazole tablets?	0	1
v	Did you take your co-trimoxazole tablets yesterday?	1	0
vi	Taking medicines every day is a real inconvenient for some people. Do you ever feel hassled about sticking to your treatment plan?	0	1
vii	How often do you have difficulty remembering to take co-trimoxazole tablets?		

☐ Never/Rarely = 1

☐ Once in a while = 0.75

☐ Sometimes = 0.5

☐ Usually = 0.25

☐ All the time = 0

TOTAL SCORE

Note: The total score of >6 was interpreted as Good adherence, 4 to 5.9 as Average Adherence and <4 as Poor Adherence.

bubbles were removed. The cuvette was placed in the device tray and the holder was pushed gently into the photometer. The results were recorded from the digital display.

Malaria testing

Malaria was tested by using *SD BIOLINE Malaria Ag P. f/Pan® MRDT* manufactured by Standard Diagnostics, Inc, Korea. The blood sample was collected by finger prick method after the tip of the middle finger was cleaned by alcohol swab. The test device was placed on a clean, flat surface. About 5 µl of whole blood were added into the 'sample well' of respective test devices using a micropipette supplied with the test device. Four drops of assay diluent were added into the 'sample diluent well'. All the test results were recorded within 30 minutes.

CD-4 count

The CD-4 Count was done at Mwananyamala Hospital by *BD FACS Count®* Machine (BD Biosciences USA). About 4 ml of whole blood (4 ml) was collected in EDTA collection tubes by standard venipuncture procedure. The collected samples were kept at room temperature (18-25°C) and then transported in a special container. All samples were processed within 30 hours from the time of collection.

Management of patients

Pregnant women who were diagnosed with malaria or anaemia during the study were managed as per the Tanzania's Standard Treatment Guidelines through the respective health facilities.

Data analysis

Data were double-entered, cleaned and analysed using computer software called IBM SPSS Statistics 20 (IBM Corp.). Dependent variables were malaria infection and anaemia. While the independent variables were the levels of adherence to co–trimoxazole prophylaxis. Other independent variables were socio-demographic factors, WHO clinical stages, CD-4 count bands, gravidity, pregnancy age (trimesters), sleeping under insecticide treated bed nets (ITN), history of episodes of malaria illness, use of iron supplements, the use of deworming agent and duration of AZT use (categorized as <3 months, 3 to <6 months and ≥6 months).

Classification of anaemia was based on the recommendation by WHO [15]; normal (Hb ≥11 g/dl), mild anaemia (Hb = 10-10.9 g/dl), moderate anaemia (Hb = 7-9.9 g/dl) and severe anaemia (Hb < 7 g/dl). CD4 count was categorized according to the four bands of HIV related immunodeficiency proposed by WHO [16]. These include: no significant immunodeficiency (≥500 cells/µL), mild immunodeficiency (350–499 cells/µL), advanced immunodeficiency (200–349 cells/µL) and severe immunodeficiency (<200 µL).

Pearson Chi-square Test and Fischer's Exact Test were used in the univariate analysis between the dependent and independent variables where applicable. Independent variables which showed a statistical significant difference with the outcome variable by univariate analysis were subjected to multivariate logistic regression to determine the predictors of the outcome. The P-value of < 0.05 was considered significant to provide evidence of significant difference or association.

Ethical considerations

Ethical approval for the study was given by the Ethical Committee of the Muhimbili University of Health and Allied sciences (MUHAS). Permission from Kinondoni Municipal Council to conduct the study in the health facilities was granted. Information about the study was delivered to the patients and a written consent was obtained before the study was conducted. Confidentiality was ensured to all individuals who participated in the study.

Results

Characteristics of the study population

From February to April 2013, a total of 420 HIV infected pregnant women in various trimesters were enrolled into the study. The mean $\pm$ SD age of the subjects was 28 $\pm$ 5.2 years. Table 2 summarizes sociodemographic characteristics of the HIV infected pregnant women who were enrolled in the study.

Prevalence of malaria

The study revealed a prevalence of malaria of 4.5% (19/420). Table 3 shows the prevalence of malaria, according to selected risk factors. A pattern was seen towards the increase in the prevalence of malaria infection as the levels of adherence to co-trimoxazole prophylaxis decreased from good to poor. Pregnant women with poor adherence to co-trimoxazole prophylaxis were 6.8 times more likely to have a malaria infection as compared to those with good adherence (AOR = 6.81, 95% CI =1.35-34.43 and P = 0.02). The

Table 2 Socio-demographic characteristics of HIV infected pregnant women who were enrolled in the study (N = 420)

Characteristics	Number of respondents(n)	%
Age group (years)		
<20	16	3.8
20-34	341	81.2
≥35	63	15.0
Marital status		
Single	35	8.33
Cohabiting	69	16.43
Married	316	75.24
Level of education		
No formal education	33	7.9
Primary	276	65.7
Secondary	87	20.7
Post-secondary	24	5.7
Employment		
Employed	123	29.29
Business/self-employed	188	44.76
Not employed	109	25.95

prevalence of malaria was statistically similar in all gravidities (P = 0.563).

Prevalence of anaemia

The prevalence of any anaemia (Hb <11 g/dl) was found to be 54% (227/420); while that of mild-to-moderate anaemia and severe anaemia were 49.3% (207/420) and 5% (21/420) respectively. The overall mean $\pm$ SD haemoglobin concentration was 10.3 $\pm$ 1.5 g/dl.

Table 4 shows the prevalence of anaemia according to various selected risk factors among HIV infected pregnant women. The prevalence of anaemia increased as the levels of adherence to co-trimoxazole prophylaxis decreased from good to poor. Subjects who had poor adherence were 1.8 times more likely to have anaemia as compared to those with good adherence (AOR = 1.75, 95% CI = 1.03-2.98 and P = 0.041).

The prevalence of anaemia among subjects with malaria infection was 94.7% (18/19) as compared to 52.1% (209/401) among malaria negative subjects. Malaria infected subjects were 10.4 times more likely to have anaemia as compared to those who had a negative malaria test (AOR = 10.36, 95% CI = 1.33–80.8, P = 0.026). Likewise, subjects who had at least one episode of malaria illness during the current pregnancy were 1.8 times more likely to have anaemia as compared with those without a history (AOR = 1.75 95% CI = 1.01-3.03, P = 0.048).

The prevalence of anaemia increased as the HIV/AIDS advanced from lower to higher WHO clinical stages (i.e. from stage I to IV). Pregnant women who were on WHO clinical stage III or IV were 2.7 times more likely to have anaemia as compared to those on WHO clinical stage I (AOR = 2.65, 95% CI = 1.18-5.95 and P = 0.018).

Discussion

This study shows that the prevalence of malaria infection was 4.5% among HIV infected pregnant women receiving co-trimoxazole prophylaxis. A similar low prevalence was obtained in a previous study that was conducted in Malawi by Kapito-Tembo et al. [17]. In that study, the prevalence of malaria among HIV infected pregnant women who were receiving co-trimoxazole prophylaxis was 2.7% and 5.5% by blood smear and real time PCR method respectively. The Malawian study differs from the present study in the method of malaria diagnosis. Real-time PCR targets parasite DNA and has a higher sensitivity than the MRDT; while the blood smear method by microscopy is less sensitive compared to MRDT [9,10,18].

The prevalence of malaria infection increased as the level of adherence to co-trimoxazole decreased from good to poor. Pregnant women with poor adherence were almost seven times more likely to have a malaria infection as compared to those with good adherence. We could not find any previous study that investigated the association between the

Table 3 Prevalence of malaria according to selected risk factors among HIV infected pregnant women receiving co-trimoxazole (N = 420)

Characteristics	N	Malaria prevalence n (%)	P-value	AOR	95% CI	P-value
WHO clinical stage						
Stage I	338	12 (3.6)		1		
Stage II	43	2 (4.7)		0.851	0.171-4.226	0.844
Stage III-IV	39	5 (12.8)	0.031[a]	2.305	0.699-7.597	0.170
CD4 count (cells/µL)*						
≥500	104	4 (3.8)		-		
350-499	85	3 (3.5)		-		
200-349	96	8 (8.3)		–		
<200	59	4 (6.8)	0.417[a]	-		
Pregnancy trimester						
1st trimester	20	1 (5)		-		
2nd trimester	206	9 (4.4)		-		
3rd trimester	194	9 (4.6)	0.986[a]	-		
Gravidity						
Primigravidae	139	6 (4.3)		-		
Secundigravidae	148	5 (3.4)		-		
Multigravidae	133	8 (6)	0.563[a]	-		
Adherence to co-trimoxazole						
Good	208	2 (1)		1		
Average	80	4 (5)		3.578	0.611-20.955	0.157
Poor	132	13 (9.8)	0.001[a]	6.806	1.346-34.429	0.02
ITN use						
Yes	380	15 (3.9)		-		
No	40	4 (10)	0.096[b]	-		
ART use category						
Prophylaxis	288	11 (3.8)		-		
Life long	132	8 (6.1)	0.305[a]	-		

[a]Calculated by Pearson Chi Square, [b]Calculated by Fischer's Exact Test, *Results of CD4 count were available for only 344 subjects out of 420 (81.9%).

malaria infection and levels of adherence to co-trimoxazole prophylaxis among similar subjects. An explanation for the pattern seen in our study could be the fact that the good adherents had higher exposure to co-trimoxazole and therefore were more protected as compared with the poor adherents.

Sleeping under insecticide treated nets (ITN) by the subjects could as well have contributed to the low prevalence of malaria in this study group as it was reported in previous studies [19-21]. ITN are freely available to all pregnant women through a voucher system at antenatal clinics [21]. The prevalence of malaria among the subjects who reported to sleep under an ITN was low at 3.9% as compared to those who did not sleep under an ITN which was 10%. The use of ITN control malaria transmission by creating a barrier between the mosquitoes and people sleeping under them [20,21]. Moreover,

the insecticides that are used for treating bed nets kill or repel the mosquitoes; consequently, the numbers of mosquitoes that enter the household and attempt to feed on people inside are reduced as well as shortening their length of life [20,21]. Nevertheless, the finding was statistically not significant. This is consistent with the study by West et al. [22], in which other factors excluding ITN were significantly associated with malaria infection in a community with high and equitable distribution of ITN.

In consistent with previous studies [2,12,17,23], malaria infection was distributed to all the gravidities. The explanation for this outcome is that HIV affects the immune memory mechanism which is responsible for the parity-dependent acquisition of antimalarial immunity in pregnancy and therefore predisposes the secundigravidae and multigravidae to a similar risk of malaria infection as the primigravidae [2].

Table 4 Prevalence of anaemia according to selected risk factors among HIV infected pregnant women receiving co-trimoxazole prophylaxis (N = 420)

Univariate analysis				Multivariate analysis		
Characteristics	n	Prevalence of anaemia n (%)	P-value	AOR	95% CI	P-value
Malaria infection						
Yes	19	18 (94.7)		10.363	1.329-80.798	0.026
No (reference)	401	209 (52.1)	0.0001[a]	1		
History of malaria illness						
Yes	107	76 (71)		1.746	1.005-3.033	0.048
No (reference)	313	151 (48.2)	0.0001[a]	1		
WHO clinical stage						
Stage I (reference)	338	165 (48.8)		1		
Stage II	43	32 (74.4)		3.076	1.458-6.491	0.003
Stage III-IV	37	30 (76.9)	0.0001[a]	2.653	1.184-5.945	0.018
CD4 count (cells/μL)*						
≥500	104	48 (46.2)		-		
350-499	85	45 (52.9)		-		
200-349	96	62 (64.6)		–		
<200	59	42 (71.2)	0.005[a]	-		
Pregnancy trimester						
1st trimester	20	9 (45)		-		
2nd trimester	206	107 (51.9)		-		
3rd trimester	194	111 (57.2)	0.404[a]	-		
Gravidity						
Primigravidae	139	72 (51.8)		-		
Secundigravidae	148	83 (56.1)		-		
Multigravidae	133	72 (54.1)	0.767[a]	-		
ITN use						
Yes	380	201 (52.9)		-		
No	40	26 (65)	0.144[a]	-		
ART category						
ARV Prophylaxis	288	146 (50.7)		-		
Life-long ART	132	81 (61.4)	0.142[a]	-		
Duration of AZT use (months)						
<3	162	93 (57.4)		-		
3-5.9	168	92 (54.8)		–		
≥6	90	42 (46.7)	0.253[a]	-		
Iron supplements						
Yes	338	185 (54.7)		-		
No	82	42 (51.2)	0.567[a]	-		
Use of de-worming drug						
Yes	327	171 (52.3)		-		
No	93	56 (60.2)	0.176[a]	-		

Table 4 Prevalence of anaemia according to selected risk factors among HIV infected pregnant women receiving co-trimoxazole prophylaxis (N = 420) *(Continued)*

Adherence to co-trimoxazole						
Good (reference)	208	92 (44.2)		1		
Average	80	47 (58.8)		1.478	0.848-2.578	0.168
Poor	132	88(66.7)	0.0001[a]	1.752	1.03-2.979	0.039

[a]Calculated by Pearson Chi Square, *Results of CD4 Count were available for only 344 subjects out of 420 (81.9%).

CD-4 Count and WHO clinical staging are parameters which are used to monitor progression of HIV/AIDS [5,24]. This study could not find an association between the prevalence of malaria infection and low CD4 count or advanced WHO clinical stages; which are known to increase the vulnerability to malaria infection [2]. This could be explained by the impact of malaria control interventions; particularly the use of co-trimoxazole prophylaxis and sleeping under an ITN among HIV infected pregnant women. Kapito-Tembo et al. [17] reported similar findings in Malawi whereby HIV infected pregnant women at all bands of CD4 counts (i.e. <200, 200–499 and ≥500 cells/μL) had a similar risk of malaria infection.

The present study showed that the prevalence of anaemia among HIV infected pregnant women receiving co-trimoxazole prophylaxis was 54%. Previous studies that were conducted in the Dar Es Salaam city reported higher prevalence compared to the present study. Finkelstein et al. [25] reported a prevalence of 83% in 1997, while Mehta et al. [26] reported a prevalence of 73% in 2003. Other studies that were conducted in different countries within Sub-Saharan Africa have reported varied values of the prevalence of anaemia among similar subjects [2,17,27,28]. In Malawi; Kapito-Tembo et al. [17] reported a prevalence of 35.6%; while Nkhoma et al. [28] reported a prevalence of 27.4%. In Nigeria, a prevalence of 83.8% was reported by Uneke et al. [27]. The reasons for these variations are not clear, but may be connected to the complexity and the multifactorial aetiology of anaemia among HIV infected pregnant women in sub-Saharan Africa, including HIV/AIDS itself, malaria, protein and micronutrient deficiency and endemic diseases like hookworm and schistosomiasis [25,27].

Good adherence to co-trimoxazole was associated with reduced prevalence of anaemia. A pattern was seen towards the increase in the prevalence of maternal anaemia as the levels of adherence to co-trimoxazole prophylaxis decreased from good to poor. Poor Adherents were almost 1.8 times more likely to have anaemia as compared with good adherents. This could be due to the fact that, well adherent subjects had more exposure to the co-trimoxazole drug and therefore they were more protected from malaria infection and its sequelae particularly anaemia as compared to the poor adherent

one. Walker et al. [29], had previously reported the benefits of co-trimoxazole in reducing morbidities among the HIV infected population; this could similarly explain the reduction in anaemia among good adherents.

In consistent with a previous study by Finkelstein et al. [25], advanced HIV/AIDS clinical stages (clinical stage III or IV) or CD4 Count of < 200 had a strong association with anaemia. The subjects who were on WHO clinical stage III or IV were 3 times more likely to have anaemia as compared with those in the WHO clinical stage I. Similarly, the prevalence of anaemia increased as the CD4 Count decreases among the subjects. This pattern could be explained by the fact that subjects with advanced clinical stages or a low CD4 count had poor immunity against malaria and other infections were therefore more vulnerable to becoming anaemic [3,4]. Furthermore, advanced HIV/AIDS is associated with local diseases along the gastrointestinal tract, which could eventually result in poor absorption of nutrients necessary for the formation of haemoglobin [26].

Low CD-4 count and advanced HIV/AIDS stages reflect the chronicity (prolonged existence) of the disease; therefore another cause of anaemia could also be the state of chronic illnesses [30,31]. The immune response mounted against such infections is required for pathogen clearance, but its persistence can cause collateral damage to the host with the occurrence of anaemia as the major pathology [30]. The inflammation triggers the release of chemicals e.g. hepcidin, that signal the iron regulation mechanism to adopt a defensive mode. This type of anaemia is usually characterized by an imbalance between erythro-phagocytosis and erythropoiesis [30,31].

Similar to previous studies [2,27,28], dually infected (HIV plus malaria infection) pregnant women were at considerably greater risk of anaemia as compared with those with HIV infection alone. HIV infected pregnant women who had positive malaria test were ten times more likely to have anaemia as compared with those who had the negative malaria test. Both HIV (particularly with advanced immunosuppression) and malaria infection are individually known causes of anaemia [2]. Anaemia associated with malaria is caused by hemolysis of the red blood cells and hypersplenism, a condition characterized by the exaggeration of inhibitory or destructive function of the spleen [15].

Pregnant women who had at least one episode of malaria illness during the current pregnancy were nearly two times more likely to have anaemia as compared with those without a history. In consistent with this study, Nkhoma et al. [28] reported a significant association between the number of previous malaria episodes and maternal anaemia; having two or more episodes were associated with increased risk of anaemia. The reason could be the fact that both HIV (particularly with advanced immunosuppression) and malaria infection are individually known causes of anaemia [2].

In disagreement with previous knowledge [32-34]; the present study could not find a significant association between anaemia and zidovudine use. This could be due to the positive role of the antiretroviral drugs and co-trimoxazole in controlling the HIV infection and other morbidities and subsequently outweighed the anaemia inducing effect of zidovudine. Furthermore, the multi-aetiologies of anaemia in HIV infected pregnant women in Sub-Saharan Africa [25] e.g. HIV infection itself, malaria infection, nutrients deficiency and worm infestations could be the reason for the high prevalence in both groups and consequently lack of significant difference. Sinha et al. [35] reported similar findings in a study conducted in India. In that study [35], pregnant women who used zidovudine were surprisingly 70% less likely to be anaemic compared with women not receiving zidovudine.

Similar to a study by Finkelstein et al. [25], anaemia prevalence was higher in both the subjects who used iron supplements and those who did not; likewise to the use of de-worming agents. Lack of significant difference between the groups could be explained by the complexity and multifactorial aetiology of anaemia apart from the iron deficiency or worm infestation among HIV infected pregnant women in Sub-Saharan Africa [25,30,31].

Our study had some limitations. We attempted to control the confounders by the multivariate logistic regression; nonetheless, there were potential residual confounding effects from the unmeasured factors like the presence of other infections or pathological conditions. Secondly, because of the cross sectional design of this study, we had only one point of measurement of both the outcomes and exposure; this made it difficult to make a causal inference from the findings. Thirdly, our results may have potentially been affected by information bias because measurement of adherence to co-trimoxazole prophylaxis was done by a self-reported method and no drug levels in the blood were measured. Likewise, the use of iron supplements, deworming drugs and sleeping under an ITN were self-reported. However, antenatal records were used to verify prescriptions of medications.

Conclusions

This study has shown a low prevalence of malaria infection among HIV infected pregnant women using the daily co-trimoxazole prophylaxis; however, a significant proportion of subjects had anaemia. Good adherence to co-trimoxazole prophylaxis was associated with reduction of both malaria infection and anaemia. Routine counselling and provision of health education on the importance of good adherence to medications and the consequences of poor adherence are paramount in addressing the existing problems. Mitigation of advanced HIV/AIDS among pregnant women is also important in combating the problem of anaemia. Approaches like early diagnosis and timely initiation of anti-retroviral treatment could be of benefit. Due to the complexity and multiple etiologies of anaemia; other measures like de-worming, schistosomiasis control and nutritional supplementation should be taken on board.

Abbreviations

95% CI: 95% confidence interval; AIDS: Acquired immunodeficiency syndrome; ANC: Antenatal clinic; AOR: Adjusted odds ratio; ART: Anti-retroviral treatment; ARV: Anti-retroviral; DNA: Deoxyribonucleic acid; EDTA: Ethylenediaminetetra acetic acid; FACS: Fluorescent activated cell sorting; Hb: Haemoglobin; HIV: Human immunodeficiency virus; HRP-2: Histidine rich protein-2; IPT: Intermittent preventive treatment; MMAS: Morisky medication adherence scale; MRDT: Malaria rapid diagnostic test; PCR: Polymerase chain reaction; pLDH: Plasmodium lactate dehydrogenase; PMTCT: Prevention of mother to child transmission of HIV infection; SD: Standard deviation; SP-IPT: Intermittent preventive treatment by sulphadoxine plus pyrimethamine; SPSS: Statistical package for social sciences; WHO: World Health Organization.

Competing interests

The authors declare that they have no any competing interests.

Authors' contributions

VM participated in study design, data collection, data analysis, data interpretation, initiated the manuscript preparation, and participated in the revision process. OM engineered the study design, coordinated data collection, data interpretation and participated in the process of manuscript writing. BN participated in the study design and interpretation of data and manuscript writing. All authors read and approved the final manuscript.

Authors' information

VM: Holder of B.Pharm (Hons): Recently completed a Master's Program in Hospital and Clinical Pharmacy at Muhimbili University of Health and Allied Sciences.
OM: Senior Lecturer at the Unit of Pharmacology and Therapeutics, School of Pharmacy, Muhimbili University of Health and Allied Sciences.
BN: Lecturer at Department of Parasitology, School of Medicine, Muhimbili University of Health and Allied Sciences.

Acknowledgements

We thank all the pregnant women who participated in this study; the office of Medical Officer of Kinondoni Municipality for accepting this study to be carried out; the member of staff of Mwananyamala Hospital, Sinza Hospital, Magomeni Health Centre, Kambangwa Dispensary, Tandale Dispensary, Kimara Dispensary, Mbezi Dispensary and Mburahati Dispensary for their support during data collection; Dr Candida Moshiro of Department of Epidemiology and Biostatistics, Muhimbili University of Health and Allied Sciences for her valuable statistical advices during analysis. This study received funding from Sida-MUHAS Malaria Project.

Author details

[1]Unit of Pharmacology and Therapeutics, Muhimbili University of Health and Allied Sciences, Dar Es Salaam, Tanzania. [2]Department of Parasitology, Muhimbili University of Health and Allied Sciences, Dar Es Salaam, Tanzania.

References

1. Steketee R, Wirima J, Bloland P, Chilima B, Mermin J: **Impairment of a pregnant woman's acquired ability to limit Plasmodium falciparum by infection with Human Immunodeficiency Virus type-1.** *Am J Trop Med Hyg* 1996, **55**(1):42–49.
2. Ter Kuile FO, Parise ME, Verhoeff FH, Udhayakumar V, Newman RD, Van Eijk AM, Rogerson SJ, Steketee RW: **The burden of co-infection with Human Immunodeficiency Virus type 1 and malaria in pregnant women in Sub-Saharan Africa.** *Am J Trop Med Hyg* 2004, **71**(2):41–54.
3. Mount AM, Mwapasa V, Elliott SR, Beeson JG: **Impairment of humoral immunity to Plasmodium falciparum malaria in pregnancy by HIV infection.** *Lancet* 2004, **363**(9424):1860–1867.
4. Ned RM, Moore JM, Chaisavaneeykorn S, Udhayakumar V: **Modulation of immune responses during HIV–malaria co-infection in pregnancy.** *Trends Parasitol* 2005, **21**(6):284–291.
5. World Health Organization: *Guideline on co-trimoxazole prophylaxis for HIV-related infections among children, adolescents and adults in resource-limited settings. Recommendations for a public health approach.* Geneva; 2006.
6. Ministry of Health and Social Welfare: *Tanzania National Guideline for Prevention of Mother-to-child Transmission of HIV/AIDS.* Dar Es Salaam; 2011.
7. De Castro MC, Yamagata Y, Mtasiwa D, Tanner M, Utzinger J, Keiser J, Singer BH: **Integrated urban malaria control: a case study in Dar Es Salaam.** *Am J Trop Med Hyg* 2004, **71**(Suppl 2):103–117.
8. Omo-Aghoja LO, Abe E, Feyi-Waboso P, Okonofua FE: **The challenges of diagnosis and treatment of malaria in pregnancy in low resource settings.** *Acta Obstet Gynecol* 2008, **87**(7):693–696.
9. Uneke CJ: **Diagnosis of Plasmoduim falciparum malaria in pregnancy in Sub-Saharan Africa: the challenges and public health implications.** *J Parasitol Res* 2008, **102**:333–342.
10. Leke RFG, Djokam RR, Mbu R, Leke RJ, Fogako J, Megnekou R, Matenou S, Sama G, Zhou Y, Cadigan T, Parra M, Taylor DW: **Detection of the Plasmodium falciparum antigen histidine-rich protein 2 in blood of pregnant women : implications for diagnosing placental malaria.** *J Clin Microbiol* 1999, **37**(9):2992–2996.
11. The Municipal Medical Officer of Health: *Kinondoni municipality profile.* Dar Es Salaam; 2008.
12. Newman PM, Wanzira H, Tumwine G, Arinaitwe E, Waldman S, Achan J, Havlir D, Rosenthal PJ, Dorsey G, Clark TD, Cohan D: **Placental malaria among HIV-infected and uninfected women receiving anti-folates in a high transmission area of Uganda.** *Malar J* 2009, **8**:254.
13. Morisky D, Green L, Levine D: **Concurrent and predictive validity of a self-reported measure of medication adherence.** *J Med Care* 1986, **24**(1):67–74.
14. Morisky DE, Ang A, Krousel-wood M: **Predictive validity of a medication adherence measure in an outpatient setting.** *J Clin Hypertesion* 2009, **10**(5):348–354.
15. World Health Organization: *Prevention and management of severe anaemia in pregnancy.* Geneva; 1993.
16. World Health Organization: *WHO, case definitions of HIV for surveillance and revised clinical staging and immunological classification of HIV-related disease in adults and children.* Geneva; 2007.
17. Kapito-tembo A, Hensbroek van B, Phiri K, Fitzgerald M, Meshnick SR, Mwapasa V: **Marked reduction in prevalence of malaria parasitemia and anemia in HIV-infected pregnant women taking cotrimoxazole with Or without Sulfadoxine-Pyrimethamine intermittent preventive therapy during pregnancy in Malawi.** *J Infect Dis* 2011, **203**:464–472.
18. World Health Organization: *Malaria rapid diagnostic tests: Test of Performance.* Geneva; 2008.
19. World Health Organization: *A strategic framework for malaria prevention and control during pregnancy in the African region.* Geneva; 2004.
20. Renggli S, Mandike R, Kramer K, Patrick F, Brown NJ, McElroy PD, Rimisho W, Msengwa A, Mnzava A, Nathan R, Ntunge R, Mgullo R, Lweikiza J, Lengeler C: **Design, implementation and evaluation of a national campaign to deliver 18 million free long-lasting insecticidal nets to uncovered sleeping spaces in Tanzania.** *Malar J* 2013, **12**:1.
21. Maxwell CA, Msuya E, Sudi M, Njunwa KJ, Carneiro IA, Curtis CF: **Effect of community-wide use of insecticide-treated nets for 3–4 years on malarial morbidity in Tanzania.** *J Trop Med Int Heal* 2002, **7**(12):1003–1008.
22. West PA, Protopopoff N, Rowland M, Cumming E, Rand A, Drakeley C, Wright A, Kivaju Z, Kirby MJ, Mosha FW, Kisinza W, Kleinschmidt I: **Malaria risk factors in North West Tanzania: the effect of spraying, nets and wealth.** *PLoS One* 2013, **8**(6):e65787.
23. Mermin J, Ekwaru JP, Liechty CA, Were W, Downing R, Ransom R, Weidle P, Lule J, Coutinho A, Solberg P: **Effect of co-trimoxazole prophylaxis, anti-retroviral therapy and insecticide-treated bednets on the frequency of malaria in HIV-1-infected adults in Uganda : a prospective cohort study.** *Lancet* 2006, **367**:1256–1261.
24. Tanzania National AIDS Control Program: *National Guideline for the Management of HIV/AIDS.* Dar Es Salaam; 2012.
25. Finkelstein JL, Mehta S, Duggan CP, Spiegelman D, Aboud S, Kupka R, Msamanga GI, Fawzi WW: **Predictors of anaemia and iron deficiency in HIV-infected pregnant women in Tanzania: a potential role for vitamin D and parasitic infections.** *Public Health Nutr* 2013, **15**(5):928–937.
26. Mehta S, Manji KP, Young AM, Brown ER, Chasela C, Taha E, Read JS, Golnberg RL, Fawzi WW: **Nutritional indicators of adverse pregnancy outcomes and mother-to-child transmission of HIV among HIV-infected women.** *Am J Clin Nutr* 2008, **87**(6):1639–1649.
27. Uneke CJ, Duhlinska DD, Igbinedion EB: **Immunodeficiency Virus infection and anaemia during pregnancy in eastern Nigeria: The public health implication.** *Infect Dis Clin Pract* 2007, **15**(4):239–244.
28. Nkhoma ET, Kalilani-phiri L, Mwapasa V, Rogerson SJ, Meshnick SR: **Effect of HIV infection and Plasmodium falciparum parasitemia on pregnancy outcomes in Malawi.** *Am J Trop Med Hyg* 2012, **87**(1):29–34.
29. Walker AS, Mulenga V, Ford D, Kabamba D, Sinyinza F, Kankasa C, Chintu C, Gibb DM: **The impact of daily co-trimoxazole prophylaxis and antiretro-viral therapy on mortality and hospital admissions in HIV-infected Zambian children.** *Clin Infect Dis* 2007, **44**:1361–1367.
30. Weiss G, Goodnough LT: **Anaemia of chronic disease.** *N Engl J Med* 2005, **352**:1011–1023.
31. Sullivan PS, Hanson DL, Chu SY, Jones JL, Ward JW, Sullivan BPS: **Epidemiology of anaemia in Human Immunodeficiency Virus (HIV)-infected persons: Results from the multistate adult and adolescent spectrum of HIV disease surveillance project.** *Blood* 1998, **91**:301–308.
32. Ziske J, Kunz A, Sewangi J, Lau I, Dugange F, Hauser A, Kirschner, Harms G, Theuring S: **Hematological changes in women and infants exposed to an AZT-containing regimen for prevention of mother-to-child transmission of HIV in Tanzania.** *PLoS One* 2013, **8**(2):e55633.
33. World Health Organization: *Antiretroviral drugs for treating pregnant women and preventing HIV infection in infants: Recommendations for a public health approach.* Geneva; 2010.
34. Sharma SK: **Zidovudine-induced anaemia in HIV/AIDS.** *Indian J Med Res* 2010, **132**:359–361.
35. Sinha G, Choi TJ, Nayak U, Gupta A, Nair S, Gupte N, Bulakh PM, Satry J, Deshmukh SD, Khandekar MM, Kulkarni V, Bhosele RA, Bharuche KE, Phadke MA, Kshirsagar AS, Bolinger RC: **Clinically significant anaemia in HIV-infected pregnant women in India is not a major barrier to Zidovudine use for prevention of maternal-to-child transmission.** *J Acquir Immune Defic Syndr* 2007, **45**:210–217.

9

Nobiletin suppresses cell viability through AKT Pathways in PC-3 and DU-145 prostate cancer cells

Jianchu Chen[1,2], Ashley Creed[2], Allen Y Chen[3], Haizhi Huang[1,2], Zhaoliang Li[2], Gary O Rankin[4], Xingqian Ye[1], Guihua Xu[1] and Yi Charlie Chen[2*]

Abstract

Background: Nobiletin is a non-toxic dietary flavonoid that possesses anti-cancer properties. Nobiletin has been reported to reduce the risk of prostate cancer, but the mechanism is not well understood. In this study, we investigated the effects of nobiletin in prostate cancer cell lines PC-3 and DU-145.

Methods: Nobiletin was isolated from a polymethoxy flavonoid mixture using HPLC, cell viability was analyzed with MTS-based assays. Protein expression was examined by ELISA and western blotting. Gene expression was examined by luciferase assay. And the pathways were examined by manipulating genetic components with plasmid transfection.

Results: Data showed that nobiletin decreased cell viability in both prostate cell lines, with a greater reduction in viability in PC-3 cells. HIF-1α expression and AKT phosphorylation were decreased in both cell lines. The VEGF expression was inhibited in PC-3 but not DU-145 cells. cMyc expression was decreased in DU-145 cells. Nobiletin down-regulated NF-κB (p50) expression in nuclei of DU145 cells but not whole cells. It also suppressed NF-κB expression in both whole cells and nuclei of PC-3 cells. Increasing HIF-1α levels reversed nobiletin's inhibitory effects on VEGF expression, and up-regulating AKT levels reversed its inhibitory effects on HIF-1α expression. We speculate that AKT influences cell viability probably by its effect on NF-κB in both prostate cells. The effect of nobiletin on VEGF expression in PC-3 cell lines was through the AKT/HIF-1α pathway.

Conclusion: Taken together, our results show that nobiletin suppresses cell viability through AKT pathways, with a more profound effect against the more metastatic PC-3 line. Due to this enhanced action against a more malignant cell type, nobiletin may be used to improve prostate cancer survival rates.

Keywords: Nobiletin, Prostate cancer, VEGF, NF-κB, HIF-1α, cMyc

Background

Prostate cancer is the second most common cancer in the United States, as well as, the second leading cause of mortality among males in the western world [1]. Approximately 25% of all newly diagnosed cancers in American men are prostate cancer [2]. Studies relating lifestyle to the risk of prostate cancer have become more prevalent in recent years due the escalating number of prostate cancer cases over the past decade [1]. Nevertheless, the etiology of prostate cancer is still uncertain because no specific carcinogen is known to cause this disease [3]. Research has found that certain risk factors, such as advancing age, African American ethnicity, and a positive family history, are associated with the likelihood of developing prostate cancer [4]. However, research has also shown that prostate cancer is not solely due to genetic factors, but is also related to lifestyle, diet, and environmental factors [4-6]. It is now believed that 90-95% of all cancers are caused by lifestyle [7]. This observation has encouraged researchers to identify dietary components, such as flavonoids like nobiletin, which may have anticancer properties.

It has been suggested that dietary intake of natural products rich in citrus flavonoids can play an important role in chemoprevention [8,9]. Flavonoids are phytochemicals found in fruits, vegetables, teas, and wines. Flavonoids display anti-carcinogenic characteristics *in vitro* and might be able to decrease cancer risk by changing

* Correspondence: chenyc@ab.edu
[2]College of Science, Technology and Mathematics, Alderson Broaddus University, Philippi, WV 26416, USA
Full list of author information is available at the end of the article

levels of sex hormones, preventing oxidation or inflammation, diminishing angiogenesis or cell proliferation, or stimulating apoptosis [10]. There are more than 400 flavonoids found in our food supply; however, in this research we focused our attention on nobiletin [11].

Nobiletin is an O-methylated flavonoid found in citrus peels with an empirical formula of $C_{21}H_{22}O_8$ and molecular weight of 402.39 [12]. An inverse relationship has been identified between nobiletin and cancer risk, which is likely due to nobiletin's anticancer, antiviral, and anti-inflammatory activities [13,14]. More specifically, recent findings have identified nobiletin as a cell differentiation modulator. Cell differentiation is a crucial step in angiogenesis and therefore could affect tumor growth and metastasis which both depend on angiogenesis [15]. Research has also shown that a diet high in flavonoids reduced oxidative damage to deoxyribonucleic acid (DNA), blocking a significant step in the onset of some types of cancers [16]. These findings support the proposition that nobiletin is functionally unique and could be a possible chemopreventive agent in inflammation-associated tumorigenesis [17].

Currently, metastatic prostate cancer is incurable and ultimately claims the life of patients [18,19]. An important factor in the relative seriousness of prostate cancer is the invasiveness of the constituent tumor cells causing metastasis [19]. Nobiletin has been reported to reduce the risk of prostate cancer, but the mechanism is not well understood. Therefore we studied the effects of nobiletin in prostate cancer cell lines PC-3 and DU-145. The pathways that affect the viability and VEGF expression of these cell lines have also been investigated in this paper. DU-145 and PC-3 are prostate cancer cell lines with moderate and high metastatic potential, respectively [20]. In the present study, we isolated nobiletin from a polymethoxy flavonoid mixture. Then we investigated the effect of nobiletin on cell viability in prostate cancer cell lines PC-3 and DU-145 and also performed western blotting and ELISA to identify changes in protein expression. Moreover, we examined the VEGF changes through transfection of AKT and HIF-1α plasmids in luciferase assays.

Methods
Cell culture and treatment
PC-3 cells were cultured in F-12K medium (ATCC, Manassas, VA) supplemented with 10% US-qualified fetal bovine serum (FBS) (Invitrogen, Grand Island, NY). DU-145 cells were cultured in Eagle's minimum essential medium (ATCC, Manassas, VA) supplemented with 10% US-qualified fetal bovine serum. All cells were cultured in a cell culture incubator with 5% CO_2 at 37°C. Nobiletin was dissolved in dimethyl sulfoxide (DMSO) to make stock solutions of 100 mM and equal amount of DMSO was included in controls for every experiment.

Cell proliferation assay
Effects of nobiletin on prostate cancer cells (PC-3 and DU-145) viability were colorimetrically determined with a "Cell Titer 96 Aqueous One Solution Cell Proliferation Assay" kit from Promega (Madison, WI). Cells (5×10^3/well) were seeded into 96-well plates and incubated for 16 h before being treated with 0 to 160 μg/ml nobiletin in triplicates for 24 h with DMSO as solvent control. After removing the medium, cells were washed with phosphate buffered saline (PBS), and then 100μL Aqueous One Reagent dilute solution (80 μL PBS +20 μL Aqueous One Reagent) was added to each well. Cells were incubated at 37°C for 1.5 h and measured for optical density (OD) values at 490 nm. Cell viability was expressed as a percentage of control from three independent experiments.

ELISA for VEGF
Secreted vascular endothelial growth factor (VEGF) protein levels were analyzed by sandwich enzyme-linked immunosorbent assay (ELISA) with a Quantikine Human VEGF Immunoassay Kit from R&D Systems (Minneapolis, MN) targeting VEGF in cell culture supernates. Cells (10^4/well) were seeded into 96-well plates and incubated for 16 h before being treated with 0 to 160 μg/ml nobiletin in triplicates for 24 h with DMSO as solvent control. Culture supernates were collected for VEGF assay. VEGF levels were determined following the manufacturer's instructions. A total of 3 independent experiments, each in triplicates, were assayed, and the mean VEGF protein level from each duplicate was used for statistical analysis.

Western blot
Prostate cancer cells (10^6) were seeded in 60-mm dishes and incubated for 16 h before treatment with nobiletin for 24 h. After washing with PBS, cells were harvested with 100 μL Mammalian Protein Extraction Reagent including 1 μL Halt Protease, 1 μL Phosphatase Inhibitor and 2 μL EDTA (Thermo Scientific, Rockford, IL). Cells were then frozen at -80°C for 30 min, melted, centrifuged at 12,000 g at 4°C for 10 min, and collected in aqueous phase for measurement. Nuclear protein was extracted by NE-PER™ Nuclear and Cytoplasmic Extraction Reagents (Thermo Scientific, Rockford, IL). Total protein levels were assayed with a BCA Protein Assay Kit (Pierce, Rockford, IL), and lysates were separated by 10% SDS-PAGE and blotted into nitrocellulose membrane. For immune detection, antibodies against HIF-1α, NF-κB (p50), PTEN, cMyc, GAPDH, p-AKT, total AKT (Santa Cruz Biotechnology, Santa Cruz, CA) and PCNA (Cell Signaling Technology, Boston, MA) were applied and signals visualized with x-ray film (Pierce Biotechnology, Rockford, IL). Protein bands were quantitated with NIH ImageJ software, normalized to corresponding GAPDH, PCNA or total AKT bands, and expressed as percentages of control. A total

of three independent experiments were carried out for statistical analysis.

Transient transfection and luciferase assay

PC-3 prostate cancer cells were seeded in 96-well plate at 10^4 cells/well and incubated overnight. The cells were then transfected with 0.05 μg VEGF (Hif-1α) luciferase reporter, 0-0.25 μg HIF-1α (AKT) or SR-α plasmids by 0.6 μL jetPRIME reagent (VWR, West Chester, PA) for 4 hours, followed by 16 hour treatment with 0 or 40 μM nobiletin. The cells were harvested and analyzed for luciferase and total protein levels, and the levels of VEGF (HIF-1α) reporter were normalized by corresponding total protein levels. Data represent Means ± SE from three independent experiments.

Statistical analysis

Results were expressed as mean ± standard error of mean (SEM). Statistical assessment was carried out with the program system of SPSS (Version 16.0 for Windows). The results were analyzed using one-way analysis of variance (ANOVA) and post hoc test (2-sided Dunnett's t) to test both overall differences and specific differences between each treatment and control. A p value of less than 0.05 was considered significant.

Results

Isolation and identification of nobiletin

Nobiletin was prepared from a polymethoxy flavonoid mixture, which was provided by Zhejiang Quzhou Tiansheng Plant Extraction Co. Ltd. in China, containing about 60% nobiletin and tangeretin. The polymethoxy flavonoid mixture was dissolved in methanol-dimethyl sulfoxide (1:1) to a concentration of 50 mg/mL. Then it was chromate graphed with high-performance liquid chromatography (HPLC), eluted with methanol-H_2O (70:30) in 8 mL/min at room temperature, separated into two fractions (Fractions I and II), collected individually, and evaporated.

Fraction I and fraction II were obtained by HPLC (Figure 1(a)). Fraction I was identified as nobiletin by HPLC-MS (Figure 1(b)), UV-vis chromatography (Figure 1(c)) and comparing peak time with that of nobiletin sample from Sigma (Figure 1(d)) and previous reports. Its purity was above 98%.

Nobiletin inhibits cell viability in prostate cancer cell lines

Cell viability steadily decreased as nobiletin concentration increased in both cell lines (Figure 2). Beginning at a concentration of 10 μM nobiletin, PC-3 cell viability consistently decreased from 95% to 40% at a concentration of 160 μM nobiletin ($p < 0.01$). Similarly, DU-145 cell viability was also inhibited with each successive doubling of concentration. At a concentration of 10 μM nobiletin cell viability was 92% ($p < 0.05$), which was

gradually inhibited to 46% by a 160 μM nobiletin treatment ($p < 0.01$). An overall inhibitory effect on cell viability was observed for both cell lines, although DU-145 (IC-50 = 137 μM nobiletin) cells appear more resistant than PC-3 cells (IC-50 = 117 μM nobiletin) to the inhibiting effect of nobiletin. It is in agreement with the cell viability determined by WST-1 assay [21].

Nobiletin inhibits VEGF expression in prostate cancer cell line PC-3

The levels of VEGF protein in PC-3 cell culture supernates were down-regulated to 70% at a concentration of 10 μM nobiletin ($p < 0.01$) and to 18% at a concentration of 160 μM nobiletin ($p < 0.01$) (Figure 3). However, the levels of VEGF protein in DU-145 cells ranged from 90-110% with no consistency with respect to nobiletin concentration. Our study revealed that VEGF expression was significantly ($p < 0.01$) reduced in PC-3 cancer cells by nobiletin treatment.

Nobiletin inhibits HIF-1α (Hypoxia inducible factor) protein expression in prostate cancer cell lines

HIF-1α protein levels in PC-3 cells showed intense and consistent down-regulation by nobiletin treatment (Figure 4). A 20 μM nobiletin treatment led to inhibition of HIF-1α protein to 70% ($p < 0.01$). Higher concentrations of nobiletin resulted in greater inhibition, with the levels of HIF-1α protein down to 48% by a 40 μM nobiletin treatment ($p < 0.05$) and 10% by a 80 μM nobiletin treatment ($p < 0.01$). HIF-1α protein levels in DU-145 cells showed consistent but gradual down-regulation by nobiletin treatment. DU-145 cells seem to be much more resistant to nobiletin treatment with down-regulation ranging from 94% at a concentration of 20 μM nobiletin to 79% at a concentration of 80 μM nobiletin ($p < 0.05$). HIF-1α expression in both cells lines (PC-3 and DU-145) was inhibited by nobiletin treatment, with a greater inhibition in PC-3 cells.

Nobiletin inhibits phosphorylation of AKT in prostate cancer cell lines

P-AKT levels were down-regulated from 65% by a 20 μM nobiletin treatment to 56% by a 80 μM nobiletin treatment ($p < 0.01$) in PC-3 cells (Figure 5). In DU-145 cells, p-AKT levels were down-regulated to 67% by a 20 μM nobiletin treatment ($p < 0.05$), to 51% by a 80 μM nobiletin treatment ($p < 0.01$). The percentage of down-regulation in each cell line was similar at each treatment concentration and indicates that nobiletin could decrease AKT phosphorylation for both PC-3 and DU-145. However, the observed down-regulation seemed to subside at 40 μM nobiletin treatment, with not much difference resulting at 80 μM nobiletin treatment for both cell lines. Therefore, higher concentrations may not be any more beneficial.

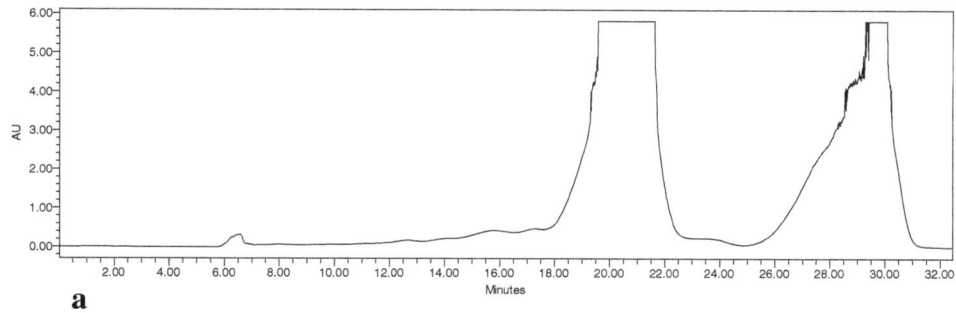

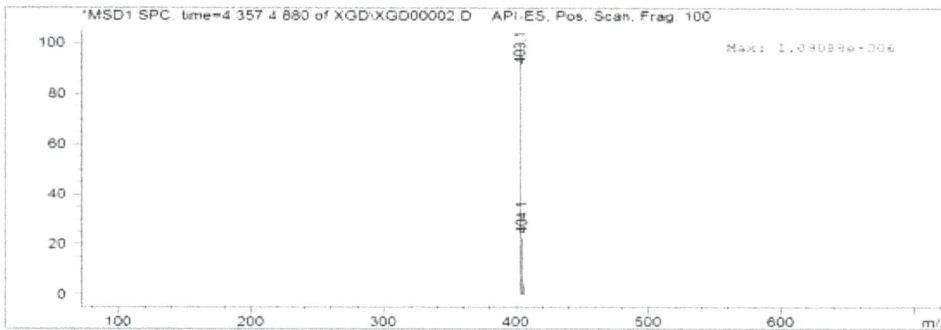

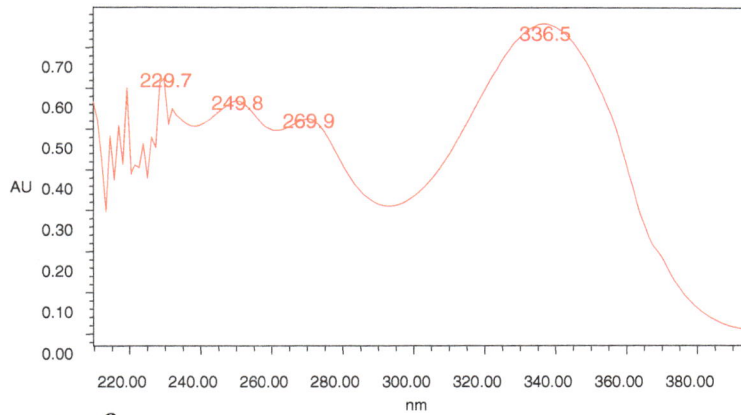

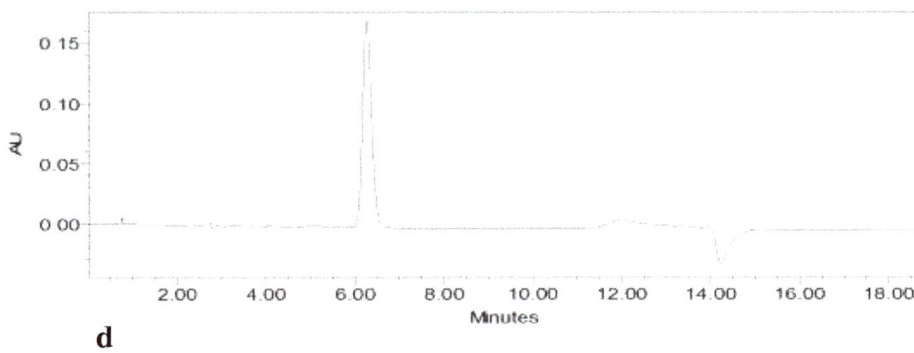

Figure 1 Isolation and identification of nobiletin. (a) Preparation HPLC graph of nobiletin and tangeretin. **(b)** HPLC-MS graph of nobiletin. **(c)** UV-vis chromatography of nobiletin. **(d)** HPLC graph of nobiletin.

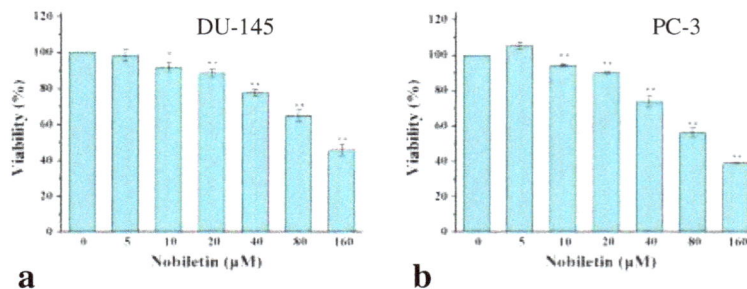

Figure 2 Effect of nobiletin on viability of PC-3 and DU-145 cells. **(a)** DU-145 cells, **(b)** PC-3 cells. Cells (5.0×10^3 /well) were seeded in 96-well plates, incubated for 16 h, and treated with nobiletin for 24 h. Cell viability was colorimetrically determined by a MTS-based method and expressed as percentages of control. Data represents mean ± SE from 3 independent experiments. *P < 0.05 as compared to control. **P < 0.01 as compared to control.

Nobiletin inhibits cMyc expression in prostate cancer cell line DU-145

In PC-3 cells, cMyc levels were slightly down regulated to 93% by a 40 μM nobiletin treatment and to 90% by a 80 μM nobiletin treatment (Figure 6). The results were very gradual, revealing that the PC-3 cells have a high level of resistance and there was no statistical significance among treatments. The cMyc levels in DU-145 cells were down-regulated to 79-84% by nobiletin treatment. Therefore, nobiletin reduced cMyc expression in DU-145 cells, but showed no evidence of inhibition in PC-3 cells.

Nobiletin inhibits NF-κB (p50) expression in nucleus of prostate cancer cell

NF-κb (p50) expression was down-regulated in both whole cells and nuclei of PC-3 cells when treated with nobiletin. At the concentration of 80 μM nobiletin, its expression was inhibited by 28% (p < 0.01) and 37% (p < 0.05) respectively in whole cells and nuclei. In nuclei of DU145 cells, p50 expression was inhibited to 42% (p < 0.01) by a 40 μM nobiletin treatment and 10% (p < 0.01) by a 80 μM nobiletin treatment (Figure 7). However, its expression in whole cells was up-regulated to 103-112% with higher concentrations of nobiletin resulting in greater promotion.

Effect of nobiletin on PTEN expression

Our study found that nobiletin had no significant effect on PTEN expression in DU-145 cells (Figure 8). PTEN was not expressed in PC-3 cells.

Nobiletin inhibits VEGF expression through regulating AKT and HIF-1α gene in prostate cancer cell line PC-3

We used PC-3 cancer cells with low levels of AKT and HIF-1α expression to test whether nobiletin affects VEGF expression. Our study found that transfected plasmid AKT and HIF-1α concentration-dependently reversed nobiletin's inhibitory effects (Figure 9). Our findings suggest that nobiletin regulates VEGF expression through down-regulating AKT and HIF-1α in prostate cancer cells.

Discussion

Approximately 25% of all newly diagnosed cancers in American men are prostate cancer [2]. The risk of developing prostate cancer is associated with advancing age, African American ethnicity, and a positive family history [4]. However, research has also shown that diet and other lifestyle factors may influence prostate cancer risk [4]. Studies relating lifestyle to the risk of prostate cancer

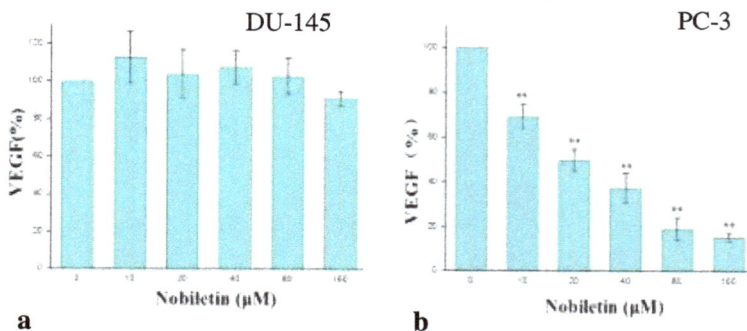

Figure 3 Effect of nobiletin on VEGF expression in PC-3 and DU-145 cells. **(a)** DU-145. **(b)** PC-3. Cells (1.0×10^4/well) were seeded into 96-well plates , incubated for 16 h, and treated with nobiletin for 24 h. Vascular endothelial growth factor (VEGF) in cellculture supernate were analyzed with a Quantikine Human VEGF Immunoassay Kit from R&D Systems (Minneapolis, MN). Data represents mean ± SE from 3 independent experiments. *P < 0.05 as compared to control. **P < 0.01 as compared to control.

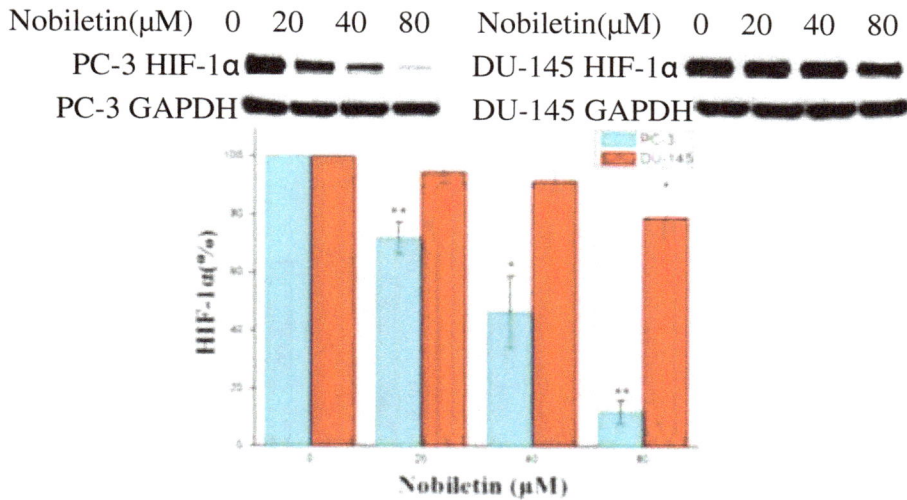

Figure 4 Nobiletin's effects on HIF-1α expression in PC-3 and DU-145 cells. Nobiletin's effect on HIF-1α expression. PC-3 and DU-145 cells (1.0×10^6) were seeded in 60-mm dishes, incubated overnight, and treated with nobiletin for 24 hours. Cells were harvested and analyzed by SDS-PAGE and Western Blotting. HIF-1α protein levels were normalized by GAPDH protein levels. Data represents means ± SE from 3 independent experiments. *P < 0.05 compared to control. **P < 0.01 compared to control.

have become more prevalent in recent years due to the escalating number of prostate cancer cases.

It has been suggested that dietary intake of natural products rich in flavonoids from citrus fruits may play a role in the prevention of cancer [8]. Tangeretin, nobiletin, hesperetin, hesperidin, naringenin, and naringin are just a few examples of citrus flavonoids that have the potential to be used as chemotherapeutic agents. Research has shown that these flavonoids possess inhibition activity on certain cancer cells' growth through various mechanisms [8].

Nobiletin, a citrus polymethoxy flavonoid, possesses anticancer, antiviral, and anti-inflammatory activities [14]. More specifically, recent findings have identified nobiletin as a cell differentiation modulator. Cell differentiation is a crucial step in angiogenesis and therefore could affect tumor growth and metastasis which both depend on angiogenesis [15]. These findings support the proposition that nobiletin is functionally unique and could be a possible chemopreventive agent in inflammation-associated tumorigenesis [17].

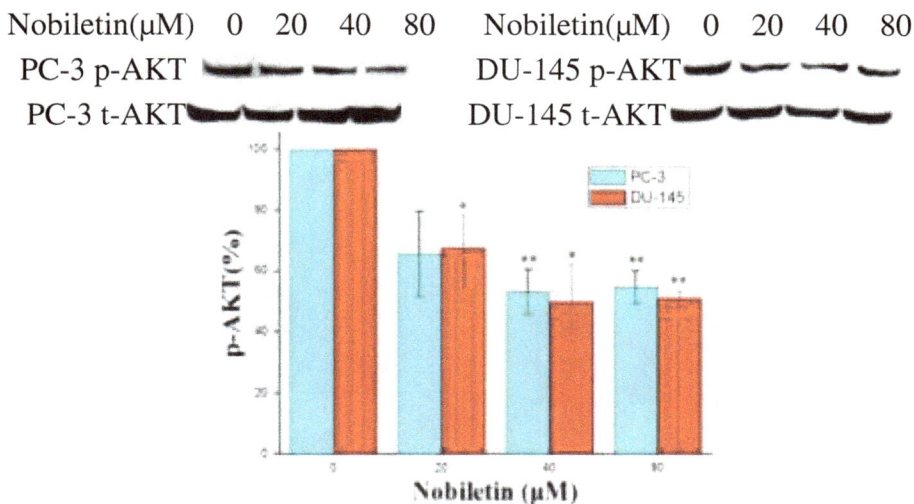

Figure 5 Nobiletin's effect on AKT phosphorylation in PC-3 and DU-145 cells. PC-3 and DU-145 cells (1.0×10^6) were seeded in 60-mm dishes, incubated overnight, and treated with nobiletin for 24 hours. Cells were harvested and analyzed by SDS-PAGE and Western Blotting. P-AKT protein levels were normalized by total AKT protein levels and expressed as percentages of control. Data represents means ± SE from 3 independent experiments. *P < 0.05 compared to control. **P < 0.01 compared to control.

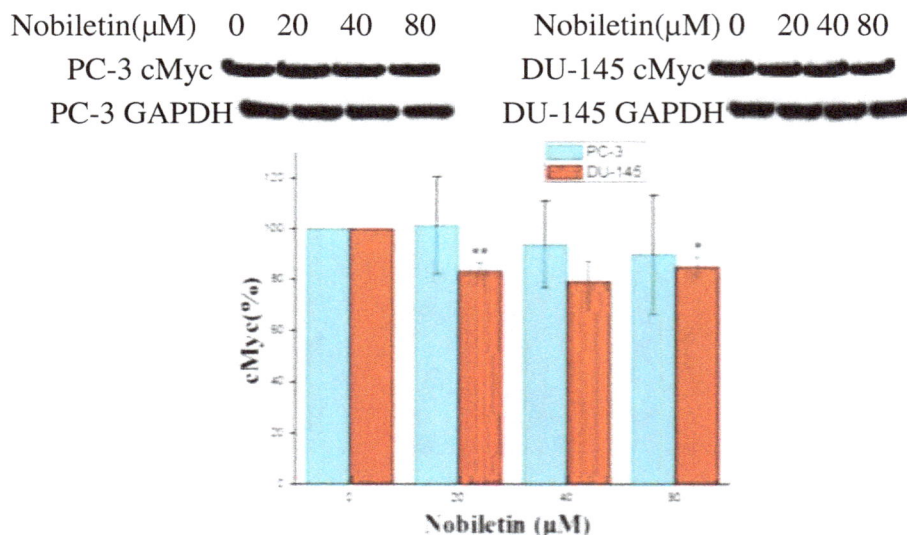

Figure 6 Nobiletin's effect on cMyc. PC-3 and DU-145 cells (1.0×10^6) were seeded in 60-mm dishes, incubated overnight, and treated with nobiletin for 24 hours. Cells were harvested and analyzed by SDS-PAGE and Western Blotting. cMyc levels were normalized by GAPDH protein levels and expressed as percentages of control. Data represents means ± SE from 3 independent experiments. *$P < 0.05$ compared to control. **$P < 0.01$ compared to control.

We tested the effectiveness of the preventive and/or treatment measures that nobiletin exhibits on PC-3 and DU-145 prostate cancer cells and showed that PC-3 and DU-145 cell viability was suppressed concentration-dependently by nobiletin treatment. Several pathways including VEGF, HIF-1α, AKT phosphorylation, cMyc, and NF-κB influence cell viability inhibition. In both cell lines, nobiletin inhibited phosphorylation of AKT, which is known to be the major signal for cell survival and proliferation [22]. Nobiletin treatment also reduced NF-κB (p50) expression in nuclei of both prostate cancer cells. NF-κB activation plays many roles when it enter into

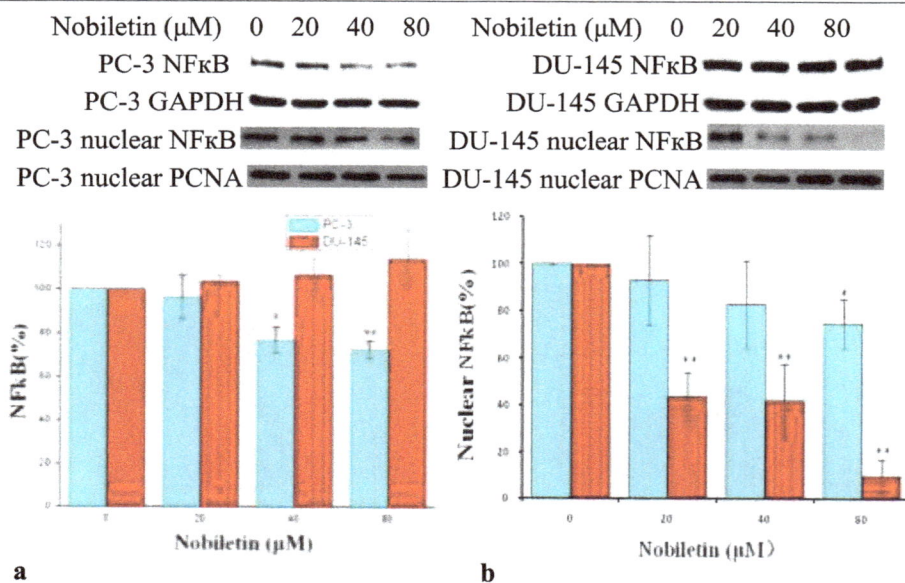

Figure 7 Nobiletin's effect on NF-κB (p50) expression. (a) Effect of nobiletin on total NF-kB expression, **(b)** Effect of nobiletin on nuclear NF-kB expression. PC-3 and DU-145 cells (1.0×10^6) were seeded in 60 mm dishes, incubated overnight, and treated with nobiletin for 24 hours. Cells were harvested and analyzed by SDS-PAGE and Western Blotting. NF-κB protein levels whole cells were normalized by GAPDH protein levels and its protein levels of nucleus were normalized by PCNA protein levels. They were expressed as percentages of control. Data represents means ± SE from 3 independent experiments. *$P < 0.05$ compared to control. **$P < 0.01$ compared to control.

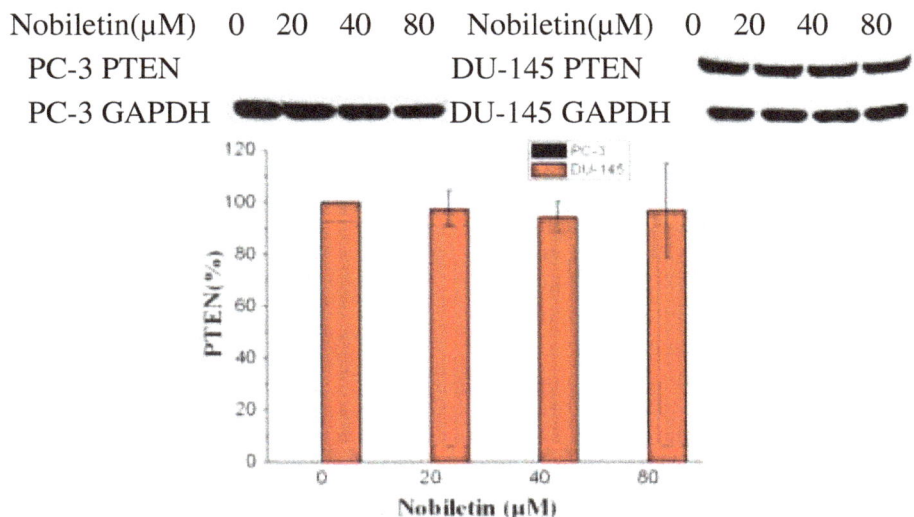

Figure 8 Nobiletin's effect on PTEN expression. PC-3 and DU-145 cells (1.0×10^6) were seeded in 60-mm dishes, incubated overnight, and treated with nobiletin for 24 hours. Cells were harvested and analyzed by SDS-PAGE and Western Blotting. PTEN protein levels were normalized by GAPDH protein levels and expressed as percentages of control. Data represents means ± SE from 3 independent experiments. *P < 0.05 compared to control. **P < 0.01 compared to control.

the nucleus, including initiating cellular transformation, mediating cellular proliferation, mediating cellular invasion and angiogenesis, mediating metastasis, and linking inflammation and cancer [23,24]. Suppression of NF-κB in tumor samples also inhibits proliferation, causes cell cycle arrest, and leads to apoptosis, indicating the crucial role of NF-κB in cell proliferation and survival [25]. Some researchers have found that the expression, activation and translocation of NF-κB were regulated by AKT pathways [26-28]. Our results showed that nobiletin treatment could decrease NF-κB expression in nuclei of both cells

and AKT phosphorylation, indicating that AKT may influence cell viability by its effect on NF-κB in both prostate cells. It was also found that HIF-1α promoter is responsive to selective NF-κB subunits, indicating that NF-κB is a direct modulator of HIF-1α expression [29]. VEGF is a signal protein produced by cells related to vasculogenesis and angiogenesis, and it is also the downstream gene of HIF-1α. Our study revealed that VEGF expression was significantly (p < 0.01) reduced in PC-3 cancer cells by nobiletin treatment. HIF-1α expression in both cells lines (PC-3 and DU-145) was also inhibited by nobiletin

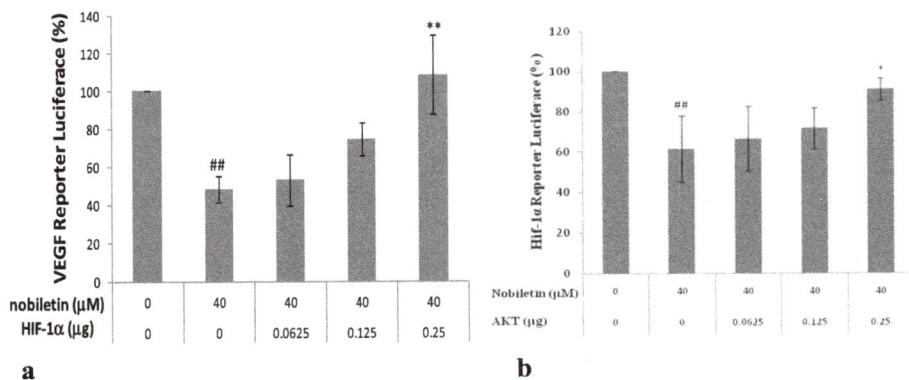

Figure 9 Nobiletin inhibits VEGF expression by regulating AKT and HIF-1α gene in PC-3 cells. (a) Nobiletin inhibits VEGF expression by regulating HIF-1 α gene, **(b)** Nobiletin inhibits VEGF expression by regulating AKT gene. PC-3 prostate cancer cells were seeded in 96-well plate at 10,000 cells/well and incubated overnight. The cells were then transfected with 0.05 ug VEGF (Hif-1α) luciferase reporter, 0-0.25 μg HIF-1α (AKT) or SR-α plasmids by 0.6 μL jetPRIME reagent for 4 hours, followed by 16 hour treatment with 0 or 40 μM nobiletin. The cells were harvested and analyzed for luciferase and total protein levels, and the levels of VEGF (Hif-1α) reporter were normalized by corresponding total protein levels. Data represent Means ± SE from 3 independent experiments. #p < 0.05 as compared to control. ##p <0.01 as compared to control. *p <0.05 as compared to nobiletin-treated control. **p <0.01 as compared to nobiletin-treated control.

treatment, with a greater inhibition in PC-3 cells. Furthermore, it was found that nobiletin inhibited VEGF expression through regulating AKT/HIF-1α pathways in prostate cancer cell line PC-3. Increasing HIF-1α levels actually reversed nobiletin's inhibitory effects on VEGF expression. Similarly up-regulating AKT levels reversed its inhibitory effects on HIF-1α expression. These results correspond to a previous study that HIF-1α/VEGF expression can be regulated by AKT pathways [30]. Nobiletin reduced cMyc expression in DU-145 cells, but showed no evidence of inhibition in PC-3 cells. PTEN has been shown to play a pivotal role in apoptosis, cell cycle arrest, and possibly cell migration. PTEN is the most frequently mutated gene in prostate cancer, loss of heterozygosity at 10q23 can be detected in approximately 50% of human prostate cancers, whereas homozygous deletions of PTEN can be detected in approximately 10% of these cases [31]. However, nobiletin appears to lower cell viability through a mechanism independent of PTEN, as it does not seem to affect PTEN concentrations.

Our research indicated that nobiletin is a good candidate for the chemoprevention of prostate cancer in humans and could be an effective measure in inhibiting prostate cancer cell viability. Nobiletin has the apparent ability to suppress cell viability through multiple pathways, thus inhibiting tumor growth. Most encouraging is its capacity to suppress the more metastatic PC-3 cell line. Since the lethality of a tumor links directly to its ability to spread, nobiletin promises to increase the prostate cancer survival rate. However, more data needs to be obtained on nobiletin's toxicity and tolerable dosages before it can become part of prostate cancer prevention and/or treatment. Also, as an in vitro model, cell culture cannot take absorption, distribution, metabolism, and excretion of nobiletin into consideration. Further studies in animal models and human trials are warranted to determine if physicians can promote this natural compound toward chemoprevention of prostate cancer cells.

Conclusion

Our research indicated that nobiletin is a good candidate for the chemoprevention of prostate cancer in humans and could be an effective measure in suppressing prostate cancer cell viability. For these two prostate cancer cell lines, nobiletin has the apparent ability to suppress cell viability concentration-dependently through multiple pathways (VEGF, HIF-1α, AKT phosphorylation, cMyc, and NF-κB). Because nobiletin seems to work better against the more dangerous PC-3 cell line, nobiletin holds real potential in improving prostate cancer outcomes. However, more data needs to be obtained on nobiletin's toxicity and tolerable dosages before it can become part of prostate cancer prevention and/or treatment. Also, as an in vitro model, cell culture cannot take absorption,

distribution, metabolism, and excretion of nobiletin into consideration. Further studies in animal models and human trials are warranted to determine if physicians can promote this natural compound toward chemoprevention of prostate cancer cells.

Competing interest
The authors state that they have no competing interest.

Authors' contributions
JC carried out the majority of experimental work. YC drafted the manuscript. All authors participated in experimental design and read and approved the final manuscript.

Acknowledgments
This research was supported by a West Virginia Experimental Program to Stimulate Competitive Research grant and an NIH grant (5P20RR016477 and 8P20GM104434) from the National Center for Research Resources awarded to the West Virginia IDeA Network of Biomedical Research Excellence.

Author details
[1]College of Biosystems Engineering and Food Science, Fuli Institute of Food Science, Zhejiang Key Laboratory for Agro-Food Processing, Zhejiang University, Hangzhou 310058, China. [2]College of Science, Technology and Mathematics, Alderson Broaddus University, Philippi, WV 26416, USA. [3]Department of Pharmaceutical Science, West Virginia University, Morgantown, WV 26506, USA. [4]Department of Pharmacology, Physiology and Toxicology, Joan C. Edwards School of Medicine, Marshall University, Huntington, WV 25755, USA.

References
1. Mohile SG, Shelke AR: **Treating prostate cancer in elderly men: how does aging affect the outcome?** *Curr Treat Options Oncol* 2011, **12**:263–275.
2. Crawford E: **Understanding the epidemiology, natural history, and key pathways involved in prostate cancer.** *Urology* 2009, **73**:4–10.
3. Bosland MC: **The role of steroid hormones in prostate carcinogenesis.** *J Natl Cancer Inst Monogr* 2000, **27**:39–66.
4. Crawford E: **Epidemiology of prostate cancer.** *Urology* 2003, **62**:3–12.
5. Gronberg H: **Prostate cancer epidemiology.** *Lancet* 2003, **361**:859–864.
6. Whittemore AS, Kolonel LN, Wu AH, John EM, Gallagher RP, Howe GR: **Prostate cancer in relation to diet, physical activity, and body size in blacks, whites, and Asians in the United States and Canada.** *J Natl Cancer Inst* 1995, **87**:652–661.
7. Gupta S, Kim J, Prasad S, Aggarwal B: **Regulation of survival, proliferation, invasion, angiogenesis, and metastasis of tumor cells through modulation of inflammatory pathways by nutraceuticals.** *Cancer and Metastasis Reviews* 2010, **29**:405–434.
8. Meiyanto E, Hermawan A, Anindyajati: **Natural products for cancer-targeted therapy: citrus flavonoids as potent chemopreventive agents.** *Asian Pac J Cancer Prev* 2012, **13**:427–436.
9. Yang C, Wang X, Lu G, Picinich S: **Cancer prevention by tea: animal studies, molecular mechanisms and human relevance.** *Nat Rev Cancer* 2009, **9**:429–439.
10. Gates M, Vitonis A, Tworoger S, Rosner B, Titus-Ernstoff L, Hankinson S, Cramer H: **Flavonoid intake and ovarian cancer risk in a population based case-control study.** *Int J Cancer* 2009, **124**:1918–1925.
11. McCann S, Freudenheim J, Marshall J, Saxon G: **Risk of human ovarian cancer is related to dietary intake of selected nutrients, phytochemicals and food groups.** *Journal of Nutrition* 2003, **133**:1937–1942.
12. Bernini R, Crisante F, Ginnasi MC: **A convenient and safe O-methylation offlavonoids with dimethyl carbonate (DMC).** *Molecules* 2011, **16**:1418–1425.
13. Knekt P, Järvinen R, Seppänen R, Heliövaara M, Teppo L, Pukkala E, Aromaa A: **Dietary flavonoids and the risk of lung cancer and other malignant neoplasms.** *Am J Epidemiol* 1997, **146**:223–230.
14. Li S, Yu H, Ho CT: **Nobiletin: efficient and large quantity isolation from orange peel extract.** *Biomed Chromatogr* 2006, **20**:133–138.
15. Kunimasa K, Ikekita M, Sato M, Ohta T, Yamori Y, Ikeda M, Kuranuki S, Oikawa T: **Nobiletin, a citrus polymethoxy flavonoid, suppresses multiple**

angiogenesis-related endothelial cell functions and angiogenesis in vivo. *Cancer Sci* 2010, **101**:2462–2469.

16. Nichenametla S, Taruscio TG, Barney DL, Exon JH: **A review of the effects and mechanisms of polyphenolics in cancer.** *Crit Rev Food Sci Nutr* 2006, **46**:161–183.

17. Murakami A, Nakamura Y, Torikai K, Tanaka T, Koshiba T, Koshimizu K, Kuwahara S, Takahashi Y, Ogawa K, Yano M, Tokuda H, Nishino H, Mimaki Y, Sashida Y, Kitanaka S, Ohigashi H: **Inhibitory effect of citrus nobiletin on phorbol ester-induced skin inflammation, oxidative stress, and tumor promotion in mice.** *Cancer Res* 2000, **60**:5059–5066.

18. Kim SJ, Uehara H, Yazici S, Langley RR, He J, Tsan R, Fan D, Killion JJ, Fidler IJ: **Simultaneous blockade of platelet-derived growth factor-receptor and epidermal growth factor-receptor signaling and systemic administration of paclitaxel as therapy for human prostate cancer metastasis in bone of nude mice.** *Cancer Res* 2004, **64**:4201–4208.

19. Kim SJ, Johnson M, Koterba K, Herynk MH, Uehara H, Gallick GE: **Reduced c-Met expression by an adenovirus expressing a c-Met ribozyme inhibits tumorigenic growth and lymph node metastases of PC3-LN4 prostate tumor cells in an orthotopic nude mouse model.** *Clin Cancer Res* 2003, **9**:5161–5170.

20. Pulukuri SM, Gondi CS, Lakka SS, Jutla A, Estes N, Gujrati M, Rao JS: **RNA interference-directed knockdown of urokinase plasminogen activator and urokinase plasminogen activator receptor inhibits prostate cancer cell invasion, survival, and tumorigenicity in vivo.** *Journal of Biological Chemisry* 2005, **280**:36529–36540.

21. Tang M, Ogawa K, Asamoto M, Hokaiwado N, Seeni A, Suzuki S, Takahashi S, Tanaka T, Ichikawa K, Shirai T: **Protective effects of citrus nobiletin and auraptene in transgenic rats developing adenocarcinoma of the prostate (TRAP) and human prostate carcinoma cells.** *Cancer Sci* 2007, **98**:471–477.

22. Fang J, Zhou Q, Shi XL, Jiang BH: **Luteolin inhibits insulin-like growth factor 1 receptor signaling in prostate cancer cells.** *Carcinogenesis* 2007, **28**:713–723.

23. Aggarwal BB: **Nuclear-factor-κB: The enemy within.** *Cancer Cell* 2004, **6**:203–206.

24. Gilmore TD: **Introduction to NF-κB: players, pathways, perspectives.** *Oncogene* 2006, **25**:6680–6684.

25. Bharti AC, Aggarwal BB: **Nuclear factor-κB and cancer: Its role in prevention and therapy.** *Biochem Pharmacol* 2002, **64**:883–888.

26. Kar S, Palit S, Ball WB, Das PK: **Carnosic acid modulates Akt/IKK/NF-κB signaling by PP2A and induces intrinsic and extrinsic pathway mediated apoptosis in human prostate carcinoma PC-3 cells.** *Apoptosis* 2012, **17**:735–747.

27. Kim MO, Moon DO, Heo MS, Lee JD, Jung JH, Kim SK, Choi YH, Kim GY: **Pectenotoxin-2 abolishes constitutively activated NF-κB, leading to suppression of NF-κB related gene products and potentiation of apoptosis.** *Cancer Letter* 2008, **271**:25–33.

28. Ozes ON, Mayo LD, Gustin JA, Pfeffer SR, Pfeffer LM, Donner DB: **NF-κB activation by tumour necrosis factor requires the Akt serine-threonine kinase.** *Nature* 1999, **401**:82–85.

29. Uden PV, Kenneth NS, Rocha S: **Regulation of hypoxia-inducible factor-1α by NF-κB.** *Biochemical Journal* 2008, **412**:477–484.

30. Shi YH, Wang YX, Bingle L, Gong LH, Heng WJ, Li Y, Fang WG: **In vitro study of HIF-1 activation and VEGF release by bFGF in the T47D breast cancer cell line under normoxic conditions: involvement of PI-3K/Akt and MEK1/ERK pathways.** *Journal of Pathology* 2005, **205**:530–536.

31. Chu EC, Tarnawski AS: **PTEN regulatory functions in tumor suppression and cell biology.** *Med Sci Monit* 2004, **10**:RA235–241.

10

A systematic review of the pathophysiology of 5-fluorouracil-induced cardiotoxicity

Anne Polk[1,2]*, Kirsten Vistisen[2], Merete Vaage-Nilsen[1] and Dorte L Nielsen[2]

Abstract

Background: Cardiotoxicity is a serious side effect to treatment with 5-fluorouracil (5-FU), but the underlying mechanisms are not fully understood. The objective of this systematic review was to evaluate the pathophysiology of 5-FU- induced cardiotoxicity.

Methods: We systematically searched PubMed for articles in English using the search terms: 5-FU OR 5-fluorouracil OR capecitabine AND cardiotoxicity. Papers evaluating the pathophysiology of this cardiotoxicity were included.

Results: We identified 27 articles of 26 studies concerning the pathophysiology of 5-FU-induced cardiotoxicity. The studies demonstrated 5-FU-induced: hemorrhagic infarction, interstitial fibrosis and inflammatory reaction in the myocardium; damage of the arterial endothelium followed by platelet aggregation; increased myocardial energy metabolism and depletion of high energy phosphate compounds; increased superoxide anion levels and a reduced antioxidant capacity; vasoconstriction of arteries; changes in red blood cell (RBC) structure, function and metabolism; alterations in plasma levels of substances involved in coagulation and fibrinolysis and increased endothelin-1 levels and N-terminal-pro brain natriuretic peptide levels. Based on these findings the proposed mechanisms are: endothelial injury followed by thrombosis, increased metabolism leading to energy depletion and ischemia, oxidative stress causing cellular damage, coronary artery spasm leading to myocardial ischemia and diminished ability of RBCs to transfer oxygen resulting in myocardial ischemia.

Conclusions: There is no evidence for a single mechanism responsible for 5-FU-induced cardiotoxicity, and the underlying mechanisms might be multifactorial. Further research is needed to elucidate the pathogenesis of this side effect.

Keywords: 5-fluorouracil, Cardiotoxicity, Pathophysiology, Systematic review

Background

5-Fluorouracil (5-FU) and capecitabine are chemotherapeutics used to treat solid cancers, including gastrointestinal cancers, breast cancer, head and neck cancer and pancreatic cancer. Capecitabine is a 5-FU pro-drug, that is converted to 5-FU inside tumour cells [1]. A severe side effect to 5-FU and capecitabine-based treatment is cardiotoxicity, which often presents as myocardial ischemia, but to a lesser extent cardiac arrhythmias, hyper- and hypotension, left ventricular dysfunction, cardiac arrest and sudden death [2-7]. The incidence of 5-FU-induced cardiotoxicity varies between 0-35% and may depend on dose, cardiac comorbidity and schedule of chemotherapy [2,3,5].

The clinical handling of 5-FU-induced cardiotoxicity is difficult as the pathophysiological mechanisms underlying this cardiotoxicity remain undefined [2,8-13]. Several mechanisms have been proposed, including vascular endothelial damage followed by coagulation, ischemia secondary to coronary artery spasm, direct toxicity on the myocardium and thrombogenicity due to altered rheological factors. The present review addresses the pathophysiology of 5-FU- and capecitabine-induced cardiotoxicity and discusses the evidence for the proposed mechanisms.

Method

This systematic review is conducted according to the PRISMA guidelines [14] (Additional file 1).

* Correspondence: anne.polk@hotmail.com
[1]Departments of Cardiology, Herlev Hospital, University of Copenhagen, Herlev Ringvej 75, DK-2730 Herlev, Denmark
[2]Departments of Oncology, Herlev Hospital, University of Copenhagen, Herlev Ringvej 75, DK-2730 Herlev, Denmark

Search strategy

We searched PubMed (1966–2013) for publications in English using the search string: (5-FU or 5-fluorouracil or capecitabine) AND cardiotoxicity. The last search was carried out in October 2013. Additionally we hand-searched reference lists of retrieved papers.

Study selection process

All citations retrieved were reviewed on full citation, abstracts and indexing terms (where provided in the databases) by two authors independently. They were rated as "relevant", "possibly relevant" or "not relevant". Full-text publications of all potentially relevant articles were reviewed for eligibility independently by the same two authors. All disagreements in rating or eligibility were resolved by discussion of the full-text articles till consensus was reached. All articles or abstracts in English exploring the pathophysiology of 5-FU or capecitabine cardiotoxicity were eligible. Case reports were excluded. Full articles were obtained, and references were checked for additional relevant articles.

Data extraction

The studies were grouped into in vitro studies (studies on cultured cells or cell lines), ex vivo animal studies (conducted on functional organs that had been removed from the intact organism), in vivo animal studies (conducted on living organisms in their normal intact state) and human studies. One author extracted the following data from all studies where provided: the type of study (in vitro, ex vivo animal, in vivo animal or human), the experimental model used, the number of tests objects, the parameters evaluated, the methods applied and the results of the performed tests.

Results

Twenty-seven papers of 26 studies were included (eight in vitro studies, two ex vivo animal studies, nine in vivo animal studies, six human studies and one study with results from both in vitro and human experiments) (Figure 1). All studies evaluated the pathophysiology of 5-FU-induced cardiotoxicity. We did not identify any studies evaluating the pathophysiology of capecitabine-induced cardiotoxicity. Additional file 2 shows a table with characteristics and results of the included studies. The positive, negative and conflicting findings from these studies are summarized in Table 1.

Histopathological studies of the myocardium

The histopathological effects of 5-FU- were examined in two animal studies [15]. In rat hearts, multifocal interstitial hemorrhages, multifocal myofiber necrosis, inflammatory reactions including perivascular involvement, pericarditis, valvulitis and vascular changes, were found [15]. The vascular changes included dilated vessels, ruptured vascular walls, extravasation of blood and microthrombosis. In rabbits, a single high intravenous dose resulted in hemorrhagic infarction of the ventricle walls, proximal spasms of the coronary arteries and lethal outcome for all rabbits within 1 day [16]. In contrast, repeated lower doses resulted in left ventricular hypertrophy due to reticular interstitial fibrosis with edema, concentric fibrous thickening of the intima of small distal coronary arteries and disseminated foci of necrotic myocardial cells [16]. Whether the differences in histopathological effects were species specific, or due to different doses, is not clear.

Histopathological studies of the arteries

Four studies [9,22-24] examined the histopathological effects of 5-FU on the arterial endothelium in rabbits. Scanning electron microscopy of the arteries showed extensive cytolysis, denudation of the underlying internal elastic lamina, platelet aggregation and fibrin formation [9,22-24]. Areas of contracted vessel walls with contracted endothelial cells were present [9,22-24]. Cell detachment was frequently seen and endothelial cells presented with a range of morphologic features compatible with cytolysis [9,22-24]. The endothelial damage was comparable in arteries exposed to direct injection of 5-FU and arteries exposed to 5-FU through systemic circulation [24]. The endothelial changes were most pronounced on day 3 after 5-FU injections and had diminished on day 7 and day 14 [9]. Concomitant treatment with probucol, a lipid-lowering drug with strong antioxidant properties, abrogated the effects of 5-FU on the endothelium [24], while concomitant treatment with dalteparin, a low-molecular-weight heparin, resulted in a somewhat different picture with endothelial damage on day 3, diminishing on day 7 but increasing again by day 14 [9]. Dalteparin prevented fibrin formation and to a lesser extent platelet aggregation [9].

Studies on cultured myocardial and endothelial cells

In vitro treatment of H9c2 rat cardiomyocytes with 5-FU induced a time- and dose-dependent growth inhibition that was enhanced by levofolene [17]. Apoptosis was more frequent in 5-FU- and levofolene-treated H9c2 cells compared with colon cancer cells, and cleavage of caspase 3, an effector caspase in the apoptotic pathways, was increased in 5-FU treated H9c2 cells [17]. Moreover, superoxide anion levels increased [17]. Comparing the toxicity of 5-FU on cardiomyocytes and endothelial cells from rat hearts, Wenzel and Cosma [36] found that 5-FU induced more severe metabolic and morphological changes in endothelial cells than in cardiomyocytes. In contrast, an in vitro study of human endothelial cells and bovine endothelial cells showed no effect on cell death of 5-FU, but decreased (^{3}H)thymidine incorporation, decreased total cellular protein levels and increased prostacyclin release

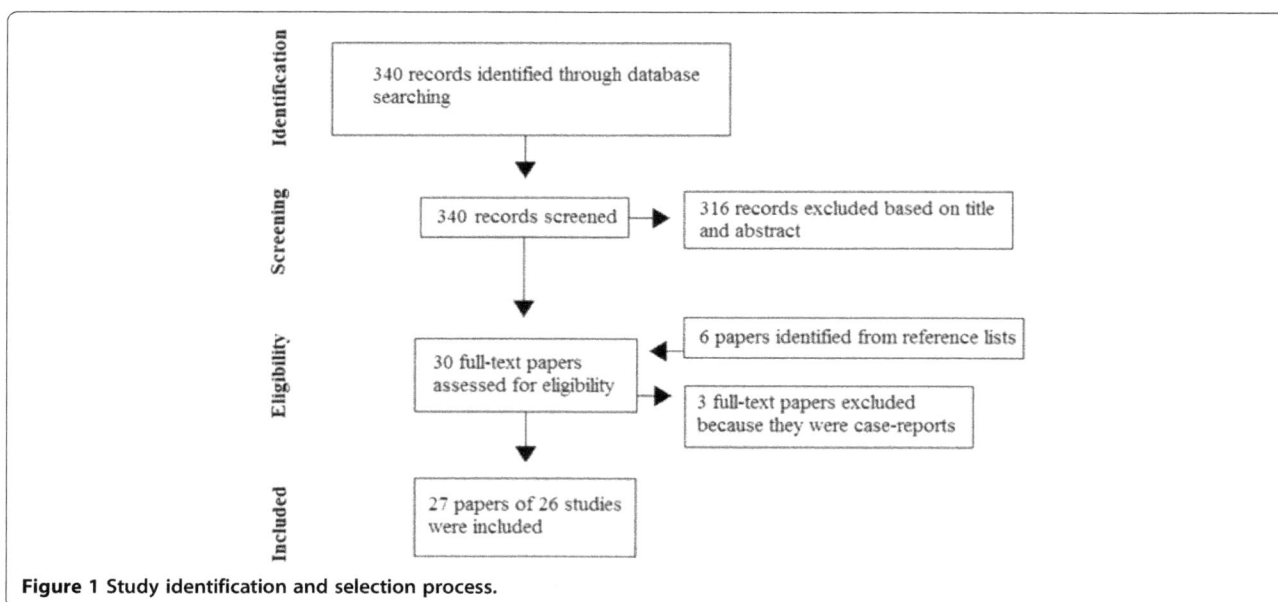

Figure 1 Study identification and selection process.

after 5-FU incubation [25]. Taken together, these findings suggest differences in susceptibility between different cell lines to the direct toxic effects from 5-FU [17,36] and possibly even different cellular responses to the same stressor [17]. The toxic effects may not be lethal for the cells, but may reflect reversible interference with cellular function [36].

Studies of myocardial metabolism and hemodynamic function

Studies of myocardial metabolism in guinea pigs showed that 5-FU induced a decrease in myocardial high energy phosphate levels [12,36,37] and accumulation of citrate in the myocardium [12] reflecting increased anaerobic metabolism. These changes were associated with electrocardiographic (ECG) changes suggestive of myocardial ischemia occurring around 3 hours after intravenous administration of 5-FU [12]. The depletion of high energy compounds was not associated with alterations in myocardial blood flow [12] as myocardial blood flow remained unchanged during 5-FU treatment. In contrast, Millart et al. [20] found that mean coronary flow was consistently increased in 5-FU-pre-treated rat hearts. This discrepancy can be due to different species, different experimental models or different methods to measure coronary flow. Likewise, Tamatsu et al. [37] showed that the experimental model used (open-chest or closed-chest) influenced the magnitude of depletion in high energy phosphate compounds [37].

Millart et al. [20] found no changes in oxygen uptake and cardiac contractility during perfusion of the isolated perfused rat heart with 1 mg/L 5-FU for 80 minutes.

However, when rats where pre-treated with 5-FU (50 mg/kg intraperitoneally for 5 days) before killing and excision of the hearts, oxygen consumption and mean coronary flow were significantly higher compared with controls [20]. Also, a negative inotropic effect was seen in 5-FU pre-treated rats. In contrast, Satoh et al. [21] reported that 5-FU had a positive inotropic effect on the atria, and a positive chronotropic effect on the sinoatrial node, in an isolated sinoatrial node and atrial model. These conflicting findings may be due to the different animal models used.

Studies of the myocardial antioxidant system

The influence of 5-FU treatment on the antioxidant system in myocardial tissue was studied by Durak et al. [18]. They found lowered activities of superoxide dismutase and glutathione peroxidase accompanied by higher catalase activity in 5-FU-treated female guinea pigs. The antioxidant potential, defined relative to malondialdehyde (MDA) levels, declined in 5-FU-treated animals compared with controls, while MDA levels increased [18]. A slight increase in intratissular MDA levels (not significant) and lower α-hydroxybutyrate dehydrogenase activity were demonstrated by Millart et al. [19].

The iron level was 20% higher in 5-FU-treated rat myocardial tissue compared with controls in one study [19], while another study of open-chest guinea pigs could not demonstrate increased iron levels in the myocardium after 5-FU infusion [18]. The two studies used comparable methods for iron content determination (flame atomic absorption spectrophotometry and atomic absorption spectroscopy), but they used different species and dosages. Magnesium, potassium, calcium and copper

Table 1 Positive, negative and conflicting findings from the included studies

Myocardium and hemodynamic function	
Positive	Hemorrhagic infarction, interstitial fibrosis and inflammatory reaction in the myocardium [15,16]
	Induction of apoptosis and increased oxidative stress [17]
	Impaired antioxidant defense system and lipid peroxidation [18,19]
	Depletion of high energy phosphate compounds and accumulation of citrate in the myocardium [12]
	Increased oxygen consumption [20]
	Positive chronotropic effect on the sinus node [21]
Conflicting or unclarified	Increased/no change in iron levels in the myocardium [18,19]
	Positive/negative inotropic effect on the heart [20,21]
	Increased/no change in myocardial blood flow [12,20]
Negative	No changes in magnesium, potassium, calcium or copper levels in the myocardium [18,19]
	No changes in blood pressure and heart rate [12]
Arteries	
Positive	Endothelial damage followed by platelet aggregation [9,22-24]
	Decreased DNA synthesis, decreased total cellular protein levels and increased prostacyclin release from endothelial cells [25]
	Vasoconstriction of arteries [26-28]
Rheological factors and RBCs	
Positive	Changes in erythrocyte structure, function and metabolism [29-32]
Negative	Decreased and not increased blood and plasma viscosity [33]
Substances in blood samples	
Positive	Rise in fibrinopeptide A activation and reduction in protein C activity compared with protein C antigen [10]
	Decrease in fibrinogen levels [33]
	Decrease in coagulation factors II + VII + X and increase in lactic acid, NT-proBNP, von Willebrand factor and fibrin D-dimer levels and urine albumin-to-creatinine-ratio [8,34]
	Increased plasma levels of endothelin-1 [35]
Conflicting or unclarified	A trend towards increased levels of big endothelin [28]
Negative	No change in angiotensin II levels [27]

levels in myocardial tissue were unaffected by 5-FU treatment in both studies [18,19].

Studies of vasoconstriction of arteries

5-FU-induced vasoconstriction has been demonstrated in three studies [26-28]. Two studies [27,28] showed that vasoconstriction of the brachial artery occurred in patients immediately after 5-FU infusion. The 5-FU-induced vasoconstriction was short-lived, reoccurred with repeated 5-FU injections and was abolished by glycerol nitrate [28]. In the study by Südhoff et al. [28] no patients had symptoms of cardiotoxicity, and in the study by Salepci et al. [27] three of 31 patients treated with 5-FU developed chest pain. ECG abnormalities were documented in five of 31 patients by Salepci et al. [27], while ECG recordings were not performed by Südhoff et al. [28].

Mosseri et al. [26] studied 5-FU-induced vasoconstriction in vitro using isolated aorta rings excised from rabbits. The prevalence of vasoconstriction correlated with the molar concentration of 5-FU and the magnitude was proportional to the concentration of 5-FU. The magnitude of vasoconstriction was similar for aorta rings, with functionally preserved endothelium and aorta rings with purposely disrupted endothelium indicating that an intact endothelium was not a prerequisite for 5-FU-induced vasoconstriction [26]. 5-FU-induced vasoconstriction was abolished by nitroglycerin, and acetylcholine-induced endothelium-dependent relaxation was unaffected by 5-FU-treatment [26], suggesting that 5-FU-induced vasoconstriction is not due to impairment of endothelial relaxation pathways. Pre-treatment with staurosporine, a protein kinase C (PK-C) inhibitor, reduced 5-FU-induced vasoconstriction, while pre-treatment with phorbol-12,13-dibutyrate, an activator of PK-C, increased the magnitude of 5-FU-induced vasoconstriction 23-fold [26]. In contrast, neomycin, an inhibitor of phosphoinositide turnover, and the cyclo-oxygenase inhibitor, indomethacin, did not alter the magnitude of 5-FU-induced vasoconstriction [26]. All of the membrane receptor blockers tested in the study [26], including the α-adrenergic receptor blocker phentolamine, the β-adrenergic receptor blocker propranolol, the H_1 receptor inhibitor diphenhydramine, the H_2 receptor inhibitor cimetidine and the Ca^{2+} channel blockers verapamil and diltiazem failed to alter the magnitude of 5-FU-induced vasoconstriction [26].

Studies on blood rheology and red blood cells

In vitro studies of red blood cells (RBCs) incubated in 5-FU showed a dose-dependent, reversible transformation of RBCs into echinocytic shape [29,30], which resulted in impaired transit through small pores [29]. Also, alterations in membrane fluidity and RBC metabolism were observed [30-32]: potassium efflux increased [30], oxygen tension ($pO2$) decreased [31,32], deoxyhemoglobin levels increased [32], intracellular ATP levels declined and the intracellular 2,3-bisphosphoglycerate (2,3-BPG) concentration rose [31,32]. Spasojevic et al. [32] measured ^{31}P-nuclear magnetic resonance (^{31}P-NMR) spectra of blood samples obtained from five patients treated with 5-FU and cisplatin, and found a downfield shift in ^{31}P-NMR spectra in vivo. However, the number of patients was too small for statistical analysis.

Baerlocher et al. [29] demonstrated a continuous decrease in blood viscosity with increasing 5-FU concentrations at low shear rates (the rate of change of velocity at which one layer of fluid passes over an adjacent layer) and increasing blood viscosity at high shear rates. 5-FU had no effect on plasma viscosity in this in vitro study [29]. In contrast, plasma viscosity and blood viscosity at both natural and standardized hematocrit decreased in blood samples from 11 patients receiving 5-FU and cisplatin [33]. These inconsistent findings may have resulted from differences in exposure to 5-FU between in vitro and human studies.

Studies of substances in blood samples from humans

Studies of the clotting-fibrinolytic system have shown increased levels of D-dimer [8] and fibrinopeptide A [10], decreased levels of fibrinogen [33] and coagulation factors II + VII + X [8], and decreased activity of the coagulation inhibitor, protein C, in blood [10]. Additionally, von Willebrand factor, which mediates the adherence and aggregation of platelets to the subendothelium, increased during 5-FU therapy [8]. However, none of the abnormalities reported in these studies was confined to patients experiencing cardiotoxicity [8,10,33]. Jensen et al. [8,34] reported that coagulation factors II + VII + X decreased during infusion, while levels of lactic acid, plasma N-terminal pro brain natriuretic peptide (NT-proBNP), von Willebrand factor, fibrin D-dimer, and the urine albumin-to-creatinine-ratio, increased. These changes were transient and only NT-proBNP levels were

higher in patients experiencing cardiotoxicity [34]. A trend towards increased levels of big endothelin, a precursor to endothelin-1, was demonstrated in one study, but a large inter-individual variation was found [28]. Thyss et al. [35] reported higher plasma levels of endothelin-1 in 5-FU-treated patients compared with cancer patients receiving non-5-FU-based chemotherapy. Also, patients experiencing cardiotoxicity during 5-FU treatment had higher endothelin-1 levels compared with patients without cardiotoxicity [35]. Angiotensin II levels remained unchanged during 5-FU treatment [27]. Thus, several substances in blood were affected by 5-FU treatment, but only NT-proBNP and endothelin-1 were associated with cardiotoxicity.

Discussion

The experimental studies and human studies included in this review showed that 5-FU induced a range of effects on the heart, on the vascular endothelium and at the cellular level of RBCs, myocardial and endothelial cells. However, to what extent these effects are involved in the pathogenesis of the clinical cardiotoxicity is more difficult to resolve. In the following, we discuss the findings and their possible role in the pathogenesis of 5-FU-induced clinical cardiotoxicity.

Histopathological changes

Animal studies showed that 5-FU induced pathological changes in the myocardium as well as on the endothelium, in arterial vessel walls. Although the endothelial studies did not involve the coronary arteries, there was evidence of systemic endothelial injury [24]. In the myocardium, the damages seemed to depend on the dose of 5-FU administered, as high doses led to more pronounced injuries [16].

It is not clear to what extent the histopathological features demonstrated in animal studies can be found in patients experiencing clinical signs of cardiotoxicity, as no biopsy studies have been performed in patients experiencing cardiotoxicity. Human myocardial biopsy samples are hard to obtain, and it is doubtful whether they will provide new and meaningful information as most cancer patients are exposed to several drugs. Therefore, the use of experimental models is necessary to obtain better insight into the mechanisms of 5-FU-cardiotoxicity. One approach is to use cellular models of isolated cardiac myocytes, which have been extensively used to study the cardiotoxic effects of anthracyclines [38-46]. Likewise, Lamberti et al. [17] used rat H9c2 cardiomyocytes to demonstrate that 5-FU toxicity in cardiomyocytes was largely due to induction of apoptosis, as opposed to cytotoxicity in colon cancer cells, which was more likely due to necrosis or autophagy. Whether this finding reflects a different mechanism of cardiotoxicity compared with the antineoplastic effect in tumor cells, or merely different cellular responses to the same stressor, is not clear.

5-FU induced endothelial injury and thrombus formation

Platelet aggregation and fibrin formation on sites of endothelial injury in scanning electron microscopy studies of rabbit vascular endothelium suggested that the pathophysiological mechanism of 5-FU-induced cardiotoxicity involved a thrombogenic effect of 5-FU, secondary to endothelial injury [9,22-24]. However, the absence of vascular occlusions in many patients undergoing coronary angiography for 5-FU-induced chest pain does not support thrombosis as a main mechanism [47-63]. On the other hand, a state of ongoing intravascular coagulation was evident from studies of the clotting-fibrinolytic system. A pro-coagulant state is common in cancer patients and is triggered by tumor-produced pro-coagulant factors and tumor-cell-derived cytokines [64]. Several studies have shown that fibrin and fibrinogen degradation products are elevated in patients with colorectal cancer [65-68]. Also, von Willebrand factor is increased in cancer patients and has been correlated to advanced tumor state [69-72]. In the study by Jensen et al. [8] 47 of 106 patients had baseline plasma levels of von Willebrand factor above the reference interval before 5-FU therapy, but 97 of 106 patients had von Willebrand factor levels above the reference interval during 5-FU therapy. Hence, it is likely that both the underlying cancer disease and exposure to 5-FU contribute to the observed alterations in plasma levels of substances involved in coagulation and fibrinolysis. However, it is unlikely that these alterations play an important role in the pathogenesis of 5-FU-induced cardiotoxicity, as they were not confined to patients experiencing cardiotoxicity.

The role of myocardial metabolism in 5-FU induced cardiotoxicity

Animal studies of myocardial metabolism demonstrated depletion of high energy phosphate compounds, citrate accumulation and increased oxygen consumption in the heart after pre-treatment with 5-FU [12,20,37]. Depletion in high energy phosphate compounds can result from increased oxygen consumption leading to insufficient oxygen supply, increased anaerobic metabolism, or to metabolic derangements produced by 5-FU. The stable and increased myocardial blood flow observed in two studies suggests that insufficient blood and oxygen supply is not a contributing factor. Instead, Suzuki et al. [73] reported that the respiratory control rate of myocardial mitochondria was significantly lower in rabbits treated with 5-FU compared with controls. Therefore, Millart et al. [20] proposed that the increase in anaerobic metabolism and the increase in oxygen uptake could be due to reduced aerobic efficiency resulting from mitochondrial uncoupling. Uncoupling of the mitochondrial respiratory chain results in increased basal oxygen consumption and decreased ATP-production. This theory should be further studied.

The theory of oxidative stress

The pathogenesis of 5-FU induced cardiotoxicity may involve oxidative stress, as increased levels of superoxide anion were demonstrated in H9c2 cells after 5-FU treatment [17]. Reactive oxygen species (ROS), like superoxide anions, are under normal physiological conditions cleared by antioxidant defense systems, such as sodium oxide dismutase (SOD) and glutathione peroxidase (GSH-Px). Superoxide anion is dismutated to hydrogen peroxide (H_2O_2) in a process catalyzed by SOD, and H_2O_2 is then eliminated by catalase or GSH-Px [74]. The activities of SOD and GSH-Px were lowered in 5-FU treated guinea pigs [18] demonstrating a reduced antioxidant capacity. If not eliminated by cellular antioxidant systems, superoxide anions can generate the highly reactive and toxic hydroxyl radicals (−OH) through the Haber–Weiss reaction, which is catalyzed by iron [74,75]. Increased ROS levels inside cells lead to oxidation of macromolecules, including lipids, nucleic acids, and proteins, thereby disturbing cellular functions [75]. MDA is a frequently used marker of lipid peroxidation [76], and MDA levels were elevated in guinea pig hearts after 5-FU-treatment [18], and slightly elevated (but not significantly) in isolated rat hearts after 5-FU-treatment [19]. These findings indicate that some degree of oxidative stress and cellular damage takes place in animal hearts during 5-FU-treatment. Likewise, Kinhult et al. [24] suggested that 5-FU-induced damage to the arterial endothelium may be due to generation of free radicals, resulting in lipid peroxidation. Their demonstration of a protective effect of probucol on arterial endothelium in rabbits treated with 5-FU supports this statement. Probucol increases SOD and GSH-Px activities in animals, thereby improving antioxidant potential [77-79].

The role of iron and other redox active metals in formation of ROS and promotion of myocardial oxidative stress during 5-FU treatment was investigated in two studies, with conflicting results [18,19]. Increased iron levels were demonstrated in the isolated perfused rat heart by Millart et al. [19], but no changes in iron levels were found in guinea pigs by Durak et al. [18]. Iron catalyzes the formation of hydroxyl radicals, promoting oxidative stress. If iron and oxidative stress plays a role in 5-FU-induced cardiotoxicity then iron-chelators could be a possible treatment option. Taken together, the role of oxidative stress in the pathogenesis of 5-FU cardiotoxicity is not well-established, and the source of ROS formation remains undefined. In vitro studies of free radical formation and animal studies investigating the role of iron-chelators may confirm or disprove this hypothesis.

The theory of vasospasm

The theory of vasospasm leading to myocardial ischemia has been proposed, because coronary angiography largely failed to show stenoses in patients with acute 5-FU-induced cardiotoxicity [47-63]. Moreover, coronary artery vasospasm has been visualized during coronary angiography in a few cases [80-82], and peripherally, vasoconstriction of the brachial artery appears immediately after 5-FU-injection [27,28]. It is anticipated that vasoconstriction measured peripherally after 5-FU-injection occurs in the coronary arteries as well. However, invasive methods such as cardiac catheterization and coronary angiography during infusion are necessary to prove vasospasm in the coronary arteries. While vasoconstriction is observed immediately after 5-FU injection, clinical cardiotoxicity often presents at the end of infusion, or hours to days later [2]. Moreover, cardiotoxicity may occur after several series of 5-FU or capecitabine. Hence, it remains to be elucidated in which circumstances 5-FU-induced vasoconstriction leads to clinical signs of cardiotoxicity.

In the search for the mechanism that leads to 5-FU-induced vasoconstriction, Mosseri et al. [26], exposed rabbit aorta rings to a range of substances that are involved in regulation of vascular tonus. The authors found preserved acetylcholine-induced relaxation of the vascular wall, and that glyceryl nitrate prevented 5-FU-induced vasoconstrictions [26]. Acetylcholine is an endothelium-dependent vasodilator that induces vasodilation through the NO-cGMP pathway [83]. Intact endothelial cells are a prerequisite for acetylcholine-induced vasodilation, and in the absence of endothelial cells acetylcholine leads to vasoconstriction [83]. As both acetylcholine-induced vascular relaxation and vascular relaxation by glyceryl nitrate were intact during 5-FU infusion, it seems unlikely that 5-FU causes functional vasoconstriction through impaired vasodilatory response. In contrast, Mosseri et al. [26] showed that PK-C might be a mediator of 5-FU-induced vasoconstriction. PK-C requires Ca^{2+} and phospholipid for its activation [84]. Diacylglycerol (DAG) considerably increases the affinity of PK-C for Ca^{2+}, and thereby fully activates PK-C without a net increase in the Ca^{2+} concentration [84]. DAG is formed from phosphatidylinositol-4,5-bisphosphate (PIP_2) cleavage, but neomycin, a competitive inhibitor of the phosphodiesterase that cleaves PIP_2, did not alter the 5-FU-induced vasoconstriction [26]. That denotes that PK-C might not be activated through cleavage of PIP_2 and DAG formation, but rather through an unknown mechanism, or directly from 5-FU. Furthermore, there was no evidence

for any modulation of 5-FU-induced vasoconstriction by membrane receptor blockers or activators of the cyclooxygenase pathway [26]. Noteworthy is that no effect of the Ca^{2+}-antagonists, verapamil and diltiazem, which are often used to treat vasospasm, were seen [26].

The high plasma levels of endothelin-1 observed by Thyss et al. [35] in 5-FU treated patients, and especially in patients experiencing 5-FU-induced cardiotoxicity, may support the hypothesis of 5-FU-induced vasoconstriction. Endothelin-1 is a potent vasoconstrictor produced by endothelial cells, cardiomyocytes and cardiac fibroblasts, but it is also produced in several noncardiac tissues such as the lungs [85,86]. Endothelin-1 is known to have a regulatory role in coronary vascular resistance and myocardial capillary blood flow in coronary artery diseases [86-88]. Hypoxia, ischemia or shear stress are stimuli that induce the synthesis and secretion of endothelin-1 in vascular endothelial cells [85]. Endothelin-1 is synthesized from the precursor peptide big endothelin [85]. A trend towards increased big endothelin levels in the plasma of 5-FU treated patients was found by Salepci et al. [27], but this trend was not confined to patients who developed vasoconstrictions. As endothelin-1 and some big endothelin-1 are secreted mainly towards the adjacent smooth-muscle layer of blood vessel wall, only smaller amounts of the peptides reach the lumen of the vessel and contribute to the plasma levels [85]. Hence, it is possible that the raised endothelin-1 in plasma may come from cellular sources other than the endothelial cells. To further elucidate the role of endothelins in 5-FU-induced cardiotoxicity, the cellular source of endothelin-1 and the contribution of endothelin-1 to vasomotor tone during 5-FU infusion should be studied.

5-FU-induced changes in rheological factors and cardiotoxicity

Reversible transformation of RBCs into echinocytic shapes, increased membrane fluidity of RBCs and altered metabolism in terms of a rapid depletion of pO_2, production of 2,3-BPG and decreased ATP levels [30-32] diminish the ability of RBCs to transfer oxygen to the heart. However, cisplatin induced almost similar changes in RBC morphology and membrane fluidity [32]. As cisplatin does not cause myocardial ischemia, which is the primary manifestation of 5-FU-induced cardiotoxicity, this finding might indicate that changes in RBC shape and membrane fluidity are not the principal cause of 5-FU-induced ischemia [32]. In contrast, significant depletion of pO_2, increase in deoxy-hemoglobin levels, increase in 2,3-BPG levels and decrease in ATP levels were only observed for erythrocytes treated with 5-FU alone and erythrocytes treated with the combination of 5-FU and cisplatin. Hence, altered RBC metabolism might be a cause of 5-FU-induced ischemia. However, it is unknown whether the changes in RBC metabolism and morphology observed in vitro also occur in vivo. Also, the link between these changes and clinical signs of cardiotoxicity in patients is not proven. It is unlikely that changes in blood viscosity are a part of the pathogenesis of 5-FU induced cardiotoxicity, as studies on blood viscosity reported conflicting results [29,33].

Other proposed mechanisms for 5-FU-induced cardiotoxicity

Few other mechanisms for 5-FU-induced cardiotoxicity have been proposed. Lemaire et al. [11] proposed that 5-FU cardiotoxicity was due to degradation products formed in the basic medium in which 5-FU is dissolved. The compound thought to be responsible for the cardiotoxicity is fluoroacetate, which is formed through alkaline hydrolysis of 5-FU and by catabolism of 5-FU in the liver [89]. However, the consistent nature of 5-FU and capecitabine-induced cardiotoxicity, regardless of the solutions or formulations used, makes it unlikely that 5-FU cardiotoxicity is due to degradation products formed in the solution of 5-FU in a basic medium. Thus, if fluoroacetate plays a role in 5-FU-induced cardiotoxicity it is likely because of metabolism of 5-FU to fluoroacetate in the liver.

Toxic myocarditis has been proposed by Sasson et al. [90], as they found biventricular dilation and diffusely scattered areas of cell necrosis associated with an inflammatory infiltrate, on autopsy of a case of 5-FU-induced fatal cardiogenic shock.

Limitations

First, the selection of studies concerning the pathophysiology of 5-FU cardiotoxicity could not be based on objective criteria, but instead relied on the author's judgments of which studies were concerned with the pathophysiology of 5-FU-induced cardiotoxicity. Still, we made a broad inclusion of studies that investigated the effects of 5-FU on any part of the cardiovascular system. Therefore, we believe that this review makes up a comprehensive and systematic synthesis of the results from the pathophysiological studies of 5-FU cardiotoxicity. However, as our literature search was restricted to English, a few studies may have been missed.

Second, most experimental studies included few animals and were only carried out once. Hence the statistical powers in these studies were low and the findings rarely confirmed in other studies, which makes those findings less consistent.

Third, extrapolation of results from in vitro and ex vivo studies to in vivo settings should be done with precaution, as isolated cells in vitro and isolated organs may not behave the same as in in vivo settings. There are also

important differences between species, and more importantly, between animals and humans.

Fourth, some in vivo animal experiments used repeated administrations of 5-FU, but numerous studies have used regimens in which animals were treated with only a single and/or a very high 5-FU dose. In clinical practice, 5-FU is often administered according to the De Gramont schedule where a short bolus infusion is given followed by a 48-hour continuous infusion. Hence, differences in administration schedules and doses may also limit the extrapolation of the results from these studies to clinical settings.

Fifth, most of the findings in the human studies were not confined to patients experiencing cardiotoxicity, as only NT-proBNP and endothelin-1 were higher in patients with cardiotoxicity. Hence, for nearly all findings, their role in the pathogenesis of cardiotoxicity is still unclear.

Finally, some types of studies that can be conducted in animals are difficult to carry out in human patients. For example, biopsy samples are hard to obtain and carry a risk of bleeding and myocardial wall perforation for the patient. Such risks may outweigh the expected benefit for the patient, and therefore make such procedures unreasonable to perform.

Conclusions

This review indicates that there is no evidence for a single mechanism responsible for 5-FU-induced cardiotoxicity, and the underlying mechanisms might be multifactorial. The proposed cardiotoxic pathways leading to myocardial and endothelial damage are not mutually exclusive, and they may each contribute to cardiovascular dysfunction resulting in the clinical picture of cardiotoxicity. Further research is needed to elucidate the pathogenesis of this side effect. Studies on cardiac and endothelial cell lines might contribute to further elucidation of the cellular response to 5-FU. A human study with continuous ECG monitoring concurrent with measurements of the brachial artery diameters could be interesting, to explore the theory of arterial vasospasm leading to myocardial ischemia. Other methods to further study the pathogenesis of 5-FU-induced cardiotoxicity could be studies of myocardial perfusion with magnetic resonance scanning or PET rubidium scanning of the heart in patients presenting with signs of cardiotoxicity.

Additional files

Additional file 1: PRISMA Checklist. The PRISMA Checklist for this systematic review.

Additional file 2: Characteristics and results of the included studies. This table shows the characteristics of the studies included in the review.

Competing interests

The authors declare that they have no competing interests.

Authors' contributions

AP participated in the design of the review, the literature search, the study selection process and the data synthesis, and drafted the manuscript. KV and MVN participated in the design of the review. DN participated in the design of the review, the literature search, the study selection process and helped with the data synthesis. All authors read and approved the final version of the manuscript.

References

1. Malet-Martino M, Jolimaitre P, Martino R: **The prodrugs of 5-fluorouracil.** *Curr Med Chem Anticancer Agents* 2002, **2:**267–310.
2. Polk A, Vaage-Nilsen M, Vistisen K, Nielsen DL: **Cardiotoxicity in cancer patients treated with 5-fluorouracil or capecitabine: A systematic review of incidence, manifestations and predisposing factors.** *Cancer Treat Rev* 2013, **39:**974–84.
3. Kosmas C, Kallistratos MS, Kopterides P, Syrios J, Skopelitis H, Mylonakis N, Karabelis A, Tsavaris N: **Cardiotoxicity of fluoropyrimidines in different schedules of administration: a prospective study.** *J Cancer Res Clin Oncol* 2008, **134:**75–82.
4. Meydan N, Kundak I, Yavuzsen T, Oztop I, Barutca S, Yilmaz U, Alakavuklar MN: **Cardiotoxicity of de Gramont's regimen: incidence, clinical characteristics and long-term follow-up.** *Jpn J Clin Oncol* 2005, **35:**265–270.
5. Meyer CC, Calis KA, Burke LB, Walawander CA, Grasela TH: **Symptomatic cardiotoxicity associated with 5-fluorouracil.** *Pharmacotherapy* 1997, **17:**729–736.
6. Ng M, Cunningham D, Norman AR: **The frequency and pattern of cardiotoxicity observed with capecitabine used in conjunction with oxaliplatin in patients treated for advanced colorectal cancer (CRC).** *Eur J Cancer* 2005, **41:**1542–1546.
7. Rezkalla S, Kloner RA, Ensley J, al-Sarraf M, Revels S, Olivenstein A, Bhasin S, Kerpel-Fronious S, Turi ZG: **Continuous ambulatory ECG monitoring during fluorouracil therapy: a prospective study.** *J Clin Oncol* 1989, **7:**509–514.
8. Jensen SA, Sorensen JB: **5-fluorouracil-based therapy induces endovascular injury having potential significance to development of clinically overt cardiotoxicity.** *Cancer Chemother Pharmacol* 2012, **69:**57–64.
9. Kinhult S, Albertsson M, Eskilsson J, Cwikiel M: **Antithrombotic treatment in protection against thrombogenic effects of 5-fluorouracil on vascular endothelium: a scanning microscopy evaluation.** *Scanning* 2001, **23:**1–8.
10. Kuzel T, Esparaz B, Green D, Kies M: **Thrombogenicity of intravenous 5-fluorouracil alone or in combination with cisplatin.** *Cancer* 1990, **65:**885–889.
11. Lemaire L, Malet-Martino MC, De ⊠ FM, Martino R, Lasserre B: **Cardiotoxicity of commercial 5-fluorouracil vials stems from the alkaline hydrolysis of this drug.** *Br J Cancer* 1992, **66:**119–127.
12. Matsubara I, Kamiya J, Imai S: **Cardiotoxic effects of 5-fluorouracil in the guinea pig.** *Jpn J Pharmacol* 1980, **30:**871–879.
13. Tsavaris N, Kosmas C, Vadiaka M, Efremidis M, Zinelis A, Beldecos D, Sakelariou G, Koufos C, Stamatelos G: **Cardiotoxicity following different doses and schedules of 5-fluorouracil administration for malignancy – a survey of 427 patients.** *Med Sci Monit* 2002, **8:**I51–I57.
14. Moher D, Liberati A, Tetzlaff J, Altman DG: **Preferred reporting items for systematic reviews and meta-analyses: the PRISMA statement.** *PLoS Med* 2009, **6:**e1000097.
15. Kumar S, Gupta RK, Samal N: **5-fluorouracil induced cardiotoxicity in albino rats.** *Mater Med Pol* 1995, **27:**63–66.
16. Tsibiribi P, Bui-Xuan C, Bui-Xuan B, Lombard-Bohas C, Duperret S, Belkhiria M, Tabib A, Maujean G, Descotes J, Timour Q: **Cardiac lesions induced by 5-fluorouracil in the rabbit.** *Hum Exp Toxicol* 2006, **25:**305–309.
17. Lamberti M, Porto S, Marra M, Zappavigna S, Grimaldi A, Feola D, Pesce D, Naviglio S, Spina A, Sannolo N, Caraglia M: **5-Fluorouracil induces apoptosis in rat cardiocytes through intracellular oxidative stress.** *J Exp Clin Cancer Res* 2012, **31:**60.
18. Durak I, Karaayvaz M, Kavutcu M, Cimen MY, Kacmaz M, Buyukkocak S, Ozturk HS: **Reduced antioxidant defense capacity in myocardial tissue from guinea pigs treated with 5-fluorouracil.** *J Toxicol Environ Health A* 2000, **59:**585–589.
19. Millart H, Kantelip JP, Platonoff N, Descous I, Trenque T, Lamiable D, Choisy H: **Increased iron content in rat myocardium after 5-fluorouracil chronic administration.** *Anticancer Res* 1993, **13:**779–783.
20. Millart H, Brabant L, Lorenzato M, Lamiable D, Albert O, Choisy H: **The effects of 5-fluorouracil on contractility and oxygen uptake of the isolated perfused rat heart.** *Anticancer Res* 1992, **12:**571–576.
21. Satoh H, Hashimoto K: **Effects of ftorafur and 5-fluorouracil on the canine sinoatrial node.** *Jpn J Pharmacol* 1983, **33:**357–362.
22. Cwikiel M, Zhang B, Eskilsson J, Wieslander JB, Albertsson M: **The influence of 5-fluorouracil on the endothelium in small arteries. An electron microscopic study in rabbits.** *Scanning Microsc* 1995, **9:**561–576.
23. Cwikiel M, Eskilsson J, Wieslander JB, Stjernquist U, Albertsson M: **The appearance of endothelium in small arteries after treatment with 5-fluorouracil. An electron microscopic study of late effects in rabbits.** *Scanning Microsc* 1996, **10:**805–818.
24. Kinhult S, Albertsson M, Eskilsson J, Cwikiel M: **Effects of probucol on endothelial damage by 5-fluorouracil.** *Acta Oncol* 2003, **42:**304–308.
25. Cwikiel M, Eskilsson J, Albertsson M, Stavenow L: **The influence of 5-fluorouracil and methotrexate on vascular endothelium. An experimental study using endothelial cells in the culture.** *Ann Oncol* 1996, **7:**731–737.
26. Mosseri M, Fingert HJ, Varticovski L, Chokshi S, Isner JM: **In vitro evidence that myocardial ischemia resulting from 5-fluorouracil chemotherapy is due to protein kinase C-mediated vasoconstriction of vascular smooth muscle.** *Cancer Res* 1993, **53:**3028–3033.
27. Salepci T, Seker M, Uyarel H, Gumus M, Bilici A, Ustaalioglu BB, Ozturk A, Sonmez B, Orcun A, Ozates M, Irmak R, Yaylaci M: **5-Fluorouracil induces arterial vasoconstrictions but does not increase angiotensin II levels.** *Med Oncol* 2010, **27:**416–420.
28. Sudhoff T, Enderle MD, Pahlke M, Petz C, Teschendorf C, Graeven U, Schmiegel W: **5-Fluorouracil induces arterial vasocontractions.** *Ann Oncol* 2004, **15:**661–664.
29. Baerlocher GM, Beer JH, Owen GR, Meiselman HJ, Reinhart WH: **The antineoplastic drug 5-fluorouracil produces echinocytosis and affects blood rheology.** *Br J Haematol* 1997, **99:**426–432.
30. Spasojevic I, Maksimovic V, Zakrzewska J, Bacic G: **Effects of 5-fluorouracil on erythrocytes in relation to its cardiotoxicity: membrane structure and functioning.** *J Chem Inf Model* 2005, **45:**1680–1685.
31. Spasojevic I, Zakrzewska J, Bacic GG: **31P NMR spectroscopy and polarographic combined study of erythrocytes treated with 5-fluorouracil: cardiotoxicity-related changes in ATP, 2,3-BPG, and O2 metabolism.** *Ann N Y Acad Sci* 2005, **1048:**311–320.
32. Spasojevic I, Jelic S, Zakrzewska J, Bacic G: **Decreased oxygen transfer capacity of erythrocytes as a cause of 5-fluorouracil related ischemia.** *Molecules* 2009, **14:**53–67.
33. Cwikiel M, Persson SU, Larsson H, Albertsson M, Eskilsson J: **Changes of blood viscosity in patients treated with 5-fluorouracil–a link to cardiotoxicity?** *Acta Oncol* 1995, **34:**83–85.
34. Jensen SA, Hasbak P, Mortensen J, Sorensen JB: **Fluorouracil induces myocardial ischemia with increases of plasma brain natriuretic peptide and lactic acid but without dysfunction of left ventricle.** *J Clin Oncol* 2010, **28:**5280–5286.
35. Thyss A, Gaspard MH, Marsault R, Milano G, Frelin C, Schneider M: **Very high endothelin plasma levels in patients with 5-FU cardiotoxicity.** *Ann Oncol* 1992, **3:**88.
36. Wenzel DG, Cosma GN: **A model system for measuring comparative toxicities of cardiotoxic drugs for cultured rat heart myocytes, endothelial cells and fibroblasts. II. Doxorubicin, 5-fluorouracil and cyclophosphamide.** *Toxicology* 1984, **33:**117–128.
37. Tamatsu H, Nakazawa M, Imai S, Watari H: **31P-topical nuclear magnetic resonance (31P-TMR) studies of cardiotoxic effects of 5-fluorouracil (5-FU) and 5'-deoxy-5-fluorouridine (5'-DFUR).** *Jpn J Pharmacol* 1984, **34:**375–379.
38. Barnabe N, Zastre JA, Venkataram S, Hasinoff BB: **Deferiprone protects against doxorubicin-induced myocyte cytotoxicity.** *Free Radic Biol Med* 2002, **33:**266–275.
39. Hasinoff BB, Patel D, Wu X: **The oral iron chelator ICL670A (deferasirox) does not protect myocytes against doxorubicin.** *Free Radic Biol Med* 2003, **35:**1469–1479.

40. Hershko C, Link G, Tzahor M, Pinson A: **The role of iron and iron chelators in anthracycline cardiotoxicity.** *Leuk Lymphoma* 1993, **11**:207–214.

41. Kang YJ, Zhou ZX, Wang GW, Buridi A, Klein JB: **Suppression by metallothionein of doxorubicin-induced cardiomyocyte apoptosis through inhibition of p38 mitogen-activated protein kinases.** *J Biol Chem* 2000, **275**:13690–13698.

42. Kim DS, Kim HR, Woo ER, Hong ST, Chae HJ, Chae SW: **Inhibitory effects of rosmarinic acid on adriamycin-induced apoptosis in H9c2 cardiac muscle cells by inhibiting reactive oxygen species and the activations of c-Jun N-terminal kinase and extracellular signal-regulated kinase.** *Biochem Pharmacol* 2005, **70**:1066–1078.

43. Kwok JC, Richardson DR: **Unexpected anthracycline-mediated alterations in iron-regulatory protein-RNA-binding activity: the iron and copper complexes of anthracyclines decrease RNA-binding activity.** *Mol Pharmacol* 2002, **62**:888–900.

44. Minotti G, Ronchi R, Salvatorelli E, Menna P, Cairo G: **Doxorubicin irreversibly inactivates iron regulatory proteins 1 and 2 in cardiomyocytes: evidence for distinct metabolic pathways and implications for iron-mediated cardiotoxicity of antitumor therapy.** *Cancer Res* 2001, **61**:8422–8428.

45. L'Ecuyer T, Horenstein MS, Thomas R, Vander HR: **Anthracycline-induced cardiac injury using a cardiac cell line: potential for gene therapy studies.** *Mol Genet Metab* 2001, **74**:370–379.

46. Sawyer DB, Fukazawa R, Arstall MA, Kelly RA: **Daunorubicin-induced apoptosis in rat cardiac myocytes is inhibited by dexrazoxane.** *Circ Res* 1999, **84**:257–265.

47. Ozturk MA, Ozveren O, Cinar V, Erdik B, Oyan B: **Takotsubo syndrome: an underdiagnosed complication of 5-fluorouracil mimicking acute myocardial infarction.** *Blood Coagul Fibrinolysis* 2013, **24**:90–94.

48. Kim SM, Kwak CH, Lee B, Kim SB, Sir JJ, Cho WH, Choi SK: **A case of severe coronary spasm associated with 5-fluorouracil chemotherapy.** *Korean J Intern Med* 2012, **27**:342–345.

49. Tsiamis E, Synetos A, Stefanadis C: **Capecitabine may induce coronary artery vasospasm.** *Hellenic J Cardiol* 2012, **53**:320–323.

50. Shah NR, Shah A, Rather A: **Ventricular fibrillation as a likely consequence of capecitabine-induced coronary vasospasm.** *J Oncol Pharm Pract* 2012, **18**:132–135.

51. Basselin C, Fontanges T, Descotes J, Chevalier P, Bui-Xuan B, Feinard G, Timour Q: **5-Fluorouracil-induced Tako-Tsubo-like syndrome.** *Pharmacotherapy* 2011, **31**:226.

52. Calik AN, Celiker E, Velibey Y, Cagdas M, Guzelburc O: **Initial dose effect of 5-fluorouracil: rapidly improving severe, acute toxic myopericarditis.** *Am J Emerg Med* 2012, **30**:257–3.

53. Atar A, Korkmaz ME, Ozin B: **Two cases of coronary vasospasm induced by 5-fluorouracil.** *Anadolu Kardiyol Derg* 2010, **10**:461–462.

54. Tajik R, Saadat H, Taherkhani M, Movahed MR: **Angina induced by 5-fluorouracil infusion in a patient with normal coronaries.** *Am Heart Hosp J* 2010, **8**:E111–E112.

55. Camaro C, Danse PW, Bosker HA: **Acute chest pain in a patient treated with capecitabine.** *Neth Heart J* 2009, **17**:288–291.

56. Gianni M, Dentali F, Lonn E: **5 flourouracil-induced apical ballooning syndrome: a case report.** *Blood Coagul Fibrinolysis* 2009, **20**:306–308.

57. Yung LT, McCrea WA: **Capecitabine induced acute coronary syndrome.** *BMJ Case Rep* 2009, **2009**.

58. Scott PA, Ferchow L, Hobson A, Curzen NP: **Coronary spasm induced by capecitabine mimicks ST elevation myocardial infarction.** *Emerg Med J* 2008, **25**:699–700.

59. Canale ML, Camerini A, Stroppa S, Porta RP, Caravelli P, Mariani M, Balbarini A, Ricci S: **A case of acute myocardial infarction during 5-fluorouracil infusion.** *J Cardiovasc Med (Hagerstown)* 2006, **7**:835–837.

60. Cardinale D, Colombo A, Colombo N: **Acute coronary syndrome induced by oral capecitabine.** *Can J Cardiol* 2006, **22**:251–253.

61. Mafrici A, Alberti A, Corrada E, Ferrari S, Marenna B: **Management of patients with persistent chest pain and ST-segment elevation during 5-fluorouracil treatment: report about two cases.** *Ital Heart J* 2003, **4**:895–899.

62. McGlinchey PG, Webb ST, Campbell NP: **5-fluorouracil-induced cardiotoxicity mimicking myocardial infarction: a case report.** *BMC Cardiovasc Disord* 2001, **1**:3.

63. Schnetzler B, Popova N, Collao LC, Sappino AP: **Coronary spasm induced by capecitabine.** *Ann Oncol* 2001, **12**:723–724.

64. Prandoni P, Falanga A, Piccioli A: **Cancer and venous thromboembolism.** *Lancet Oncol* 2005, **6**:401–410.

65. Okholm M, Iversen LH, Thorlacius-Ussing O, Ejlersen E, Boesby S: **Fibrin and fibrinogen degradation products in plasma of patients with colorectal adenocarcinoma.** *Dis Colon Rectum* 1996, **39**:1102–1106.

66. Oya M, Akiyama Y, Okuyama T, Ishikawa H: **High preoperative plasma D-dimer level is associated with advanced tumor stage and short survival after curative resection in patients with colorectal cancer.** *Jpn J Clin Oncol* 2001, **31**:388–394.

67. Blackwell K, Hurwitz H, Lieberman G, Novotny W, Snyder S, Dewhirst M, Greenberg C: **Circulating D-dimer levels are better predictors of overall survival and disease progression than carcinoembryonic antigen levels in patients with metastatic colorectal carcinoma.** *Cancer* 2004, **101**:77–82.

68. Iversen LH, Okholm M, Thorlacius-Ussing O: **Pre- and postoperative state of coagulation and fibrinolysis in plasma of patients with benign and malignant colorectal disease–a preliminary study.** *Thromb Haemost* 1996, **76**:523–528.

69. Damin DC, Rosito MA, Gus P, Roisemberg I, Bandinelli E, Schwartsmann G: **Von Willebrand factor in colorectal cancer.** *Int J Colorectal Dis* 2002, **17**:42–45.

70. Rohsig LM, Damin DC, Stefani SD, Castro CG Jr, Roisenberg I, Schwartsmann G: **von Willebrand factor antigen levels in plasma of patients with malignant breast disease.** *Braz J Med Biol Res* 2001, **34**:1125–1129.

71. Gil-Bazo I, Catalan G,V, Alonso GA, Rodriguez RJ, Paramo Fernandez JA, de la Camara GJ, Hernandez Lizoain JL, Garcia-Foncillas LJ: **Impact of surgery and chemotherapy on von Willebrand factor and vascular endothelial growth factor levels in colorectal cancer.** *Clin Transl Oncol* 2005, **7**:150–155.

72. Wang WS, Lin JK, Lin TC, Chiou TJ, Liu JH, Yen CC, Chen PM: **Plasma von Willebrand factor level as a prognostic indicator of patients with metastatic colorectal carcinoma.** *World J Gastroenterol* 2005, **11**:2166–2170.

73. Suzuki T, Nakanishi H, Hayashi A: **Cardiac toxicity of 5-fluorouracil in rabbits.** *Jpn J Pharmacol* 1977, **27 s**:137. Ref Type: Abstract.

74. Sterba M, Popelova O, Vavrova A, Jirkovsky E, Kovarikova P, Gersl V, Simunek T: **Oxidative stress, redox signaling, and metal chelation in anthracycline cardiotoxicity and pharmacological cardioprotection.** *Antioxid Redox Signal* 2013, **18**:899–929.

75. Kehrer JP: **The Haber-Weiss reaction and mechanisms of toxicity.** *Toxicology* 2000, **149**:43–50.

76. Nielsen F, Mikkelsen BB, Nielsen JB, Andersen HR, Grandjean P: **Plasma malondialdehyde as biomarker for oxidative stress: reference interval and effects of life-style factors.** *Clin Chem* 1997, **43**:1209–1214.

77. Li T, Danelisen I, Bello-Klein A, Singal PK: **Effects of probucol on changes of antioxidant enzymes in adriamycin-induced cardiomyopathy in rats.** *Cardiovasc Res* 2000, **46**:523–530.

78. Siveski-Iliskovic N, Kaul N, Singal PK: **Probucol promotes endogenous antioxidants and provides protection against adriamycin-induced cardiomyopathy in rats.** *Circulation* 1994, **89**:2829–2835.

79. Kaul N, Siveski-Iliskovic N, Thomas TP, Hill M, Khaper N, Singal PK: **Probucol improves antioxidant activity and modulates development of diabetic cardiomyopathy.** *Nutrition* 1995, **11**:551–554.

80. Alter P, Herzum M, Soufi M, Schaefer JR, Maisch B: **Cardiotoxicity of 5-fluorouracil.** *Cardiovasc Hematol Agents Med Chem* 2006, **4**:1–5.

81. Shoemaker LK, Arora U, Rocha Lima CM: **5-fluorouracil-induced coronary vasospasm.** *Cancer Control* 2004, **11**:46–49.

82. Luwaert RJ, Descamps O, Majois F, Chaudron JM, Beauduin M: **Coronary artery spasm induced by 5-fluorouracil.** *Eur Heart J* 1991, **12**:468–470.

83. Schwartz BG, Economides C, Mayeda GS, Burstein S, Kloner RA: **The endothelial cell in health and disease: its function, dysfunction, measurement and therapy.** *Int J Impot Res* 2010, **22**:77–90.

84. Nishizuka Y: **Studies and perspectives of protein kinase C.** *Science* 1986, **233**:305–312.

85. Levin ER: **Endothelins.** *N Engl J Med* 1995, **333**:356–363.

86. Khimji AK, Rockey DC: **Endothelin–biology and disease.** *Cell Signal* 2010, **22**:1615–1625.

87. MacCarthy PA, Pegge NC, Prendergast BD, Shah AM, Groves PH: **The physiological role of endogenous endothelin in the regulation of human coronary vasomotor tone.** *J Am Coll Cardiol* 2001, **37**:137–143.

88. Kinlay S, Behrendt D, Wainstein M, Beltrame J, Fang JC, Creager MA, Selwyn AP, Ganz P: **Role of endothelin-1 in the active constriction of human atherosclerotic coronary arteries.** *Circulation* 2001, **104**:1114–1118.

89. Arellano M, Malet-Martino M, Martino R, Gires P: **The anti-cancer drug
     5-fluorouracil is metabolized by the isolated perfused rat liver and in rats
     into highly toxic fluoroacetate.** *Br J Cancer* 1998, **77**:79–86.
90. Sasson Z, Morgan CD, Wang B, Thomas G, MacKenzie B, Platts ME:
     **5-Fluorouracil related toxic myocarditis: case reports and pathological
     confirmation.** *Can J Cardiol* 1994, **10**:861–864.

11

Retrospective evaluation of cotrimoxazole use as preventive therapy in people living with HIV/AIDS in Boru Meda Hospital

Berhanu Geresu[1*], Desye Misganaw[1] and Yeshiwork Beyene[2]

Abstract

Background: Drug use evaluation is a performance improvement method that focuses on evaluating and improving drug use process to achieve optimal patient outcomes. Drug use evaluation helps in identifying, preventing or resolving actual and potential drug related problems. The objective of the study was to evaluate the use of cotrimoxazole as preventive therapy in people living with HIV/AIDS in Boru Meda Hospital, Northeast Ethiopia.

Methods: A retrospective drug use evaluation was conducted on patients' medical history records based on a validated drug use evaluation criteria according to the national guideline. Medical history records of 248 patients were selected using systematic sampling method.

Results: The result showed that 49.6% of the patients were at WHO clinical stage III at the start of cotrimoxazole preventive therapy. In this study, the use of cotrimoxazole preventive therapy was consistent with the guideline in the rationale for indication (97.98%), dose (96.77%), and its use despite the presence of contraindications (91.93%). Problems regarding drug-drug interaction were identified in 49.59% of cases, and 20.97% of patients discontinued cotrimoxazole preventive therapy due to different reasons.

Conclusions: In most patients cotrimoxazole preventive therapy was consistent with the national guideline regarding the rationale for indication, dose, discontinuation and its use in the presence of contraindications.

Keywords: Drug use evaluation, Cotrimoxazole, Preventive therapy, HIV/AIDS, Boru Meda

Background

Rational drug use is concerned with promoting quality of care and cost- effective therapy, preventing unnecessary exposure to side effects, maximizing therapeutic benefits, and improving patient compliance [1]. Drug use evaluation (DUE) is one of the methods used in combating the development of bacterial resistant to anti-microbial agents and improving therapy [2].

Cotrimoxazole (CTX), a fixed dose combination of sulfamethoxazole and trimethoprim, is a broad spectrum antimicrobial agent that targets a range of aerobic gram positive and gram negative organisms, fungi and protozoa [3,4]. CTX is preferable for both primary and secondary prophylaxis of pneumocystis jirvoeic pneumonia (PCP) in adults and adolescents [5,6]. The World Health Organization (WHO) and the Joint United Nations Programme on HIV/AIDS (UNAIDS) have recently recommended the use of co-trimoxazole prophylaxis for HIV-infected adults in Africa with symptomatic HIV disease (stage II, III or IV of the WHO classification of HIV infection and disease) and for asymptomatic individuals who have a CD4 T-lymphocyte count of $\leq 500 \times 10^6/l$ or total lymphocyte count (TLC) equivalent [7].

The recommended dose for adult and Adolescents is two single strength tablets of CTX (tablets of 80 mg Trimethoprim and 400 mg Sulphamethoxazole) or one double strength tablet (1 tablet of 160 mg Trimethoprim and 800 mg sulfamethoxazole) daily or three times per week. In addition, children in the age range

* Correspondence: berhanu.grs@gmail.com
[1]Department of Pharmacy, College of Medicine and Health Sciences, Wollo University, Dessie, Ethiopia
Full list of author information is available at the end of the article

6 months-5 years or (5-15 kg) take (200 mg/40 mg) CTX, 6 years-14 years or (15-30 kg) take (400 mg/80 mg) CTX and >14 years or >30 kg take (800/60 mg) CTX. Adverse conditions that lead to discontinuation of CTX are itching (with mucocutaneous lesion and or fever), significant rash, fever, Steven Johnson syndrome and sever anemia [4].

CTX preventive therapy (CPT) is a simple well tolerated and cost effective intervention which can extend and improve the quality of life for people living with HIV/AIDS (PLWHA) including those on antiretroviral therapy (ART). CPT is associated with a 25-46% reduction in mortality among individuals infected with HIV in sub-Saharan Africa even in areas of high bacterial resistance to the antibiotic [7,8].

Despite the proven clinical benefits of CTX and recommendation by WHO, its routine use in developing countries particularly in sub-Saharan Africa has remain limited [8]. CPT is effective at preventing a number of opportunistic infections (OIs) among HIV positive individuals initiating ART. Although the drug is cheap and widely available, many countries failed to implement policies to provide nation wide coverage of the drug [9]. Use of judiciously selected drugs with a valid set of guidelines will bring success not only to health care system of the country but also to the whole socio-economic development [6].

Antibiotics represent approximately 30% of the acute hospital care expenditure and they are prescribed for 20-50% of patients. The development of drug resistant organisms may emerge as a result of many factors including irrational use of drugs [2]. The inevitable consequences of the emergence of antimicrobial resistant pathogens fuels an ever increasing need for new drugs and contribute to the rising cost of medical care [10].

Retrospective DUE addresses issues of indications, contra indications, drug interactions, dosage, therapeutic duplications and patient monitoring patterns. In addition it provides information that opens ways to provide feedback for prescribers on their performance in implementing treatment protocols and their compliance with preset approved guidelines for the use of each medication. In dealing with the fight against health problems like HIV/AIDS, that have deep rooted socio-economic impact, it is quite useful to evaluate the effectiveness of programs for better outcomes. Thus DUE should be incorporated as one of such monitoring systems in the health care system of the country in response to the issue of AIDS epidemic and OPIs [11]. Therefore, the aim of this study was to evaluate the use of cotrimoxazole as preventive therapy in PLWHA Boru Meda Hospital.

Methods

A retrospective drug use evaluation was conducted on patients' medical history records in Boru Meda Hospital

(BMH), Northeast Ethiopia from May 22-30/2012. The hospital is a rural hospital located 4 kilo meters away from Dessie town and comprised of 6 general practitioners, 40 nurses, 16 pharmacy technicians and 4 X-ray technicians with a total beds of 80. A total of 701 patients were receiving CPT before February 2012. Medical history records of 248 patients out 701 were selected using systematic sampling method from sequentially arranged medical records.

The independent variables were age, sex, patients' clinical condition and laboratory results. Whereas the dependent variables include indication, contraindication, drug-drug interaction, dosage and discontinuation of CPT.

Data collection format containing the variables to be measured was developed and used to collect data. The collected data were filtered, categorized and the results were analyzed using SPSS version 15, interpreted and presented using tables and charts.

Ethical clearance was obtained from College of Medicine and Health Sciences, Wollo University Institutional Review Committee (IRC), and permission was sought from BMH.

Results

Out of 248, 123 (49.60%) patients were at WHO clinical stage III HIV infection at the start of CPT. Even though co morbid illnesses were not documented for most (67%) of the patients, the prevalence of tuberculosis (TB) and fungal infections were 11.69% and 12.50%, respectively. Majority of the patients 221 (89.11%) were found to have CD4 count of less than 350cell/mm^3 (Table 1).

The result also showed that 243 (97.98%) patients were in line with the national CPT guideline regarding to

Table 1 Baseline characteristics of PLWHA at the start of CPT on BMH before February 2012

Conditions	Variables	Number (%)
HIV infection clinical stage	I	37 (14.92)
	II	66 (26.61)
	III	123 (49.60)
	IV	22 (8.87)
Co morbid illness	TB	29 (11.69)
	Fungal infection	31 (12.75)
	PCP	2 (0.8)
	Others	18 (7.26)
Laboratory results	CD4 count <350 cell/mm^3	221 (89.11)
	Hemoglobin <7 g/dl	4 (1.61)
	Platelet count < 50,000 cells/dl	4 (1.61)
	Neutrophil count < 750 cells/dl	3 (1.2)
	ALT > 115 IU/L (for males) >90 IU/L (for females)	3 (1.2)

ALT- alanine transaminase, IU- international unit.

indication to start and 240 (96.77%) patients received correct dose of CTX (Table 2). The medical history cards showed that 20 (8.06%) patients were using CTX against contraindications out of which 5 (25%) developed sever anemia (Table 3).

In 123 (49.6%) cases CTX interaction with zidovudine (AZT) was documented and there were no other drug-drug interactions involving CTX. Among 52 patients who discontinued CPT, 10 (19.25%) and 14 (26.92%) were due to improvement of CD4 (>350 cells/mm^3) and peptic ulcer disease, respectively (Table 4).

Discussion

One of the most pressing problems facing health providers and administers in many countries is insuring rational drug use, which implies an individual approach to patient treatment. The presence of standard treatment guidelines and drug formularies for selected drugs in a health facility does not ensure that drugs are prescribed and used correctly. One mechanism to ensure correct use of drug is DUE [2].

In this study the use of CTX among PLWHA was consistent with the national guideline in the rationale for indication in most (97.98%) patients. In 2% of the patients (who were WHO clinical stage I and CD4 level >350 cells/ml) CPT was started without any symptomatic disease. The CTX dosage prescribed for most patients were appropriate except in 1.6% of patients in the age range 6 months to 14 years. This might leads to insufficient and inappropriate treatment.

The finding on the rationale for indication and appropriate dose were in line with the study conducted in Jimma University Specialized Hospital in which all cases of the indication to start and dose were according to the national guideline [12]. On the contrary, the result for CTX dose was slightly different from the study done in Hawasa referral hospital in which 87% of the cases on usage of CTX dose were according to the national guideline [10].

Table 2 Cotrimoxazole dosage prescribed for PLWHA in BMH before February 2012

Age distribution	Number (%) of cases		
	Appropriate dose, number (%)	Inappropriate dose, number (%)	Total
<6 month	3 (1.2)	–	3 (1.2)
6 month-5 yr	4 (1.61)	4 (1.61)	8 (3.23)
6-14 yr	14 (5.64)	4 (1.61)	18 (7.25)
15-49 yr	202 (81.45)	–	202 (81.45)
>50 yr	17 (6.85)	–	17 (6.85)
Total	240 (96.77)	8 (3.23)	248 (100)

Table 3 Cotrimoxazole use despite the presence of contraindications among PLWHA in BMH before February 2012

Condition evidence for contra use of CPT	Number (%)
Severe anemia (Hg < 7 g/dl of blood)	5 (25)
Elevated liver enzymes (SGPT > 115 IU/L for males and 90 IU/L for female)	3 (15)
Severe neutrophil (<750 cell/dl)	3 (15)
Severe thrombocytopenia (<50,000 cells/dl)	4 (20)
1st trimester of pregnancy	5 (25)
Sulfa allergy	–
Total	20 (8.06)

CTX was used despite contra indications in cases of 8.06% and in 91.93% of cases the drug was used without any contraindications. This is in agreement with a research done in Jimma [12], which showed 98.3% of the cases were in accordance with the guideline. The national guideline suggests the importance of monitoring drug usage for patients with severe anemia taking CTX and AZT [1]. In 49.59% of cases CPT had interactions with AZT, which is far from 98.3% of patients in Jimma [12]. The interaction of these drugs causes bone marrow suppression and thereby hematological abnormalities [13]. This in turn results in lack of adherence and poor patient outcomes.

WHO and the Federal Ministry of Health of Ethiopia recommended the reasons for discontinuation of CPT in PLWHA for better treatment outcome and for preventing potential drug related problems [6,8]. Among 52 patients who discounted CPT, 25% of them were without any documented data for their discontinuation and 23% of them discontinued due to both skin rash and pregnancy. Most patients discontinued CPT due to peptic ulcer (19.25%) and CD4 improvement (26.92%). The result for discontinuation of CPT (75%) which was in agreement with the national guideline and with the study done in Jimma University Specialized Hospital [12].

Table 4 Common reasons for discontinuation of CPT among PLWHA in BMH before February 2012

Reason for discontinuation	Number (%)
Peptic ulcer	10 (19.21)
Skin rash	6 (11.53)
Sever anemia	3 (5.77)
Pregnancy	6 (11.53)
CD4 > 350 cells/mm^3	14 (26.92)
Others (not recorded)	13 (25.00)
Total	52 (20.97)

Patients discontinue CPT when their CD4 count was restored to the recommended level and this in turn decreases pill burden in patients taking ART and thereby increases treatment adherence. If discontinuation is not according to the guideline, it may lead to antimicrobial resistance, fuelling an ever increasing need for new drugs and contributing the rising cost of medical care.

To date, there are no published studies conducted on evaluation of cotrimoxazole use for prophylaxis in PLWHA outside Ethiopia and hence it was not possible to compare the practice of this hospital with practices of other clinical settings. The findings were discussed in relation to the 2005 CPT guideline of Ethiopia and few studies done in Ethiopia.

Conclusions

In summary the use of CPT among PLWHA was consistent with the national guideline regarding to rationale for indication, dose, discontinuation and its use despite the presence of contraindications in most patients, however, problems regarding drug- drug interaction were identified in more than half of the patients.

Competing interests
The author(s) declare(s) that they have no conflicts of interest to disclose.

Authors' contribution
All have been involved in the design and conceptual framework of the study. BG worked on analyzing the data; DM was involved in drafting the manuscript, and the role of YB was crucial in data collection and manipulation. All the authors have read and approved the final manuscript.

Authors' information
BG is a pharmacologist working at Wollo University as instructor, researcher and head of department of pharmacy. DM and YB are a pharmacist and a nurse working at Wollo University as an instructor and a researcher, respectively.

Acknowledgements
This work has been supported by Research Office of Wollo University.

Author details
[1]Department of Pharmacy, College of Medicine and Health Sciences, Wollo University, Dessie, Ethiopia. [2]Department of Nursing, College of Medicine and Health Sciences, Wollo University, Dessie, Ethiopia.

References
1. Drug Administration and Control Authority of Ethiopia (DACA): *Training Modules on Operation and Management of Special Pharmacies.* 2nd edition. Addis Ababa: DACA; 2002.
2. Management sciences for health (MSH): *Managing Drug Supply.* 2nd edition. West Hart Ford Conn, USA: Kumarian press; 1997.
3. Chambers F: **Sulfonamides-Trimethoprim and Quinoloes.** In *Basic and Clinical Pharmacology.* 9th edition. Edited by K. B. New York, USA: Mc Graw Hill; 2004:775.
4. Date A, *et al*: **Implementation of cotrimoxazole prophylaxis and isoniazide preventive therapy for people living with HIV.** *Bull WHO* 2009, **88**:253–259.
5. Vilar FJ, Khoo SH, Walley T: **The management of *Pneumocystis carini* pneumonia.** *Br J Clin Pharmacol* 1999, **47**:605–609.
6. Ethiopian Ministry of Health (MOH): *Guidelines for use of Cotrimoxazole as Preventive Therapy Among People Living with HIV AIDS in Ethiopia.* 2nd edition. Addis Ababa, Ethiopia: FMOH; 2006.
7. Badri M, Ehrlich R, Wood R, Maartens G: **Initiating co-trimoxazole prophylaxis in HIV-infected patients in Africa: an evaluation of the provisional WHO/UNAIDS recommendations.** *AIDS* 2001, **15**:1143–1148.
8. WHO: *Guideline on Cotrimoxazole Prophylaxis for HIV Related Infections Among Children, Adolescent & Adults.* 2nd edition. Geneva: WHO press; 2009.
9. Nunn A, *et al*: **Role of co-trimoxazole prophylaxis in reducing mortality in HIV infected adults being treated for tuberculosis: randomised clinical trial.** *BMJ* 2008, **337**:a257.
10. Deresse D, Alemayehu T: **Evaluation of prophylactic use of cotrimoxazole in people living with HIV/AIDS in Hawassa hospital: a retrospective evaluation.** *Asian J Med Sci* 2009, **1**(3):88–90.
11. WHO: *The Rational use of Drugs: Report of the Conference of Experts.* 2nd edition. Geneva: WHO press; 1985.
12. Dirba L, Worku F, Girma T: **Evaluation of prophylactic use of cotrimoxazole for people living with HIV/AIDS in Jimma University specialized hospital, South West Ethiopia.** *Ethio J Health Sci* 2008, **18**(3):59–64.
13. Gilman AG: *The Pharmacological Basis of Therapeutics.* 11th edition. Dallas, Texas: Mc Graw Hill; 2006.

12

Determinants of saxagliptin use among patients with type 2 diabetes mellitus treated with oral anti-diabetic drugs

M Elle Saine[1,2], Dena M Carbonari[1,2], Craig W Newcomb[1], Melissa S Nezamzadeh[1,2], Kevin Haynes[1,2,3], Jason A Roy[1,2], Serena Cardillo[4], Sean Hennessy[1,2], Crystal N Holick[3], Daina B Esposito[3], Arlene M Gallagher[5], Harshvinder Bhullar[6], Brian L Strom[1,2,7] and Vincent Lo Re III[1,2,4]*

Abstract

Background: The patterns and determinants of saxagliptin use among patients with type 2 diabetes mellitus (T2DM) are unknown in real-world settings. We compared the characteristics of T2DM patients who were new initiators of saxagliptin to those who were new initiators of non-dipeptidyl peptidase-4 (DPP-4) inhibitor oral anti-diabetic drugs (OADs) and identified factors associated with saxagliptin use.

Methods: We conducted a cross-sectional study within the Clinical Practice Research Datalink (CPRD), The Health Improvement Network (THIN), US Medicare, and the HealthCore Integrated Research Database (HIRD^SM) across the first 36 months of saxagliptin availability (29 months for US Medicare). Patients were included if they were: 1) ≥18 years old, 2) newly prescribed saxagliptin or a non-DPP-4 inhibitor OAD, and 3) enrolled in their respective database for 180 days. For each saxagliptin initiator, we randomly selected up to ten non-DPP-4 inhibitor OAD initiators matched on age, sex, and geographic region. Conditional logistic regression was used to identify determinants of saxagliptin use.

Results: We identified 64,079 saxagliptin initiators (CPRD: 1,962; THIN: 2,084; US Medicare: 51,976; HIRD^SM: 8,057) and 610,660 non-DPP-4 inhibitor OAD initiators (CPRD: 19,484; THIN: 19,936; US Medicare: 493,432; HIRD^SM: 77,808). Across all four data sources, prior OAD use, hypertension, and hyperlipidemia were associated with saxagliptin use. Saxagliptin initiation was also associated with hemoglobin A1c results >8% within the UK data sources, and a greater number of hemoglobin A1c measurements in the US data sources.

Conclusions: In these UK and US data sources, initiation of saxagliptin was associated with prior poor glycemic control, prior OAD use, and diagnoses of hypertension and hyperlipidemia.

Trial registration: ClinicalTrials.gov identifiers NCT01086280, NCT01086293, NCT01086319, NCT01086306, and NCT01377935

Keywords: Diabetes mellitus, Saxagliptin, Dipeptidyl peptidase IV inhibitor, Pharmacoepidemiology

* Correspondence: vincentl@mail.med.upenn.edu
[1]Department of Biostatistics and Epidemiology, Center for Clinical Epidemiology and Biostatistics, Perelman School of Medicine at the University of Pennsylvania, 423 Guardian Drive, Philadelphia, PA, USA
[2]Department of Biostatistics and Epidemiology, Center for Pharmacoepidemiology Research and Training, Perelman School of Medicine at the University of Pennsylvania, Philadelphia, PA, USA
Full list of author information is available at the end of the article

Background

Type 2 diabetes mellitus (T2DM) is a global public health problem, affecting 347 million people worldwide [1,2]. Current estimates suggest that more than 29.1 million adults and children in the United States (US) and 3.2 million adults and children in the United Kingdom (UK) have T2DM, representing more than 9.3% and 6% of these populations, respectively [3-5]. Oral anti-diabetic drugs (OADs), along with diet and exercise, can help to control T2DM-associated hyperglycemia in adults [6].

Saxagliptin, a relatively new dipeptidyl peptidase-4 (DPP-4) inhibitor [7], was approved by the US Food and Drug Administration (FDA) in July 2009 and the European Medicines Agency in October 2009 to be used with diet and exercise to control hyperglycemia in adults with T2DM. In clinical trials, saxagliptin was shown to be efficacious in lowering fasting plasma glucose, 2-hour postprandial glucose, and hemoglobin A1c when used as monotherapy [8], in combination with metformin in treatment-naive patients [9], or as add-on therapy to metformin [10], sulfonylureas [11], thiazolidinediones [12], or insulin [13]. Because of its recent market introduction, prescribing patterns associated with saxagliptin's use in real-world settings remain unknown. Determining how OADs are prescribed in clinical practice can provide valuable information on healthcare decision-making [14,15]. Further, since the effectiveness and safety of saxagliptin and other OAD therapies may be affected by demographic characteristics, medical comorbidities, and additional medications prescribed to T2DM patients, identifying the factors associated with the use of particular OADs in real-world settings can provide important information needed for the future conduct of studies evaluating the comparative effectiveness and safety of anti-diabetic drugs. In particular, such variables can be incorporated within propensity scores to help to minimize confounding by indication [16,17].

The objectives of this study were to: 1) compare the characteristics of patients with T2DM who newly initiate saxagliptin to those who newly initiate OADs in classes other than DPP-4 inhibitors, and 2) identify determinants of saxagliptin use during the first years of its availability in the UK and US. We hypothesized that T2DM patients with poor glycemic control, a higher prevalence of microvascular and macrovascular complications, and prior OAD use would be more likely to initiate saxagliptin.

Methods

Data sources

Four data sources, two each in the UK and US, were used in this study. Within the UK, data from the Clinical Practice Research Datalink (CPRD; formerly General Practice Research Database) and The Health Improvement Network (THIN) were evaluated over the first 36 months of saxagliptin availability (5 October 2009 to 30 September 2012). Within the US, data from US Medicare were evaluated across all 50 states over the first 29 months of saxagliptin availability (1 August 2009 to 31 December 2011), due to the lag in availability of these data. The HealthCore Integrated Research Database (HIRD[SM]) data were examined over the first 36 months of saxagliptin availability (1 August 2009 to 31 July 2012). These four databases were selected because they include large numbers of T2DM patients across all age groups and utilize health records (UK) and claims data (US) from both private and public insurance plans, providing broadly representative study samples.

Details on the data available within each of these data sources for the purpose of evaluating OAD use have been previously described [18]. At the time of data collection, CPRD contains electronic medical records of over 15 million UK patients across 684 practices [19], and THIN contained primary medical records for over 11 million UK patients across over 550 practices [20,21]. CPRD and THIN collect demographic information, medical diagnoses and surgical procedures (recorded using Read codes), outpatient laboratory results, and general practitioner-issued prescriptions [22,23]. Since some UK practices contribute data to both CPRD and THIN [24], we excluded overlapping patients from THIN data to ensure that these patients were not counted twice. US Medicare is the largest national health insurance program administered by the US federal government, serving approximately 47.5 million people as of 2010 [25]. Medicare is available to US citizens aged 65 years or older and those under 65 years with certain disabilities. The HIRD[SM] is one of the largest longitudinal commercial health insurance databases in the US, serving 23.2 million members as of 2010 [26-28]. Both Medicare and the HIRD[SM] contain demographic information, inpatient and outpatient medical diagnoses (recorded using International Classification of Diseases, Ninth Revision, Clinical Modification diagnosis codes), surgical procedures (recorded with Current Procedural Terminology codes), and dispensed medications (recorded by National Drug Codes). Although codes for ordered laboratory tests can be identified within Medicare and the HIRD[SM], the results of these tests are not recorded in Medicare and are only available in a subset of HIRD[SM] patients. To avoid the possibility of double-counting patients concurrently enrolled in both of these US data sources, we only included HIRD[SM] data for persons aged 18–64 years and censored HIRD[SM] enrollees at age 65 years.

The study was approved by the University of Pennsylvania and Rutgers University Institutional Review Boards, the Quorum Review Institutional Review Board (HIRD[SM]), and the Independent Scientific Advisory Committees for

CPRD and THIN. A data use agreement was obtained from the Centers for Medicare and Medicaid Services (US Medicare).

Study patients

Patients were eligible for study inclusion if they were: 1) newly prescribed (in the UK) or dispensed (in the US) either saxagliptin, as a single agent or in combination with other OADs, or an OAD in a class other than DPP-4 inhibitors ("index drug"); 2) ≥18 years old; and 3) enrolled in their respective data source for at least 180 days prior to initiation of their index drug. The rationale for selecting new initiators of other OADs as the comparator group was to study patients with diabetes who required initiation of new OAD therapy. Given that we wished to identify factors specifically associated with saxagliptin use, we did not include new initiators of other DPP-4 inhibitors within the comparator OAD group.

All eligible patients prescribed saxagliptin were included. Within each data source, a random sample (without replacement) of up to ten new initiators of non-DPP-4 inhibitor OADs was selected for each saxagliptin initiator. These patients were matched on age (within 5-year age groups), sex, and geographic region (i.e., country within UK data sources; census region within US data sources).

Main study outcome

The main study outcome was a new prescription (UK data source) or pharmacy claim (US data source) for either saxagliptin or a non-DPP-4 inhibitor OAD. The index date was defined as the date of first prescription of saxagliptin or comparator OAD in the respective data source.

Determinants of saxagliptin use

The following variables were evaluated as determinants of use of saxagliptin compared to other OADs: calendar year of initiation, medical comorbidities, surgical procedures, and medications of interest (listed in Table 1). In clinical practice, primary care physicians and endocrinologists likely select and prescribe oral anti-diabetic drugs based on consideration of at least many of these factors. We included a variety of medications and drug classes as potential determinants of saxagliptin because concerns for drug-drug interactions or exacerbation of medication toxicities might influence decisions to prescribe saxagliptin.

Comorbidities were identified based on the presence of diagnoses recorded in the 180 days prior to the index date within US Medicare and HIRD[SM], and at any time prior to the index date within CPRD and THIN. General practitioners in the UK do not have a financial incentive to record pre-existing diagnoses at each visit and only utilizing diagnoses recorded in the 180 days prior to

the index date could lead to incomplete comorbidity ascertainment within the UK data sources. Within all data sources, pre-existing microvascular and macrovascular T2DM complications were determined based on diagnoses and surgical procedures recorded within 180 days prior to the index date and categorized according to the Diabetes Complications Severity Index [29].

Within the UK data sources, we collected the closest hemoglobin A1c result recorded in the 180 days prior to the index date. Smoking history and obesity, defined as body mass index (calculated as height in meters/[body weight in kg]^2) >30 kg/m^2, were also extracted from CPRD and THIN. Within the US data sources, we collected the number of claims for hemoglobin A1c tests recorded in the 180 days prior to the index date, since patients with unmanaged and/or severe T2DM typically have hemoglobin A1c measured more frequently [30].

Across all data sources, patients were considered exposed to a particular drug if a prescription or pharmacy claim for that drug was recorded within 180 days prior to the index date. Particularly, prior OAD use within the 180 days preceding the index date was determined. Patients whose prescriptions or claims for their existing OAD therapy continued for 90 days before and after the initiation of their index drug were considered to have "added on" saxagliptin or the comparator OAD to their current therapy. Patients whose prescriptions or claims for their existing OAD therapy were recorded 90 days before, but not after, the initiation of the index drug were considered to have "switched to" saxagliptin or a comparator OAD.

Statistical analysis

Baseline characteristics of new initiators of saxagliptin or other OADs were compared using standardized differences, of which a value exceeding 0.1 is generally considered meaningful [31]. For the purpose of these analyses, standardized difference was calculated as the difference in mean (or proportion for binary variables) divided by the standard deviation (pooled standard deviation for the continuous variables). Conditional logistic regression was used to determine adjusted odds ratios with 95% confidence intervals of saxagliptin use associated with demographic variables, comorbidities, and drug therapies. To explore whether the determinants of saxagliptin use were different between first-time OAD initiators and those who were previously treated with OADs, we re-ran analyses in each database, stratified by whether patients received prior OAD therapy. Because the conditional logistic regression is conditioned on the matched group, initiators who no longer had a matched comparator in the stratified cohorts were removed from this analysis. Data were analyzed using SAS 9.4 (SAS Institute Inc., Cary, NC).

Table 1 Demographic characteristics of type 2 diabetes mellitus patients within United Kingdom data sources

Characteristic[*]	Clinical Practice Research Datalink			The Health Improvement Network		
	Saxagliptin	Other OAD	Standardized difference	Saxagliptin	Other OAD	Standardized difference
	(n = 1,962)	(n = 19,484)		(n = 2,084)	(n =19,936)	
Mean (SD) age, years[†]	52.7 (10.6)	52.2 (10.6)	0.01	64.7 (12.9)	64.6 (12.9)	0.01
Male sex[†]	58.2%	58.2%	<0.01	57.7%	57.0%	0.01
UK country[†]						
England	60.4%	60.6%	<0.01	63.1%	65.7%	0.05
Northern Ireland	7.1%	7.0%	<0.01	5.3%	5.0%	0.01
Scotland	11.4%	11.5%	<0.01	12.3%	12.8%	0.01
Wales	21.0%	20.9%	<0.01	19.2%	16.5%	0.07
Other OAD initiated at index date						
Alpha-glucosidase inhibitors: Acarbose	0%	0.2%	-	0%	0.2%	-
Biguanide: Metformin	0%	63.1%	-	0%	62.1%	-
Meglitinides	0%	0.4%	-	0%	0.4%	-
Nateglinide	0%	0.1%	-	0%	0.0%	-
Repaglinide	0%	0.3%	-	0%	0.3%	-
Sulfonylureas	0%	27.9%	-	0%	29.1%	-
Glibenclamide (Glyburide in US data sources)	0%	0.2%	-	0%	0.2%	-
Gliclazide	0%	24.9%	-	0%	26.1%	-
Glimepiride	0%	2.1%	-	0%	1.9%	-
Glipizide	0%	0.6%	-	0%	0.7%	-
Tolbutamide	0%	0.1%	-	0%	0.2%	-
Thiazolidinediones	0%	8.3%	-	0%	8.2%	-
Pioglitazone	0%	8.1%	-	0%	8.0%	-
Rosiglitazone	0%	0.2%	-	0%	0.2%	-
On glucagon-like peptide-1 receptor agonist	3.1%	1.9%	0.08	2.4%	1.9%	0.03
On insulin	5.4%	7.3%	0.08	7.7%	7.2%	0.02
Hemoglobin A1c measurements						
Mean (SD)	8.7 (1.6)	8.6 (1.8)	0.06	8.8 (1.6)	8.6 (1.8)	0.08
Hemoglobin A1c >8%	57.6%	39.8%	0.36	56.2%	40.8%	0.31
Mean body mass index (SD)	32.4 (6.5)	31.5 (6.7)	0.14	-	-	-
Missing values	42.9%	41.4%	0.03	0.7%	2.0%	0.11
Underweight (15–18.5 kg/m^2)	0.2%	0.4%	0.03	0.0%	0.4%	0.08
Normal (18.5-24.9 kg/m^2)	4.4%	6.7%	0.10	7.9%	11.4%	0.12
Overweight (25.0-29.9 kg/m^2)	15.9%	17.8%	0.05	29.0%	31.5%	0.05
Obese (30–60 kg/m^2)	36.7%	33.9%	0.06	62.3%	54.7%	0.15
Smoking	36.5%	36.5%	<0.01	63.5%	61.0%	0.05
Severity of type 2 diabetes mellitus (prior 180 d)						
Cerebrovascular disease	0.5%	0.7%	0.02	0.9%	0.7%	0.02
Coronary artery disease, congestive heart failure, ventricular tachycardia/fibrillation	1.3%	1.5%	0.01	1.9%	1.5%	0.03
Diabetic coma	0%	0.1%	-	0%	0.1%	-
Nephropathy	0.3%	0.2%	0.02	0.6%	0.2%	0.06
Neuropathy	0.8%	0.6%	0.02	0.9%	0.6%	0.03
Peripheral vascular disease	1.1%	0.9%	0.02	1.2%	0.9%	0.03

Table 1 Demographic characteristics of type 2 diabetes mellitus patients within United Kingdom data sources
(*Continued*)

Retinopathy	5.7%	3.7%	0.09	5.5%	3.5%	0.10
Unspecified additional diabetic complications	0%	0.0%	-	0%	0.0%	-
Medical comorbidities						
Allergic rhinitis/hay fever	8.8%	10.0%	0.04	9.1%	9.4%	0.01
Asthma	16.0%	15.8%	<0.01	16.4%	15.9%	0.01
Chronic obstructive pulmonary disease/bronchitis	12.1%	10.0%	0.07	13.1%	10.7%	0.07
Dermatologic disorder						
Eczema	17.0%	15.2%	0.05	16.9%	14.2%	0.08
Psoriasis/psoriatic arthritis	6.4%	5.1%	0.06	5.8%	5.3%	0.02
Gastrointestinal disease						
Cirrhosis	0.3%	0.4%	0.01	0.2%	0.4%	0.03
Gallbladder disease	6.2%	5.6%	0.02	6.3%	5.9%	0.02
Hemochromatosis	0.1%	0.1%	0.02	0%	0.2%	0.04
Hyperlipidemia	16.0%	12.0%	0.12	15.9%	12.2%	0.11
Hypertension	56.7%	50.9%	0.12	61.0%	56.1%	0.10
Infectious disease						
Hepatitis B virus infection	0.3%	0.2%	0.02	0.2%	0.2%	0.01
Hepatitis C virus infection	0%	0.1%	-	0%	0.1%	-
Malignancy						
Hematologic	0.8%	1.0%	0.03	0.9%	1.0%	<0.01
Solid organ	23.5%	22.9%	0.02	22.9%	23.9%	0.02
Obesity	17.8%	14.6%	0.09	17.0%	13.4%	0.10
Rheumatoid arthritis	2.7%	2.4%	0.02	1.3%	1.7%	0.03
Medications						
Acetaminophen/paracetamol	31.7%	28.7%	0.06	32.0%	30.1%	0.04
Anti-asthmatic agents	18.6%	17.7%	0.02	18.8%	18.1%	0.02
Antibacterials	35.5%	33.9%	0.03	32.1%	30.7%	0.03
Anticonvulsants	8.8%	7.8%	0.04	6.2%	5.1%	0.05
Antifungals	3.0%	2.6%	0.02	2.9%	3.4%	0.03
Antihistamines	7.2%	7.1%	<0.01	7.5%	6.9%	0.02
Anti-hyperlipidemic agents	80.6%	58.5%	0.49	81.1%	61.9%	0.43
Antihypertensive agents						
Angiotensin-converting enzyme inhibitors	46.5%	36.1%	0.21	46.1%	38.4%	0.16
Angiotensin receptor blockers	19.2%	13.2%	0.16	22.5%	15.0%	0.19
Beta blockers	24.7%	20.7%	0.09	28.0%	23.2%	0.11
Calcium channel blockers	28.2%	23.8%	0.10	29.9%	26.9%	0.07
Loop diuretics	12.4%	11.0%	0.04	17.3%	11.4%	0.17
Other antihypertensive agents	9.2%	6.8%	0.09	10.0%	6.8%	0.11
Thiazide diuretics	19.9%	16.1%	0.10	25.1%	20.8%	0.10
Antivirals	0.7%	0.8%	0.02	0.8%	0.9%	0.02
Non-aspirin non-steroidal anti-inflammatory	13.4%	13.0%	0.01	12.5%	13.0%	0.02
Other antiplatelet/anticoagulant agents						
Aspirin	38.3%	29.7%	0.18	42.1%	32.2%	0.21
Clopidogrel	4.9%	3.7%	0.06	5.0%	3.7%	0.06

Table 1 Demographic characteristics of type 2 diabetes mellitus patients within United Kingdom data sources
(Continued)

Low-molecular-weight heparin	0.2%	0.3%	0.03	0.5%	0.3%	0.02
Warfarin	5.4%	4.9%	0.02	6.9%	5.6%	0.05
Other medications						
Allopurinol	3.2%	3.5%	0.02	5.1%	3.7%	0.07
Anti-arrhythmics	3.4%	2.6%	0.05	3.1%	3.0%	<0.01
Immune modulators/immunosuppressants	1.2%	1.2%	<0.01	1.2%	1.2%	0.01
Nitroglycerin	5.6%	5.1%	0.02	6.3%	4.9%	0.06
Urinary anti-spasmodics	4.3%	3.3%	0.05	4.7%	3.6%	0.06
Psychotropic agents						
Antidepressants	22.1%	19.6%	0.06	20.6%	19.6%	0.03
Antipsychotics	4.3%	4.4%	0.01	4.9%	4.8%	0.01
Prior OAD Therapy[‡]	93.7%	35.8%	1.53	92.1%	36.8%	1.41
Alpha-glucosidase inhibitors: Acarbose	0.3%	0.1%	0.03	0.2%	0.1%	0.03
Biguanide: Metformin	83.4%	73.7%	0.24	77.7%	73.1%	0.11
Meglitinides	1.1%	0.4%	0.09	1.2%	0.3%	0.10
Nateglinide	0.2%	0.0%	0.04	0.2%	0.1%	0.04
Repaglinide	0.9%	0.3%	0.08	1.0%	0.2%	0.10
Sulfonylureas	47.9%	12.2%	0.84	46.4%	12.8%	0.79
Glibenclamide	0.4%	0.5%	0.01	0.5%	0.6%	0.01
Gliclazide	41.4%	12.6%	0.69	39.3%	13.4%	0.61
Glimepiride	4.5%	1.5%	0.18	4.1%	1.4%	0.17
Glipizide	1.1%	0.7%	0.04	1.7%	0.8%	0.09
Tolbutamide	0.7%	0.1%	0.09	1.1%	0.2%	0.11
Thiazolidinediones	16.6%	5.3%	0.37	17.7%	5.1%	0.40
Pioglitazone	14.1%	3.5%	0.38	15.4%	3.4%	0.42
Rosiglitazone	2.7%	2.1%	0.03	2.5%	2.0%	0.03

Abbreviations: OAD = oral anti-diabetic drug; SD = standard deviation.
[*]Characteristics are presented as percentages unless otherwise indicated.
[†]Matching criteria for which a random sample (without replacement) of up to ten new initiators of non-DPP-4 inhibitor OADs were selected for each saxagliptin initiator.
[‡]Defined as use of an oral anti-diabetic drug within the 180 days prior to the initiation of the index drug. Denominator adjusted to exclude those on index drug.

Results
Patient characteristics
UK data sources

Within THIN and CPRD, respectively, we identified, 1,962 and 2,084 new initiators of saxagliptin (Figure 1a and b) as well as 19,484 and 19,936 matched new initiators of non-DPP-4 inhibitor OADs. The characteristics of these patients are presented in Table 1. Approximately 6% of saxagliptin initiators in each UK data source had not received treatment for T2DM with another OAD within 180 days prior to the index date.

Within both UK data sources, saxagliptin initiators were more likely to have had prior OAD therapy and hemoglobin A1c results >8% in the 180 days preceding the index prescription compared to initiators of other non-DPP-4 inhibitor OADs. Saxagliptin users also more frequently had hyperlipidemia, hypertension, and obesity and were more commonly prescribed aspirin, anti-hyperlipidemic agents, and anti-hypertensive drugs. Within THIN, diagnoses of retinopathy were more prevalent among saxagliptin initiators.

US data sources

During the initial 29 months of saxagliptin availability within US Medicare, 51,976 new initiators of saxagliptin and 493,432 matched new initiators of non-DPP-4 inhibitor OADs were identified (Figure 1c). During the initial 36 months of saxagliptin availability within the HIRD[SM], 8,057 new initiators of saxagliptin and 77,808 matched new initiators of non-DPP-4 inhibitor OADs were identified (Figure 1d). The characteristics of these patients are presented in Table 2. Approximately 22% of saxagliptin initiators in US Medicare and 33% of saxagliptin initiators in the HIRD[SM] had not

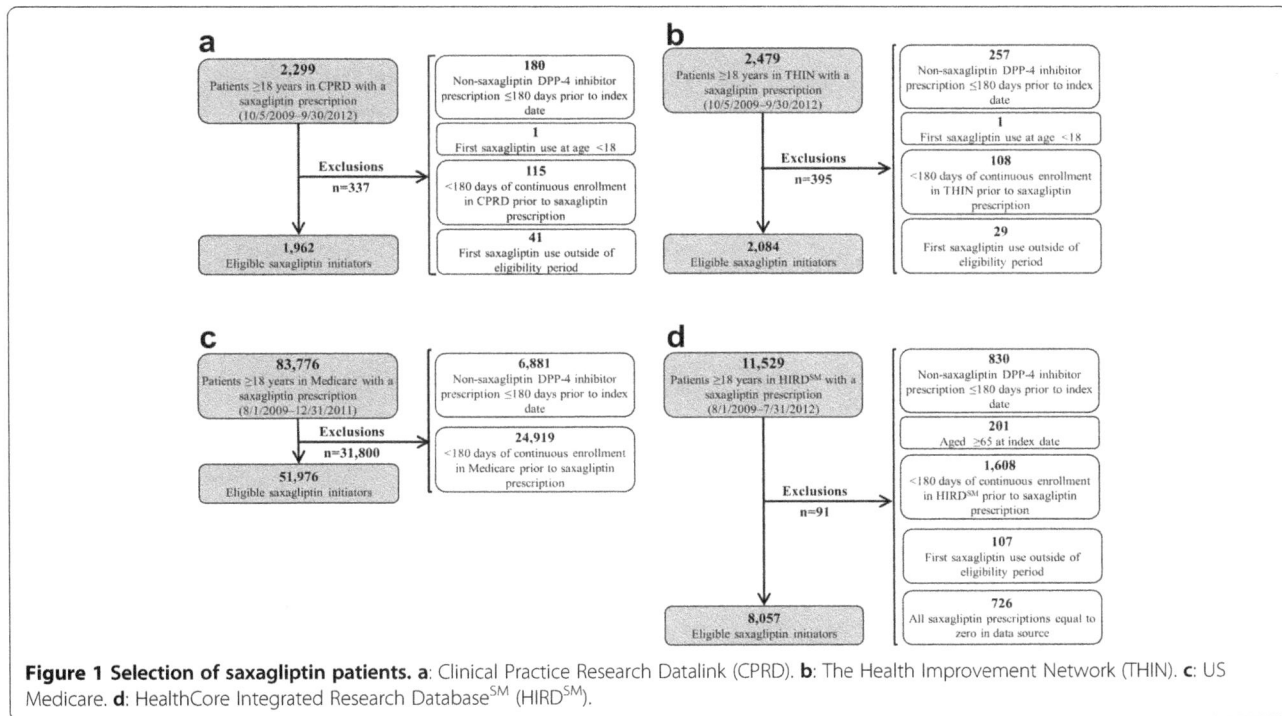

Figure 1 Selection of saxagliptin patients. a: Clinical Practice Research Datalink (CPRD). **b**: The Health Improvement Network (THIN). **c**: US Medicare. **d**: HealthCore Integrated Research Database^{SM} (HIRD^{SM}).

received treatment for T2DM with another OAD within 180 days prior to the index date.

Within both US databases, saxagliptin initiators more frequently received prior OAD therapy and had higher mean numbers of hemoglobin A1c measurements in the 180 days prior to the index date. Saxagliptin initiators were also more frequently diagnosed with hyperlipidemia and hypertension and more commonly received anti-hyperlipidemic drugs, angiotensin-converting enzyme inhibitors, and angiotensin receptor blockers. Within US Medicare, diagnoses of microvascular T2DM complications, including nephropathy and neuropathy, were more prevalent among saxagliptin initiators.

Factors associated with saxagliptin use
UK data sources
Factors associated with saxagliptin initiation within CPRD and THIN are presented in Table 3. Prior OAD use in the 180 days preceding the index date was strongly associated with saxagliptin initiation in CPRD and THIN. Within THIN, diabetic nephropathy and obesity were also associated with a higher likelihood of saxagliptin initiation.

After stratifying on prior OAD use within CPRD, results were similar to those in the primary analysis. However, prescriptions for antihyperlipidemic agents and diagnoses of chronic obstructive pulmonary disease and bronchitis were associated with saxagliptin initiation among patients without prior OAD use (Table 3).

After stratifying on prior OAD use within THIN, results were also similar to those in the primary analysis. However, obesity and diabetic nephropathy were more strongly associated with saxagliptin initiation among those with prior OAD use. Additionally, among patients with no prior OAD use, prescriptions for antihyperlipidemics and diagnoses of retinopathy were associated with saxagliptin initiation (Table 3).

US data sources
Factors associated with saxagliptin initiation in US Medicare and the HIRD^{SM} are presented in Table 4. Saxagliptin initiation was associated with prior OAD use and a greater number of hemoglobin A1c measurements in the 180 days preceding the index date in Medicare and the HIRD^{SM}. Additionally, within Medicare, saxagliptin initiators were more likely to receive angiotensin-receptor blockers.

After stratifying on prior OAD use within US Medicare, results were similar to those in the primary analysis. However, use of angiotensin-receptor blockers was more strongly associated with saxagliptin use among those without prior OAD use (Table 4).

After stratifying on prior OAD use within the HIRD^{SM}, results remained similar to those within the primary analyses (Table 4).

Table 2 Demographic characteristics of type 2 diabetes mellitus patients within United States data sources

Characteristic[*]	US Medicare			HealthCore Integrated Reseach Database[SM]		
	Saxagliptin	Other OAD	Standardized difference	Saxagliptin	Other OAD	Standardized difference
	(n = 51,976)	(n = 493,432)		(n = 8,057)	(n = 77,808)	
Mean (SD) age, years[†]	70.4 (11.1)	69.9 (11.0)	0.04	52.9 (8.4)	52.9 (8.4)	0.01
Male sex[†]	42.1%	42.8%	0.01	60.0%	59.5%	0.01
US census region[†]						
East North Central	12.7%	12.8%	<0.01	20.7%	21.2%	0.01
East South Central	10.0%	10.0%	<0.01	10.0%	10.1%	<0.01
Middle Atlantic	16.0%	15.9%	<0.01	9.0%	8.9%	<0.01
Mountain	3.1%	3.1%	<0.01	1.9%	1.9%	<0.01
New England	2.8%	2.8%	<0.01	5.7%	5.9%	<0.01
Pacific	12.8%	13.1%	<0.01	14.6%	14.8%	<0.01
South Atlantic	24.1%	24.0%	<0.01	30.5%	29.9%	0.01
West North Central	5.2%	5.0%	<0.01	5.3%	5.4%	<0.01
West South Central	13.2%	13.2%	<0.01	2.2%	1.9%	0.02
Other OAD initiated at index date						
Alpha-glucosidase inhibitors	0%	0.6%	-	0%	0.4%	-
Acarbose	0%	0.5%	-	0%	0.3%	-
Miglitol	0%	0.0%	-	0%	0.0%	-
Biguanide: Metformin	0%	51.5%	-	0%	69.1%	-
Meglitinides	0%	2.4%	-	0%	0.9%	-
Nateglinide	0%	1.0%	-	0%	0.4%	-
Repaglinide	0%	1.3%	-	0%	0.5%	-
Sulfonylureas	0%	33.8%	-	0%	22.0%	-
Chlorpropamide	0%	0.0%	-.	0%	0.0%	-
Glimepiride	0%	11.0%	-	0%	8.1%	-
Glipizide	0%	14.3%	-	0%	8.3%	-
Glyburide (glibenclamide in UK data sources)	0%	8.5%	-	0%	5.6%	-
Tolazamide	0%	0.0%	-	0%	0.0%	-
Tolbutamide	0%	0.0%	-	0%	0.0%	-
Thiazolidinediones	0%	11.7%	-	0%	7.7%	-
Pioglitazone	0%	11.0%	-	0%	7.3%	-
Rosiglitazone	0%	0.8%	-	0%	0.4%	-
On glucagon-like peptide-1 receptor agonist	2.1%	1.1%	0.07	3.8%	2.9%	0.05
On insulin	15.9%	14.9%	0.03	9.7%	8.3%	0.05
Mean (SD) number of hemoglobin A1c measures	1.3 (0.9)	0.9 (0.9)	0.51	1.1 (0.8)	0.8 (0.8)	0.50
Severity of type 2 diabetes mellitus (prior 180 d)						
Cerebrovascular disease	10.5%	10.6%	<0.01	2.4%	2.4%	<0.01
Coronary artery disease, congestive heart failure, ventricular tachycardia/fibrillation	40.8%	38.2%	0.05	11.8%	11.1%	0.02
Metabolic (ketoacidosis, hyperosmolar,coma)	1.3%	1.3%	<0.01	0.7%	0.7%	<0.01
Nephropathy	20.2%	15.7%	0.11	5.0%	3.6%	0.07
Neuropathy	22.9%	18.1%	0.12	8.3%	6.8%	0.06
Peripheral vascular disease	18.4%	16.6%	0.05	3.9%	3.4%	0.03

Table 2 Demographic characteristics of type 2 diabetes mellitus patients within United States data sources *(Continued)*

Retinopathy	13.3%	10.5%	0.09	5.3%	3.9%	0.07
Unspecified additional diabetic complications	7.9%	6.9%	0.04	3.8%	2.7%	0.06
Medical comorbidities						
Allergic rhinitis/hay fever	7.1%	5.6%	0.06	5.2%	4.6%	0.03
Asthma	7.7%	7.9%	0.01	3.8%	4.3%	0.02
Chronic obstructive pulmonary disease/bronchitis	12.5%	13.4%	0.03	2.7%	3.0%	0.02
Dermatologic disorders						
Eczema	3.5%	3.0%	0.02	2.2%	1.9%	0.02
Psoriasis/psoriatic arthritis	0.9%	0.9%	<0.01	0.9%	0.9%	0.01
Gastrointestinal disease						
Cirrhosis	0.8%	0.8%	<0.01	0.3%	0.4%	0.01
Gallbladder disease	2.2%	2.3%	0.01	1.1%	1.1%	<0.01
Hemochromatosis	0.3%	0.2%	0.01	0.2%	0.2%	<0.01
Hyperlipidemia	77.1%	66.3%	0.24	62.0%	48.7%	0.27
Hypertension	85.3%	78.1%	0.18	60.9%	50.9%	0.20
Infections						
Hepatitis B virus infection	0.2%	0.2%	<0.01	0.2%	0.2%	0.01
Hepatitis C virus infection	0.8%	0.9%	0.02	0.5%	0.5%	<0.01
Human immunodeficiency virus	0.2%	0.4%	0.02	0.1%	0.2%	0.03
Malignancy						
Hematologic	1.3%	1.3%	0.01	0.6%	0.6%	0.01
Solid organ	8.2%	8.6%	0.01	3.3%	3.3%	<0.01
Obesity	11.1%	10.7%	0.01	9.3%	9.4%	<0.01
Rheumatoid arthritis	2.8%	2.5%	0.02	0.9%	0.9%	<0.01
Medications						
Acetaminophen/paracetamol	28.1%	26.3%	0.04	20.2%	19.8%	0.01
Anti-asthmatic agents	14.4%	12.5%	0.05	8.3%	7.9%	0.01
Antibacterials	46.3%	40.3%	0.12	38.1%	35.7%	0.05
Anticonvulsants	5.4%	5.6%	0.01	7.2%	7.5%	0.01
Antifungals	10.1%	8.1%	0.07	6.8%	5.7%	0.05
Antihistamines	11.8%	9.4%	0.08	6.4%	5.7%	0.03
Anti-hyperlipidemic agents	69.2%	52.8%	0.34	53.5%	38.6%)	0.30
Antihypertensive agents						
Angiotensin-converting enzyme inhibitors	43.1%	37.2%	0.12	35.8%	28.0%	0.17
Angiotensin receptor blockers	28.5%	18.0%	0.25	20.1%	14.1%	0.16
Beta blockers	44.0%	36.1%	0.16	21.2%	18.4%	0.07
Calcium channel blockers	31.7%	26.3%	0.12	16.0%	13.9%	0.06
Loop diuretics	23.1%	18.1%	0.12	5.1%	4.7%	0.02
Other antihypertensive agents	11.9%	9.0%	0.10	4.8%	3.9%	0.04
Thiazide diuretics	21.7%	15.6%	0.16	18.2%	15.0%	0.09
Antivirals	2.3%	2.0%	0.02	1.9%	2.5%	0.04
Non-aspirin non-steroidal anti-inflammatory	17.4%	14.7%	0.08	13.9%	12.9%	0.03
Other antiplatelet/anticoagulant agents						
Aspirin	0.8%	0.6%	0.02	0.1%	0.1%	0.01
Clopidogrel	13.7%	10.4%	0.10	4.0%	3.6%	0.02

Table 2 Demographic characteristics of type 2 diabetes mellitus patients within United States data sources (Continued)

Low-molecular-weight heparin	0.5%	0.7%	0.02	0.4%	0.4%	0.01
Warfarin	7.4%	7.0%	0.02	2.1%	1.7%	0.03
Other medications						
Allopurinol	5.4%	4.1%	0.06	2.5%	2.4%	<0.01
Anti-arrhythmics	13.6%	12.2%	0.04	4.7%	4.6%	0.01
Immune modulators/immunosuppressants	4.5%	4.1%	0.02	2.2%	2.4%	0.01
Nitroglycerin	4.6%	3.8%	0.04	1.3%	1.3%	<0.01
Urinary anti-spasmodics	5.4%	4.5%	0.04	0.9%	1.2%	0.03
Psychotropic agents						
Antidepressants	27.4%	25.3%	0.05	19.1%	18.9%	<0.01
Antipsychotics	7.5%	7.8%	0.01	2.1%	2.3%	0.01
Prior OAD Therapy[‡]	77.6%	36.1%	0.92	66.7%	23.2%	0.97
Alpha-glucosidase inhibitors	0.8%	0.3%	0.08	0.4%	0.1%	0.05
Acarbose	0.7%	0.2%	0.07	0.4%	0.1%	0.05
Miglitol	0.1%	0.0%	0.03	0.0%	0.0%	0.02
Biguanide: Metformin	51.4%	37.4%	0.29	51.9%	42.6%	0.19
Meglitinides	3.0%	1.1%	0.13	1.4%	0.4%	0.10
Nateglinide	1.5%	0.5%	0.10	0.8%	0.2%	0.08
Repaglinide	1.6%	0.7%	0.09	0.7%	0.2%	0.07
Sulfonylureas	42.5%	16.8%	0.59	28.0%	8.7%	0.51
Chlorpropamide	0.0%	0.0%	<0.01	0.0%	0.0%	0.01
Glimepiride	16.5%	5.3%	0.37	12.3%	3.2%	0.34
Glipizide	17.7%	8.8%	0.27	11.0%	4.3%	0.26
Glyburide	9.5%	5.2%	0.16	5.2%	2.0%	0.17
Tolazamide	0.0%	0.0%	0.01	0%	0%	-
Tolbutamide	0.0%	0.0%	<0.01	0%	0%	-
Thiazolidinediones	24.2%	8.4%	0.44	15.0%	5.5%	0.32
Pioglitazone	21.4%	7.3%	0.41	13.6%	5.0%	0.30
Rosiglitazone	3.2%	1.9%	0.08	1.5%	0.9%	0.05

Abbreviations: OAD = oral anti-diabetic drug; SD = standard deviation.
[*]Characteristics are presented as percentages unless otherwise indicated.
[†]Matching criteria for which a random sample (without replacement) of up to ten new initiators of non-DPP-4 inhibitor OADs were selected for each saxagliptin initiator.
[‡]Defined as use of an oral anti-diabetic drug within the 180 days prior to the initiation of the index drug. Denominator adjusted to exclude those on index drug.

Discussion

Drug utilization studies can reveal how medications are administered in clinical practice, identify determinants of drug use, ensure robust prescribing practices [32], and establish topics for further study of drug effectiveness and safety [14]. This study found that across two UK and two US data sources, prior OAD use, hypertension, and hyperlipidemia were associated with initiation of saxagliptin rather than other OADs. Saxagliptin initiation was also associated with hemoglobin A1c results >8% within the UK data sources, and a greater number of hemoglobin A1c measurements in the US data sources. Interestingly, saxagliptin was the first OAD utilized for approximately 6% of patients within the UK data

sources, 22% of patients within US Medicare, and 33% of patients within the HIRD[SM]. Results from US Medicare and THIN suggest that saxagliptin may be a preferred treatment in patients with more severe (advanced) T2DM, as evidenced by increased diagnoses for microvascular complications. According to these findings, patients prescribed saxagliptin had higher prevalence of comorbid conditions, poor glycemic control, inadequate response to prior OAD therapy, or contraindications to OADs in other classes.

Stratifying our analyses on prior OAD use demonstrated that some determinants were more strongly associated with saxagliptin initiation among patients who had not received prior OAD therapy, particularly within

Table 3 Determinants of saxagliptin use among type 2 diabetes mellitus patients within United Kingdom data sources

Characteristic	Adjusted odds ratio (95% confidence interval)*					
	Clinical Practice Research Datalink			The Health Improvement Network		
	Overall	Prior OAD use	No Prior OAD use	Overall	Prior OAD use	No Prior OAD use
	(n = 21,446)	(n = 8,332)	(n = 890)	(n = 22,020)	(n = 8,621)	(n = 1,137)
Hemoglobin A1c >8%	1.26 (1.13-1.39)	1.21 (1.08-1.35)	1.66 (1.05-2.63)	1.17 (1.06-1.30)	1.12 (1.01-1.25)	1.39 (0.95-2.03)
Overweight vs. < 25 kg/m^2	0.91 (0.78-1.07)	0.87 (0.73-1.03)	1.32 (0.67-2.62)	1.38 (1.15-1.67)	1.44 (1.17-1.76)	0.95 (0.48-1.87)
Obese vs. < 25 kg/m^2	1.13 (0.99-1.29)	1.12 (0.97-1.30)	1.61 (0.88-2.94)	1.74 (1.45-2.09)	1.83 (1.50-2.22)	0.86 (0.44-1.68)
Smoking	0.93 (0.81-1.06)	0.94 (0.81-1.08)	0.73 (0.43-1.26)	1.03 (0.93-1.15)	1.03 (0.92-1.16)	0.86 (0.57-1.30)
Severity of type 2 diabetes mellitus						
Cardiovascular	1.05 (0.90-1.23)	1.03 (0.87-1.22)	1.49 (0.74-3.00)	0.97 (0.84-1.13)	1.01 (0.86-1.18)	0.74 (0.43-1.28)
Cerebrovascular	0.79 (0.64-0.98)	0.80 (0.64-1.01)	0.52 (0.20-1.38)	0.87 (0.72-1.05)	0.89 (0.72-1.09)	0.65 (0.31-1.40)
Nephropathy	1.08 (0.78-1.50)	1.05 (0.74-1.50)	1.40 (0.41-4.80)	1.75 (1.33-2.30)	1.77 (1.32-2.39)	1.79 (0.61-5.23)
Peripheral vascular disease	0.88 (0.73-1.07)	0.90 (0.74-1.10)	0.54 (0.21-1.35)	0.83 (0.69-1.00)	0.83 (0.68-1.01)	1.32 (0.65-2.68)
Retinopathy	1.11 (0.98-1.25)	1.06 (0.93-1.20)	2.25 (1.27-3.99)	1.20 (1.06-1.35)	1.14 (1.00-1.29)	2.63 (1.64-4.22)
Diagnoses						
Allergic rhinitis/hay fever	0.83 (0.69-1.00)	0.88 (0.73-1.07)	0.36 (0.13-0.97)	0.92 (0.77-1.11)	0.99 (0.82-1.21)	0.52 (0.25-1.07)
Asthma	0.99 (0.83-1.17)	0.96 (0.80-1.15)	1.35 (0.63-2.86)	0.99 (0.84-1.17)	0.96 (0.80-1.15)	1.44 (0.79-2.64)
Chronic obstructive pulmonary disease	1.23 (1.03-1.46)	1.18 (0.98-1.42)	2.64 (1.34-5.18)	1.21 (1.03-1.43)	1.21 (1.01-1.44)	1.48 (0.79-2.77)
Collagen vascular disease/autoimmune disorders	0.96 (0.82-1.13)	0.94 (0.79-1.11)	1.40 (0.64-3.07)	1.01 (0.86-1.17)	1.03 (0.88-1.22)	1.11 (0.59-2.12)
Dermatologic disorders	1.08 (0.96-1.22)	1.12 (0.99-1.27)	0.50 (0.28-0.89)	1.10 (0.98-1.24)	1.14 (1.00-1.29)	0.97 (0.62-1.52)
Hyperlipidemia	1.19 (1.03-1.37)	1.14 (0.98-1.33)	2.08 (1.14-3.81)	1.21 (1.05-1.39)	1.18 (1.02-1.37)	1.04 (0.59-1.83)
Hypertension	0.86 (0.75-0.98)	0.83 (0.73-0.96)	1.14 (0.67-1.93)	0.88 (0.78-1.00)	0.86 (0.75-0.99)	1.39 (0.87-2.22)
Infectious diseases	1.16 (1.01-1.33)	1.14 (0.99-1.32)	1.63 (0.97-2.76)	1.10 (0.96-1.25)	1.08 (0.94-1.24)	1.30 (0.79-2.13)
Malignancy	0.98 (0.87-1.11)	0.95 (0.84-1.08)	1.78 (1.08-2.95)	0.95 (0.85-1.07)	0.96 (0.84-1.09)	0.83 (0.53-1.29)
Obesity	1.07 (0.93-1.23)	0.99 (0.85-1.15)	1.47 (0.83-2.60)	1.00 (0.87-1.16)	0.96 (0.83-1.13)	1.76 (1.03-3.02)
Other diseases	1.08 (0.94-1.25)	1.08 (0.93-1.26)	0.77 (0.40-1.46)	1.12 (0.97-1.28)	1.06 (0.92-1.23)	1.31 (0.78-2.19)
Drugs						
Acetaminophen/paracetamol	0.95 (0.84-1.07)	0.96 (0.84-1.09)	0.80 (0.44-1.46)	0.92 (0.82-1.03)	0.88 (0.78-1.00)	1.18 (0.74-1.87)
Anti-asthmatic agents	0.96 (0.81-1.13)	1.03 (0.86-1.23)	0.50 (0.23-1.07)	0.92 (0.79-1.09)	0.96 (0.81-1.14)	0.78 (0.43-1.44)
Antibacterial agents	1.03 (0.92-1.16)	1.00 (0.89-1.13)	1.36 (0.82-2.26)	0.99 (0.88-1.11)	0.98 (0.87-1.10)	1.08 (0.69-1.69)
Anticonvulsants	1.16 (0.96-1.40)	1.19 (0.98-1.46)	0.87 (0.32-2.37)	1.07 (0.86-1.33)	1.05 (0.83-1.33)	0.95 (0.39-2.35)
Antihistamines	0.93 (0.76-1.14)	0.91 (0.73-1.12)	1.57 (0.61-4.04)	1.01 (0.83-1.23)	0.98 (0.79-1.22)	1.35 (0.65-2.77)
Antihyperlipidemic agents	1.33 (1.16-1.52)	1.21 (1.04-1.39)	2.79 (1.60-4.85)	1.32 (1.15-1.51)	1.19 (1.03-1.38)	2.41 (1.50-3.88)
Antihypertensive agents						
Angiotensin-converting enzyme inhibitors	1.11 (0.98-1.26)	1.12 (0.99-1.28)	0.80 (0.44-1.47)	1.00 (0.88-1.12)	0.98 (0.86-1.11)	0.88 (0.55-1.41)
Angiotensin receptor blockers	1.35 (1.16-1.57)	1.36 (1.16-1.60)	1.34 (0.65-2.75)	1.32 (1.14-1.52)	1.29 (1.11-1.51)	1.46 (0.83-2.58)
Beta blockers	1.04 (0.90-1.19)	1.03 (0.89-1.18)	1.46 (0.78-2.72)	1.09 (0.96-1.24)	1.05 (0.92-1.21)	1.49 (0.90-2.45)
Calcium channel blockers	1.00 (0.88-1.13)	1.04 (0.91-1.19)	0.29 (0.15-0.58)	0.94 (0.84-1.06)	0.99 (0.88-1.13)	0.51 (0.31-0.86)
Loop diuretics	0.95 (0.80-1.12)	0.91 (0.76-1.09)	1.00 (0.46-2.19)	1.40 (1.20-1.63)	1.31 (1.11-1.55)	1.94 (1.07-3.52)
Other antihypertensive agents	1.12 (0.97-1.29)	0.98 (0.81-1.19)	2.03 (0.82-5.03)	1.18 (1.02-1.36)	0.91 (0.74-1.12)	1.73 (0.76-3.95)
Thiazide diuretics	1.01 (0.84-1.22)	1.18 (1.02-1.37)	0.39 (0.17-0.94)	0.97 (0.80-1.18)	1.27 (1.10-1.48)	0.54 (0.28-1.02)
Anti-infective agents	0.97 (0.74-1.28)	1.00 (0.75-1.34)	0.59 (0.13-2.64)	0.78 (0.60-1.02)	0.72 (0.54-0.95)	0.80 (0.29-2.26)
Antiplatelet/anticoagulant agents	0.91 (0.81-1.03)	0.90 (0.79-1.02)	1.16 (0.65-2.07)	1.05 (0.93-1.18)	1.01 (0.89-1.14)	1.53 (0.94-2.50)

Table 3 Determinants of saxagliptin use among type 2 diabetes mellitus patients within United Kingdom data sources *(Continued)*

Non-steroidal anti-inflammatory agents	0.98 (0.84-1.14)	0.90 (0.79-1.02)	0.71 (0.30-1.69)	0.98 (0.84-1.15)	1.05 (0.89-1.24)	0.48 (0.24-0.96)
Other medications	1.03 (0.89-1.19)	1.03 (0.89-1.20)	0.63 (0.31-1.29)	1.09 (0.95-1.25)	1.12 (0.97-1.30)	0.79 (0.44-1.41)
Psychotropic agents	0.94 (0.83-1.07)	0.99 (0.87-1.13)	0.51 (0.25-1.05)	0.95 (0.83-1.07)	0.97 (0.85-1.11)	0.58 (0.34-1.00)

Abbreviations: OAD = oral anti-diabetic drug.
*Odds ratios adjusted for all other variables in this table.

the UK data sources. One exception was the finding that within THIN, obesity and diabetic nephropathy were more strongly associated with saxagliptin initiation among those with prior OAD use. However, stratifying on prior OAD use reduced the overall sample sizes within each stratum, particularly for patients without prior OAD use. As a result, these findings should be interpreted with caution.

These findings contribute to a growing body of research evaluating the characteristics of patients prescribed DPP-4 inhibitors. In three studies within the Ingenix (now Optum) administrative claims database [33-35], patients treated with sitagliptin, another DPP-4 inhibitor, were more likely to have medical comorbidities (i.e., cardiovascular disease, chronic kidney disease, hypertension, lipid disorders, and neuropathy) and were more frequently prescribed cardiovascular medications and insulin. In two additional studies within the General Electric Healthcare's Clinical Data Services electronic medical records database, patients prescribed sitagliptin were older and had a higher prevalence of preexisting comorbid conditions than patients prescribed other OAD therapies [36]. Patients prescribed sitagliptin were also more likely to have baseline microvascular and macrovascular complications of T2DM than patients receiving exenatide [37]. Our results expand understanding of the DPP-4 drug class by providing new data on determinants associated with saxagliptin initiation and including large samples of T2DM patients within the US and UK.

The observation that saxagliptin was prescribed to a large proportion of T2DM patients without prior OAD use in the US data sources (22% within US Medicare; 33% within HIRD[SM]) compared to the UK data sources (6%) is surprising given current guidelines recommending use of metformin as first-line OAD therapy [38]. A recent study utilizing the IMS Health Vector One National and Total Patient Tracker databases, a compilation of large commercial outpatient prescription and patient databases in the US, similarly found that 28% of non-insulin OAD users were not prescribed metformin and that DPP-4 inhibitors were the most commonly prescribed new drug class of agents [39]. The reasons why saxagliptin was more commonly prescribed as initial OAD treatment among T2DM patients within the US data

sources remain unclear. Decreased metformin use may be due, in part, to contraindications to the medication (e.g. renal insufficiency, active liver disease) [40-45]. Further studies are needed to evaluate the reasons for this deviation from recommended prescribing practices.

Since baseline characteristics of patients with T2DM have been shown to influence the efficacy of antidiabetic therapy [46,47], it will be important to evaluate the determinants of saxagliptin use identified in this study as effect modifiers and confounders in future comparative effectiveness and safety studies. Our results also provide valuable information on variables that should be considered for inclusion within propensity score analyses of saxagliptin use for future pharmacoepidemiologic studies evaluating the comparative effectiveness and safety of saxagliptin compared to other OADs [18].

A particular strength of our analysis was the inclusion of data from US Medicare. Prior studies that evaluated the characteristics of OAD initiators within the US [33-35,37], but did not include Medicare coverage, likely underrepresented T2DM patients over the age of 65 and may have incompletely captured claims among patients also co-enrolled in Medicare. By examining initiators of saxagliptin and other non-DPP-4 inhibitor OADs within four data sources (including US Medicare) and across two continents, our analyses ensured adequate capture and representation of elderly T2DM patients.

Our study has several potential limitations. First, we were unable to determine the duration of T2DM due to the use of administrative data (US data sources) and incomplete electronic health data from patients who may have switched practices (UK data sources). Second, actual exposure to saxagliptin and other OADs cannot be confirmed. However, minimal misclassification of medication use is expected since prescribing records within the UK data sources and pharmacy claims within the US data sources were used to determine drug exposure. Additionally, all relevant diagnosis and procedure codes were included and reviewed by clinical and pharmacoepidemiology experts to minimize misclassification of medical comorbidities examined as determinants of saxagliptin use. Third, some potentially important variables, including alcohol and illicit drug use,

Table 4 Determinants of saxagliptin use among type 2 diabetes mellitus patients within United States data sources

Characteristic	Adjusted odds ratio (95% confidence interval)*					
	US Medicare			HealthCore Integrated Research Database[SM]		
	Overall	Prior OAD use	No prior OAD use	Overall	Prior OAD use	No prior OAD use
	(n = 545,408)	(n = 177,791)	(n = 82,840)	(n = 85,865)	(n = 17,177)	(n = 22,803)
Number of hemoglobin A1c measurements						
1 vs. 0 measured	2.10 (2.04-2.16)	2.09 (2.02-2.16)	2.02 (1.91-2.12)	1.67 (1.56-1.78)	1.40 (1.27-1.54)	1.96 (1.77-2.17)
2+ vs. 0 measured	2.93 (2.85-3.01)	2.87 (2.77-2.97)	2.95 (2.78-3.12)	2.33 (2.16-2.51)	1.91 (1.72-2.12)	1.96 (1.77-2.17)
Severity of type 2 diabetes mellitus						
Cardiovascular	0.95 (0.93-0.97)	0.95 (0.93-0.98)	0.95 (0.90-1.00)	0.96 (0.88-1.05)	0.97 (0.86-1.10)	1.00 (0.76-1.32)
Cerebrovascular	0.90 (0.88-0.93)	0.92 (0.88-0.95)	0.87 (0.82-0.94)	0.92 (0.78-1.09)	0.93 (0.74-1.17)	0.90 (0.77-1.06)
Metabolic (ketoacidosis, hyperosmolar, coma)	0.95 (0.87-1.03)	0.91 (0.82-1.01)	1.06 (0.89-1.27)	-	-	-
Nephropathy	1.12 (1.09-1.15)	1.08 (1.05-1.12)	1.25 (1.18-1.32)	1.04 (0.93-1.18)	0.87 (0.75-1.02)	1.40 (1.14-1.72)
Neuropathy	1.11 (1.08-1.14)	1.08 (1.05-1.11)	1.22 (1.15-1.28)	1.01 (0.92-1.11)	1.05 (0.92-1.19)	1.03 (0.87-1.22)
Peripheral vascular disease	0.97 (0.94-1.00)	0.97 (0.94-1.01)	0.96 (0.91-1.02)	1.06 (0.92-1.21)	0.92 (0.77-1.11)	1.30 (1.03-1.63)
Retinopathy	1.03 (1.00-1.06)	1.01 (0.97-1.04)	1.09 (1.02-1.16)	1.02 (0.91-1.14)	0.95 (0.82-1.10)	1.11 (0.90-1.37)
Unspecified additional diabetic complications[†]	0.96 (0.92-0.99)	0.91 (0.82-1.01)	1.12 (1.04-1.22)	1.01 (0.89-1.14)	0.98 (0.83-1.16)	1.17 (0.93-1.47)
Diagnoses						
Allergic rhinitis/hay fever	1.16 (1.12-1.21)	1.19 (1.13-1.25)	1.14 (1.05-1.23)	1.12 (1.00-1.26)	1.29 (1.09-1.52)	0.95 (0.78-1.15)
Asthma	0.91 (0.87-0.94)	0.89 (0.85-0.94)	0.94 (0.87-1.02)	0.83 (0.72-0.95)	0.92 (0.76-1.13)	0.80 (0.63-1.02)
Chronic obstructive pulmonary disease	0.92 (0.89-0.95)	0.92 (0.88-0.95)	0.89 (0.83-0.95)	0.93 (0.79-1.08)	0.88 (0.70-1.09)	0.93 (0.72-1.21)
Collagen vascular disease/ autoimmune disorders	1.01 (0.95-1.08)	1.05 (0.97-1.14)	0.93 (0.82-1.06)	0.90 (0.79-1.03)	0.94 (0.79-1.12)	0.82 (0.66-1.03)
Rheumatoid arthritis[‡]	1.10 (1.03-1.16)	1.08 (1.00-1.17)	1.17 (1.04-1.32)	-	-	-
Spondyloarthritis[‡]	1.04 (1.00-1.09)	1.05 (1.00-1.10)	1.03 (0.95-1.12)	-	-	-
Dermatologic disorders	1.04 (0.99-1.10)	1.02 (0.96-1.09)	1.08 (0.98-1.20)	1.07 (0.93-1.23)	1.10 (0.90-1.34)	1.14 (0.90-1.44)
Psoriasis[‡]	0.97 (0.88-1.08)	0.99 (0.87-1.12)	0.86 (0.70-1.06)	-	-	-
Hyperlipidemia	1.11 (1.08-1.14)	1.11 (1.08-1.15)	1.11 (1.05-1.17)	1.17 (1.10-1.24)	1.17 (1.08-1.27)	1.11 (1.01-1.22)
Hypertension	1.00 (0.97-1.03)	1.01 (0.97-1.04)	0.99 (0.93-1.05)	1.13 (1.07-1.20)	1.17 (1.08-1.27)	1.18 (1.07-1.31)
Infectious diseases	0.86 (0.79-0.94)	0.88 (0.79-0.99)	0.85 (0.71-1.02)	0.89 (0.79-1.01)	1.17 (1.08-1.27)	0.95 (0.78-1.16)
Cellulitis[‡]	0.92 (0.88-0.95)	0.91 (0.87-0.95)	0.92 (0.85-1.00)	-	-	-
Malignancy	0.93 (0.90-0.97)	0.95 (0.91-0.99)	0.89 (0.83-0.96)	1.02 (0.90-1.17)	1.17 (1.08-1.27)	1.03 (0.83-1.27)
Obesity	0.94 (0.91-0.97)	0.96 (0.92-0.99)	0.90 (0.84-0.97)	0.88 (0.81-0.96)	0.95 (0.84-1.07)	0.76 (0.65-0.88)
Other diseases	-	-	-	0.92 (0.77-1.09)	0.94 (0.74-1.20)	0.93 (0.69-1.24)
Alcohol diseases[‡]	0.68 (0.61-0.76)	0.71 (0.62-0.81)	0.90 (0.84-0.97)	-	-	-
Gastrointestinal diseases[‡]	1.01 (0.95-1.06)	0.98 (0.91-1.05)	1.07 (0.95-1.20)	-	-	-
Neurological diseases[‡]	0.76 (0.63-0.93)	0.86 (0.68-1.08)	0.53 (0.35-0.82)	-	-	-
Drugs						
Acetaminophen/paracetamol	0.97 (0.94-0.99)	0.97 (0.94-1.00)	0.96 (0.91-1.01)	0.97 (0.91-1.04)	1.02 (0.93-1.12)	0.87 (0.78-0.98)
Anti-asthmatic agents	1.08 (1.05-1.12)	1.09 (1.05-1.14)	1.08 (1.01-1.16)	1.02 (0.93-1.13)	1.02 (0.88-1.17)	1.06 (0.89-1.25)
Antibacterial agents	1.08 (1.06-1.10)	1.08 (1.05-1.11)	1.08 (1.03-1.13)	1.07 (1.01-1.13)	1.12 (1.04-1.21)	0.95 (0.87-1.04)
Anticonvulsants	0.89 (0.85-0.93)	0.91 (0.87-0.96)	0.81 (0.74-0.90)	0.96 (0.87-1.06)	1.01 (0.88-1.16)	0.89 (0.75-1.07)
Antihistamines	1.10 (1.07-1.14)	1.10 (1.06-1.15)	1.09 (1.01-1.17)	1.05 (0.94-1.16)	1.05 (0.91-1.22)	1.11 (0.93-1.32)
Antihyperlipidemic agents	1.22 (1.19-1.24)	1.15 (1.12-1.19)	1.35 (1.29-1.41)	1.13 (1.07-1.19)	1.11 (1.03-1.20)	1.16 (1.06-1.28)
Antihypertensive agents						
Angiotensin-converting enzyme inhibitors	0.98 (0.96-1.01)	0.96 (0.94-0.99)	1.00 (0.96-1.05)	0.97 (0.91-1.02)	0.92 (0.85-1.00)	1.01 (0.90-1.12)
Angiotensin receptor blockers	1.39 (1.36-1.43)	1.32 (1.28-1.36)	1.59 (1.51-1.68)	1.22 (1.13-1.31)	1.07 (0.97-1.19)	1.44 (1.26-1.65)

Table 4 Determinants of saxagliptin use among type 2 diabetes mellitus patients within United States data sources (Continued)

Beta blockers	1.04 (1.02-1.06)	1.05 (1.02-1.08)	1.02 (0.98-1.07)	0.99 (0.93-1.06)	1.10 (1.00-1.20)	0.86 (0.76-0.97)
Calcium channel blockers	1.02 (0.99-1.04)	1.01 (0.98-1.04)	1.02 (0.97-1.07)	0.97 (0.90-1.04)	1.04 (0.94-1.14)	0.86 (0.76-0.99)
Loop diuretics	1.10 (1.07-1.13)	1.09 (1.05-1.12)	1.13 (1.07-1.20)	0.94 (0.83-1.06)	0.92 (0.79-1.08)	0.99 (0.80-1.22)
Other antihypertensive agents	1.11 (1.07-1.14)	1.11 (1.07-1.15)	1.09 (1.02-1.17)	1.06 (0.94-1.20)	1.05 (0.96-1.16)	0.99 (0.79-1.24)
Thiazidediuretics	1.14 (1.11-1.17)	1.14 (1.11-1.18)	1.14 (1.08-1.21)	0.99 (0.93-1.07)	1.05 (0.96-1.16)	0.83 (0.73-0.95)
Anti-infective agents	-	-	-	1.04 (0.95-1.14)	1.00 (0.88-1.14)	1.01 (0.86-1.18)
Antifungals[‡]	1.10 (1.06-1.14)	1.06 (1.02-1.10)	1.21 (1.13-1.30)	-	-	-
Antivirals[‡]	1.09 (1.02-1.16)	1.10 (1.02-1.19)	1.07 (0.93-1.23)	-	-	-
Antiplatelet/anticoagulant agents	0.94 (0.86-1.02)	0.97 (0.87-1.07)	0.91 (0.75-1.10)	0.98 (0.88-1.10)	0.98 (0.84-1.13)	1.07 (0.87-1.32)
Clopidogrel[†]	1.13 (1.10-1.17)	1.12 (1.08-1.16)	1.18 (1.11-1.26)	-	-	-
Warfarin[†]	0.96 (0.92-0.99)	0.99 (0.94-1.04)	0.85 (0.78-0.93)	-	-	-
Non-steroidal anti-inflammatory agents	1.06 (1.03-1.09)	1.05 (1.02-1.09)	1.09 (1.03-1.15)	1.02 (0.95-1.10)	1.05 (0.94-1.16)	0.99 (0.87-1.12)
Other medications	1.06 (1.01-1.12)	1.08 (1.01-1.15)	1.08 (0.96-1.22)	0.88 (0.81-0.96)	0.83 (0.75-0.93)	0.99 (0.85-1.14)
Allopurinol[‡]	1.05 (1.01-1.10)	1.06 (1.00-1.11)	1.07 (0.97-1.18)	-	-	-
Anti-arrhythmics[‡]	0.99 (0.96-1.02)	0.99 (0.95-1.02)	1.00 (0.94-1.08)	-	-	-
Immune modulators/ suppressants[‡]	1.05 (1.00-1.10)	1.01 (0.95-1.07)	1.16 (1.04-1.28)	-	-	-
Nitroglycerin[‡]	0.98 (0.94-1.03)	0.97 (0.92-1.03)	1.01 (0.92-1.13)	-	-	-
Urinary anti-spasmodics[‡]	1.03 (0.98-1.07)	1.03 (0.98-1.09)	1.05 (0.96-1.16)	-	-	-
Psychotropic agents	0.93 (0.91-0.95)	0.92 (0.89-0.94)	0.92 (0.87-0.96)	0.94 (0.88-1.00)	0.95 (0.87-1.04)	0.87 (0.77-0.97)

Abbreviations: OAD = oral anti-diabetic drug.

[*]Odds ratios adjusted for all other variables in this table.

[†]For HIRD[SM], due to low prevalence, metabolic complications are included in the analyses of unspecified additional diabetic complications.

[‡]Medications and diseases were evaluated separately within US Medicare because of the large sample size within this data source.

diet, exercise, family history of diseases, and nonprescription drug use, were not recorded within the data sources. Finally, our results may not be generalizable to all settings. However, our analyses have expanded the populations to which these findings can be generalized by examining results from four different data sources within the US and UK [48], which contain claims and medical records data from both private and public health insurance plans.

Conclusion

In summary, this study found that saxagliptin initiation was more common in patients with prior complications associated with T2DM, prior OAD use, and diagnoses and receipt of treatment for hyperlipidemia and hypertension. These variables should be considered in future studies evaluating the comparative safety and effectiveness of saxagliptin and other OADs.

Abbreviations

CPRD: Clinical Practice Research Datalink; DPP-4: Dipeptidyl peptidase-4; FDA: US Food and Drug Administration; HIRD[SM]: HealthCore Integrated Research Database[SM]; OAD: Oral anti-diabetic drug; T2DM: Type 2 diabetes mellitus; THIN: The Health Improvement Network; UK: United Kingdom; US: United States.

Competing interests

These series of studies are funded by AstraZeneca and Bristol-Myers Squibb. The study's sponsors approved the protocol and have the right to provide non-binding comments on resulting reports and manuscripts. All authors receive funding from AstraZeneca and Bristol-Myers Squibb through their employers. Further, Dr. Lo Re has received grant support (through the University of Pennsylvania) from Gilead Sciences, unrelated to oral anti-diabetic drugs. Dr. Hennessy has done consulting for AstraZeneca, unrelated to saxagliptin. Dr. Haynes, Dr. Holick, and Ms. Esposito are employed by HealthCore, Inc., and Ms. Bhullar is employed by CSD Medical Research. Each of these individuals' respective organizations conducts research for and receives funding from pharmaceutical manufacturers for its research services. Dr. Strom has done consulting for AstraZeneca and Bristol-Myers Squibb.

Authors' contributions

MES, DMC, CWN, JAR, MSN, KH, BLS, and VLR participated in the conception and design of the study. CNH, DBE, AG, and HB participated in data collection. CWN and JAR performed data management and analysis. MES, DMC, CWN, MSN, KH, and VLR collaborated on the initial drafts of the manuscript. All other authors contributed further to interpretation of the results and manuscript edits. All authors read and approved the final manuscript.

Acknowledgements

The authors would like to thank Jennifer Wood, PhD, MPH of Bristol-Myers Squibb and Laura Horne, MHS of AstraZeneca for their assistance with the HeathCore Integrated Research Database[SM], Clinical Practice Research Datalink, and The Health Improvement Network data sources. Industry sponsors were excluded from all analyses involving US Medicare data. The authors would also like to thank Cristin P. Freeman, MPH, MBE for her assistance in the ascertainment and use of US Medicare Data.

Author details

[1]Department of Biostatistics and Epidemiology, Center for Clinical Epidemiology and Biostatistics, Perelman School of Medicine at the University of Pennsylvania, 423 Guardian Drive, Philadelphia, PA, USA. [2]Department of Biostatistics and Epidemiology, Center for Pharmacoepidemiology Research and Training, Perelman School of Medicine at the University of Pennsylvania, Philadelphia, PA, USA. [3]HealthCore, Inc, Wilmington, DE, USA. [4]Department of Medicine, Perelman School of Medicine at the University of Pennsylvania, Philadelphia, PA, USA. [5]Clinical Practice Research Datalink, Medicines and Healthcare Products Regulatory Agency, London, UK. [6]Cegedim Strategic Data Medical Research, London, UK. [7]Rutgers Biomedical & Health Sciences, Rutgers, the State University of New Jersey, Newark, NJ, USA.

References

1. Danaei G, Finucane MM, Lu Y, Singh GM, Cowan MJ, Paciorek CJ, et al. National, regional, and global trends in fasting plasma glucose and diabetes prevalence since 1980: systematic analysis of health examination surveys and epidemiological studies with 370 country-years and 2.7 million participants. Lancet. 2011;378:31–40.
2. Wild S, Roglic G, Green A, Sicree R, King H. Global prevalence of diabetes: estimates for the year 2000 and projections for 2030. Diabetes Care. 2004;27:1047–53.
3. Gonzalez EL, Johansson S, Wallander MA, Rodriguez LA. Trends in the prevalence and incidence of diabetes in the UK: 1996–2005. J Epidemiol Community Health. 2009;63:332–6.
4. Centers for Disease Control and Prevention. National Diabetes Statistics Report: Estimates of Diabetes and Its Burden in the United States, 2014. Atlanta, GA: U.S. Department for Health and Human Services; 2014.
5. Huang ES, Basu A, O'Grady M, Capretta JC. Projecting the future diabetes population size and related costs for the U.S. Diabetes Care. 2009;32:2225–9.
6. Bolen S, Feldman L, Vassy J, Wilson L, Yeh HC, Marinopoulos S, et al. Systematic review: comparative effectiveness and safety of oral medications for type 2 diabetes mellitus. Ann Intern Med. 2007;147:386–99.
7. Tahrani AA, Piya MK, Barnett AH. Saxagliptin: a new DPP-4 inhibitor for the treatment of type 2 diabetes mellitus. Adv Ther. 2009;26:249–62.
8. Rosenstock J, Sankoh S, List JF. Glucose-lowering activity of the dipeptidyl peptidase-4 inhibitor saxagliptin in drug-naive patients with type 2 diabetes. Diabetes Obes Metab. 2008;10:376–86.
9. Jadzinsky M, Pfutzner A, Paz-Pacheco E, Xu Z, Allen E, Chen R. Saxagliptin given in combination with metformin as initial therapy improves glycaemic control in patients with type 2 diabetes compared with either monotherapy: a randomized controlled trial. Diabetes Obes Metab. 2009;11:611–22.
10. DeFronzo RA, Hissa MN, Garber AJ, Luiz Gross J, Yuyan Duan R, Ravichandran S, et al. The efficacy and safety of saxagliptin when added to metformin therapy in patients with inadequately controlled type 2 diabetes with metformin alone. Diabetes Care. 2009;32:1649–55.
11. Chacra AR, Tan GH, Apanovitch A, Ravichandran S, List J, Chen R. Saxagliptin added to a submaximal dose of sulphonylurea improves glycaemic control compared with uptitration of sulphonylurea in patients with type 2 diabetes: a randomised controlled trial. Int J Clin Pract. 2009;63:1395–406.
12. Hollander P, Li J, Allen E, Chen R, Investigators C. Saxagliptin added to a thiazolidinedione improves glycemic control in patients with type 2 diabetes and inadequate control on thiazolidinedione alone. J Clin Endocrinol Metab. 2009;94:4810–9.
13. Barnett AH, Charbonnel B, Donovan M, Fleming D, Chen R. Effect of saxagliptin as add-on therapy in patients with poorly controlled type 2 diabetes on insulin alone or insulin combined with metformin. Curr Med Res Opin. 2012;28:513–23.
14. SC Pradhan DGS, CH Shashindran, JS Bapna. Drug utilization studies. Natl Med J India 1988, 1:185–189.
15. Khan GH, Aqil M, Pillai KK, Ahmad MA, Kapur P, Ain MR, et al. Therapeutic adherence: a prospective drug utilization study of oral hypoglycemic in patients with type 2 diabetes mellitus. Asian Pac J Trop Dis. 2014;4(Supplement 1):S347–52.
16. Walker AM. Confounding by indication. Epidemiology. 1996;7:335–6.
17. Glynn RJ, Schneeweiss S, Stürmer T. Indications for propensity scores and review of their use in pharmacoepidemiology. Basic Clin Pharmacol Toxicol. 2006;98:253–9.
18. Lo Re V 3rd, Haynes K, Ming EE, Wood Ives J, Horne LN, Fortier K, et al. Safety of saxagliptin: rationale for and design of a series of postmarketing observational studies. Pharmacoepidemiol Drug Saf. 2012;21(11):202–15.
19. Williams T, van Staa T, Puri S, Eaton S. Recent advances in the utility and use of the General Practice Research Database as an example of a UK Primary Care Data resource. Ther Adv Drug Saf. 2012;3:89–99.
20. Horsfall LJ, Nazareth I, Petersen I. Serum uric acid and the risk of respiratory disease: a population-based cohort study. Thorax. 2014;69:1021–6.
21. Fett N, Haynes K, Propert KJ, Margolis DJ. Five-year malignancy incidence in patients with chronic pruritus: a population-based cohort study aimed at limiting unnecessary screening practices. J Am Acad Dermatol. 2014;70:651–8.
22. Lewis JD, Schinnar R, Bilker WB, Wang X, Strom BL. Validation studies of the health improvement network (THIN) database for pharmacoepidemiology research. Pharmacoepidemiol Drug Saf. 2007;16:393–401.
23. Lo Re V 3rd, Haynes K, Forde KA, Localio AR, Schinnar R, Lewis JD. Validity of The Health Improvement Network (THIN) for epidemiologic studies of hepatitis C virus infection. Pharmacoepidemiol Drug Saf. 2009;18:807–14.
24. Cai B, Xu W, Bortnichak E, Watson DJ. An algorithm to identify medical practices common to both the General Practice Research Database and The Health Improvement Network database. Pharmacoepidemiol Drug Saf. 2012;21:770–4.
25. Chan KA, Truman A, Gurwitz JH, Hurley JS, Martinson B, Platt R, et al. A cohort study of the incidence of serious acute liver injury in diabetic patients treated with hypoglycemic agents. Arch Intern Med. 2003;163:728–34.
26. Bullano MF, McNeeley BJ, Yu YF, Quimbo R, Burawski LP, Yu EB, et al. Comparison of costs associated with the use of etanercept, infliximab, and adalimumab for the treatment of rheumatoid arthritis. Manag Care Interface. 2006;19:47–53.
27. Sarawate C, Sikirica MV, Willey VJ, Bullano MF, Hauch O. Monitoring anticoagulation in atrial fibrillation. J Thromb Thrombolysis. 2006;21:191–8.
28. Kamat SA, Gandhi SK, Davidson M. Comparative effectiveness of rosuvastatin versus other statin therapies in patients at increased risk of failure to achieve low-density lipoprotein goals. Curr Med Res Opin. 2007;23:1121–30.
29. Young BA, Lin E, Von Korff M, Simon G, Ciechanowski P, Ludman EJ, et al. Diabetes complications severity index and risk of mortality, hospitalization, and healthcare utilization. Am J Manag Care. 2008;14:15–23.
30. American Diabetes Association. Standards of medical care in diabetes-2014. Diabetes Care. 2014;37(Supplement 1):S14–S280.
31. Mamdani M, Sykora K, Li P, Normand S-LT, Streiner DL, Austin PC, et al. Reader's guide to critical appraisal of cohort studies: 2. Assessing potential for confounding. BMJ: British Medical Journal. 2005;330:960–2.
32. Lee D, Bergman U. Studies of Drug Utilization. Pharmacoepidemiology. Fifth edn. Oxford, UK: John Wiley & Sons, Ltd.; 2012.
33. Dore DD, Seeger JD, Arnold Chan K. Use of a claims-based active drug safety surveillance system to assess the risk of acute pancreatitis with exenatide or sitagliptin compared to metformin or glyburide. Curr Med Res Opin. 2009;25:1019–27.
34. Cai B, Katz L, Alexander CM, Williams-Herman D, Girman CJ. Characteristics of patients prescribed sitagliptin and other oral antihyperglycaemic agents in a large US claims database. Int J Clin Pract. 2010;64:1601–8.
35. Brodovicz KG, Kou TD, Alexander CM, O'Neill EA, Senderak M, Engel SS, et al. Recent trends in the characteristics of patients prescribed sitagliptin and other oral antihyperglycaemic agents in a large U.S. claims database. Int J Clin Pract. 2013;67:449–54.
36. Zhang Q, Rajagopalan S, Mavros P, Engel SS, Davies MJ, Yin D, et al. Baseline characteristic differences between patients prescribed sitagliptin vs. other oral antihyperglycemic agents: analysis of a US electronic medical record database. Curr Med Res Opin. 2010;26:1697–703.
37. Zhang Q, Rajagopalan S, Mavros P, Engel SS, Davies MJ, Yin D, et al. Differences in baseline characteristics between patients prescribed sitagliptin versus exenatide based on a US electronic medical record database. Adv Ther. 2010;27:223–32.
38. Inzucchi SE, Bergenstal RM, Buse JB, Diamant M, Ferrannini E, Nauck M, et al. Management of hyperglycemia in type 2 diabetes: a patient-centered approach: position statement of the American Diabetes Association (ADA) and the

European Association for the Study of Diabetes (EASD). Diabetes Care. 2012;35:1364–79.

39. Hampp C, Borders-Hemphill V, Moeny DG, Wysowski DK. Use of antidiabetic drugs in the U.S., 2003–2012. Diabetes Care. 2014;37:1367–74.

40. Flory JH, Hennessy S. Metformin Use Reduction in Mild to Moderate Renal Impairment: Possible Inappropriate Curbing of Use Based on Food and Drug Administration Contraindicaitons. JAMA Intern Med. 2014.

41. Sulkin TV, Bosman D, Krentz AJ. Contraindications to metformin therapy in patients with NIDDM. Diabetes Care. 1997;20:925–8.

42. Calabrese AT, Coley KC, DaPos SV, Swanson D, Rao RH. Evaluation of prescribing practices: risk of lactic acidosis with metformin therapy. Arch Intern Med. 2002;162:434–7.

43. Kennedy L, Herman WH. Renal status among patients using metformin in a primary care setting. Diabetes Care. 2005;28:922–4.

44. Vasisht KP, Chen SC, Peng Y, Bakris GL. Limitations of metformin use in patients with kidney disease: are they warranted? Diabetes Obes Metab. 2010;12:1079–83.

45. Horlen C, Malone R, Bryant B, Dennis B, Carey T, Pignone M, et al. Frequency of inappropriate metformin prescriptions. JAMA. 2002;287:2504–5.

46. Bloomgarden ZT, Dodis R, Viscoli CM, Holmboe ES, Inzucchi SE. Lower baseline glycemia reduces apparent oral agent glucose-lowering efficacy: a meta-regression analysis. Diabetes Care. 2006;29:2137–9.

47. Chapell R, Gould AL, Alexander CM. Baseline differences in A1C explain apparent differences in efficacy of sitagliptin, rosiglitazone and pioglitazone. Diabetes Obes Metab. 2009;11:1009–16.

48. Hall GC, Sauer B, Bourke A, Brown JS, Reynolds MW, Casale RL. Guidelines for good database selection and use in pharmacoepidemiology research. Pharmacoepidemiol Drug Saf. 2012;21:1–10.

13

Genetic variability in drug transport, metabolism or DNA repair affecting toxicity of chemotherapy in ovarian cancer

Sandrina Lambrechts[1*†], Diether Lambrechts[2,3†], Evelyn Despierre[1], Els Van Nieuwenhuysen[1], Dominiek Smeets[2,3], Philip R Debruyne[4], Vincent Renard[5], Philippe Vroman[6], Daisy Luyten[7], Patrick Neven[1], Frédéric Amant[1], Karin Leunen[1], Ignace Vergote[1] and on behalf of the Belgian and Luxembourg Gynaecological Oncology Group (BGOG)

Abstract

Background: This study aimed to determine whether single nucleotide polymorphisms (SNPs) in genes involved in DNA repair or metabolism of taxanes or platinum could predict toxicity or response to first-line chemotherapy in ovarian cancer.

Methods: Twenty-six selected SNPs in 18 genes were genotyped in 322 patients treated with first-line paclitaxel-carboplatin or carboplatin mono-therapy. Genotypes were correlated with toxicity events (anemia, neutropenia, thrombocytopenia, febrile neutropenia, neurotoxicity), use of growth factors and survival.

Results: The risk of anemia was increased for variant alleles of rs1128503 (*ABCB1, C > T*; $p = 0.023$, OR = 1.71, 95% CI = 1.07-2.71), rs363717 (*ABCA1, A > G*; $p = 0.002$, OR = 2.08, 95% CI = 1.32-3.27) and rs11615 (*ERCC1, T > C*; $p = 0.031$, OR = 1.61, 95% CI = 1.04-2.50), while it was decreased for variant alleles of rs12762549 (*ABCC2, C > G*; $p = 0.004$, OR = 0.51, 95% CI = 0.33-0.81). Likewise, increased risk of thrombocytopenia was associated with rs4986910 (*CYP3A4, T > C*; $p = 0.025$, OR = 4.99, 95% CI = 1.22-20.31). No significant correlations were found for neurotoxicity. Variant alleles of rs2073337 (*ABCC2, A > G*; $p = 0.039$, OR = 0.60, 95% CI = 0.37-0.98), rs1695 (*ABCC1, A > G*; $p = 0.017$, OR = 0.55, 95% CI 0.33-0.90) and rs1799793 (*ERCC2, G > A*; $p = 0.042$, OR = 0.63, 95% CI 0.41-0.98) associated with the use of colony stimulating factors (CSF), while rs2074087 (*ABCC1, G > C*; $p = 0.011$, OR = 2.09, 95% CI 1.18-3.68) correlated with use of erythropoiesis stimulating agents (ESAs). Homozygous carriers of the rs1799793 (*ERCC2, G > A*) G-allele had a prolonged platinum-free interval ($p = 0.016$).

Conclusions: Our data reveal significant correlations between genetic variants of transport, hepatic metabolism, platinum related detoxification or DNA damage repair and toxicity or outcome in ovarian cancer.

Keywords: Ovarian cancer, Chemotherapy, Toxicity, SNPs, Pharmacogenetics

Background

Ovarian cancer is the fifth most common cause of cancer death in women and the leading cause of gynaecological cancer-related death in the developed world [1]. Despite optimization of debulking surgery and chemotherapy regimens, the overall 5-year survival in advanced stage disease is only 29% [2]. The current standard first-line chemotherapy is a combination of paclitaxel and carboplatin. This treatment is associated with serious hematologic toxicities including grade 3–4 anemia (incidence 4.3-6.6%), grade 3–4 thrombocytopenia (4.7-12.9%), grade 3–4 neutropenia (37-89%), febrile neutropenia (2.3-8%) [3-6] and grade 2–4 peripheral neuropathies (32-36%), resulting in dose reductions, treatment delays and representing an important physical, psychological and financial burden for the patient and society. Inter-individual differences in both toxicity and outcome related to treatment with paclitaxel-

* Correspondence: sandrina.lambrechts@uzleuven.be
†Equal contributors
[1]Division of Gynaecologic Oncology and Leuven Cancer Institute, University Hospitals Leuven, KU Leuven, Herestraat 49, 3000 Leuven, Belgium
Full list of author information is available at the end of the article

carboplatin are reported. A few patient-related risk factors for toxicity have been identified, such as elderly age (≥65 years), poor performance status and poor nutritional status [7]. Furthermore, tumor-related factors including advanced stage at diagnosis, high-grade serous disease and residual tumor after debulking surgery are associated with poor survival. Genetic variability represents another potential factor explaining this inter-individual variability.

Genes related to drug transport, metabolism, detoxification and DNA repair could influence the cytotoxic effects associated with chemotherapy, including those involved in the transport (e.g., *ABCB1, ABCC1, ABCC2, ABCG2,* and *SLCO1B3*) [8-24], hepatic metabolism (*CYP3A4, CYP3A5, CYP2C8, CYP1B1*) [8-12,14,18,25-27] and pharmacodynamics (e.g., *MAPT, TUBB, TP53*) [28,29] of paclitaxel. Likewise, genes involved in detoxification (e.g., *GSTP1, GSTT1, GSTM1*) [30-33] and base-excision DNA repair (e.g., *ERCC1, ERCC2, XRCC1*) [34,35] have previously been linked with cytotoxicity of platinum agents. In particular, genetic variants in these genes, which generally are supposed to reduce the function of the affected gene, have been proposed to underlie the inter-individual differences in chemotherapy related hematologic and neurotoxicity. Likewise, variants in other genes, including *SLC12A6, SERPINB2, PPARD* and *ICAM* have been proposed to contribute to chemotherapy-induced peripheral neurotoxicity [36]. Most studies identifying these candidate genes, however, have been performed in small study populations and were limited to testing only a few variants. Consequently, most of the reported associations have failed to be replicated in subsequent large-scale validation studies. Furthermore, most studies did not correlate genotypes with detailed clinical toxicity data.

In the current study, we therefore aimed to assess prior associations for 26 selected genetic variants in 18 genes, in a large cohort of 322 ovarian cancer patients treated with paclitaxel-carboplatin combination therapy or carboplatin mono-therapy of whom detailed clinical toxicity data were available.

Methods

Study population

All ovarian cancer patients presenting in participating hospitals of the Belgian and Luxembourg Gynaecological Oncology Group (BGOG) were recruited for this study. Collection of germ-line DNA and baseline patient characteristics were collected for each patient. Disease characteristics were recorded after histologic examination with registration of tumor stage according to the International Federation of Gynecology and Obstetrics (FIGO) classification, residual disease after debulking surgery, measurement of tumor size on computed tomography (CT) scans and determination of cancer antigen 125 (CA125) before, during and after chemotherapy. Response to treatment

and disease progression were evaluated based on radiologic examination according to the Response Evaluation Criteria in Solid Tumors Group (RECIST) criteria [37]. Paclitaxel was administered at a starting dose of 175 mg/m^2 and carboplatin at a starting area under the plasma concentration-versus time curve (AUC) of 5–7 mg/ml/min, with possible dose reductions after the occurrence of severe toxicity. During treatment, the use of erythropoiesis stimulating agents (ESAs) and colony stimulating factors (CSFs) was conform to uniform institutional standards; ESAs are given during treatment with chemotherapy in symptomatic patients with a hemoglobin level below 11 g/dl while CSFs are given if (1) neutropenia grade 4 (ANC <500/mm^3) together with fever > 38°C *or* (2) neutropenia grade 4 (ANC < 500/mm^3) during minimum 5 consecutive days. Toxicity during chemotherapy was systematically and routinely scored according to the Common Terminology for Adverse Events (CTCAE) version 4.0. Hematological toxicity was scored based on routinely performed weekly complete blood counts during treatment and before each cycle to determine the nadir of anemia, neutropenia and thrombocytopenia of each administered cycle, neurotoxicity was scored at each clinical-physical examination before each cycle. The scored toxicities for each patient together with all events of neutropenic fever and use of growth factors were systematically recorded in medical electronic records and for the purpose of the present study retrospectively collected by two independent investigators. The highest grade of toxicity over all courses within a patient was reported, if weekly performed blood counts were not available for each administered cycle or if neurotoxicity was not scored for every cycle, the patient was excluded from the analysis. The primary objective of this study was the correlation of genetic variation with the occurrence of hematologic toxicity or neurotoxicity in patients treated with first-line carboplatin with or without paclitaxel. Secondary objectives included the relation between genetic variation and the need for growth factors during treatment with chemotherapy, platinum-free interval (PFI) defined as the time between the last first-line platinum dose and progression, and overall survival (OS). Analyses for PFI and OS were performed in the population receiving a combination of carboplatin and paclitaxel (n = 266) with exclusion of the more favorable prognostic population receiving carboplatin alone, based on clinical prognostic parameters such as FIGO stage, tumor grade and histological subtype. All included patients provided written informed consent before enrollment. The Medical Ethics Committee of the Leuven University Hospitals approved the study (ML6541), serving as central site with the authority to approve the study for all participating sites.

Genotyping

We performed an extensive literature search before start of enrolment to identify genes associated with treatment outcome or toxicity after platinum and/or paclitaxel administration [8-34,36]. We then selected common missense or synonymous mutations in these genes, as well as a number of SNPs that were located in the promoter region of these genes, but have previously been correlated with toxicity after platinum. In addition, we selected 5 additional SNPs previously associated with thalidomide-related neuropathy to investigate their role in repair mechanisms and inflammation in the peripheral nervous system leading to altered neurotoxicity, rather than having a thalidomide-specific contribution to correlated neurotoxicity [36]. Genomic DNA was extracted from the leucocyte fraction of whole blood samples (Qiagen DNeasy blood and tissue kit). All selected SNPs were genotyped using Sequenom MassARRAY technology (Sequenom Inc., CA, USA), as reported previously [38]. Overall 26 SNPs in 18 genes (Table 1) were genotyped with an individual call rate >95% and an overall success rate >98.5%. We genotyped 15 duplicate samples revealing a genotype accuracy exceeding 99%.

Statistical analysis

We calculated median values and inter-quartile ranges for all continuous variables, while frequencies and percentages were calculated for categorical variables. Genotype frequencies were tested for Hardy-Weinberg equilibrium using a 1°-of-freedom $\chi 2$-test and considered significant at P < 0.05. Each of the variants were correlated with toxicity events (i.e., the primary objective) using binary logistic regression, while assuming an additive genotypic model. Per-allele odds ratios (OR) and their respective 95% confidence intervals (CI) are reported. Regression analyses were performed without correction for covariates and after correction for relevant covariates, including age and BMI at the time of treatment, dose of carboplatin per cycle (AUC), number of administered cycles and treatment regimen (paclitaxel/carboplatin versus carboplatin alone). For anemia, an additional covariate was included, i.e., use of ESAs, whereas for neutropenia and febrile neutropenia, use of CSFs was included as an additional covariate. Secondary objectives, PFI and OS, were analyzed for 26 variants using Cox-regression analysis, adjusted for age at diagnosis only or fully adjusted for age at diagnosis, FIGO stage, tumor grade, tumor histology and residual disease after debulking surgery and PFS and OS estimates were calculated using Kaplan-Meier method. Additionally, we investigated which of the variants could predict the need for ESAs or CSFs during treatment. All tests were two-sided and statistical significance was set at p = 0.05. The Bonferroni p-value threshold correcting for the multiple testing of 26

SNPs was p < 0.0019. Statistical analyses were performed using SPSS version 19 (SPSS for Windows, Rel. 19.0.0. 2010. Chicago, Illinois, USA: SPSS Inc.)

Results

Study population

Between January 2009 and December 2011 (pre-specified period of 2 years), we recruited 322 ovarian cancer patients treated with 3–6 cycles paclitaxel-carboplatin combination therapy (n = 266) or 3–6 cycles carboplatin mono-therapy (n = 56) (Additional file 1: Figure S1). Of all recruited patients, 99% was Caucasian (Table 2). Hematological toxicity was analyzed in 290 patients, after exclusion of patients for which weekly blood examinations were not available (n = 32). For neurotoxicity, 56 patients treated with carboplatin monotherapy were excluded since the incidence of sensory neuropathy was significantly lower in this population (p < 0.001). One patient with pre-existing sensory neuropathy before start of chemotherapy was additionally excluded, bringing the total number of patients eligible up to 265. For the secondary objectives, PFI and OS, all patients treated with paclitaxel-carboplatin (n = 266) were included. Patient, disease and toxicity characteristics are summarized in Table 2. Briefly, grade 3–4 anemia was present in 57 patients (19.7%), grade 3–4 thrombocytopenia in 57 patients (19.7%), grade 4 neutropenia in 202 patients (69.7%), whereas only 23 patients (7.9%) presented with grade 3–4 febrile neutropenia. In the group of patients selected for neurotoxicity analysis, 48 patients (18.1%) developed grade 2–3 sensory and none motor neuropathy following combination treatment with paclitaxel-carboplatin. Minor allele frequencies (MAF) were similar to those reported previously in Caucasians and adhered to Hardy-Weinberg equilibrium. Allele frequencies of all genotyped SNPs are shown in Additional file 2: Table S1.

Association with anemia, thrombocytopenia, neutropenia and sensory neuropathy

Among the 290 patients eligible for the hematological toxicity analysis, we observed significant associations for 5 variants (Table 3). In particular, rs1128503 (*ABCB1, C > T*), rs12762549 (*ABCC2, C > G*), rs363717 (*ABCA1, A > G*) and rs11615 (*ERCC1, T > C*) were significantly associated with grade 3–4 anemia (p = 0.035, OR 1.58; p = 0.005, OR 0.55; p = 0.001, OR 1.31 and p = 0.024, OR = 1.58). After correction for relevant covariates (as explained in the statistical methods), these variants were still significantly associated with toxicity (p = 0.023, OR 1.71; p = 0.004, OR 0.51; p = 0.002, OR 2.08; and p = 0.031, OR 1.61 respectively). Another variant rs4986910 (*CYP3A4, T > C*) correlated with thrombocytopenia grade 3–4, before and after correction for relevant covariates (p = 0.012, OR 5.61 and p = 0.025, OR 4.99 respectively; Table 3).

Table 1 Overview of the 26 genotyped single nucleotide polymorphisms (SNPs)

Gene	Name	Function of the gene product	Variant allele (rs number, nucleotide, amino acid change)	Effect of the polymorphism on the toxicity or clinical outcome
ABCB1	Multidrug resistance 1, P-glycoprotein	ATP binding membrane transporter implicated in efflux of cytotoxic agents	rs1128503, c.1236C>T, Gly412Gly	Homozygous carriers of the variant allele: docetaxel clearance decreased [9].
			rs1045642, c.3435C>T, Ile1145Ile	Variant allele carriers: more pronounced neutrophil depression following treatment with paclitaxel ± carboplatin [18] and increased AUC of the paclitaxel metabolite 3'-p-hydroxypaclitaxel [8].
				Homozygous carriers of the variant allele: decreased risk of neutropenia and neurotoxicity [11]
				No correlation was found with pharmacokinetics, toxicity or outcome in OC patients in different other studies [9,10,12,13,15,17].
			rs2229109,c.1199G>A, Ser400Asn	Variant allele carriers: correlation with in vitro resistance to paclitaxel [22].
ABCC1	Multidrug resistance-associated protein 1	ATP binding membrane transporter implicated in efflux of cytotoxic drugs	rs2230671, c.4002G>A, Ser1334Ser	In vitro evidence: over-expression of ABCC1 protein has been associated with a low degree of resistance to paclitaxel [23].
			rs2074087, c.2284-30G>C	No correlation of variants in rs2230671 and rs2074087 with toxicity and outcome after platinum/taxane treatment in OC patients [12].
ABCC2	Multidrug resistance-associated protein 2	ATP binding membrane transporter implicated in efflux of cytotoxic drugs	rs2073337, c.1668+148A>G	In vitro evidence: paclitaxel and docetaxel are ABCC2 substrates in cell lines [24]. No correlation was found with toxicity or treatment outcome with platinum-taxane treatment in OC patients [12,17].
			rs12762549, g.101620771C>G	Variant allele carriers from Japan: increased risk for severe neutropenia following treatment with docetaxel [19].
ABCG2	ATP-binding cassette sub-family G member 2	ATP binding membrane transporter implicated in efflux of cytotoxic drugs	rs2231142, c.421C>A, Gln141Lys	Variant allele carriers in OC: 6-month longer median PFS following platinum/taxane-based chemotherapy [17].
ABCA1	ATP-binding cassette sub-family A member 1	ATP binding membrane transporter, efflux pump for S1P and cholesterol	rs363717, c.*1896 A>G	Variant allele carriers: decreased risk on thalidomide related neuropathy grade ≥2 [36].
SCLO1B3	Solute carrier organic anion transporter family member 1B3	Hepatocyte membrane transporter involved in the transport of cytotoxic drugs	rs4149117, 334T>G, Ser112Ala	Docetaxel and paclitaxel transport by SCLO1B3-expressing oocytes was higher compared to controls in vitro [20].
			rs11045585, c.1683-5676A>G	Variant allele carriers from Japan: increased docetaxel induced leukopenia/neutropenia [19], higher docetaxel clearance and lower AUC in nasopharyngeal carcinoma patients [21].
CYP1B1	Cytochrome P450 family 1, subfamily B, polypeptide 1	Enzyme in the oxidative metabolic pathway of exogenous chemicals including taxanes and estrogens	rs1056836, 4326C>G, Val432Leu (CYP1B1*3)	Homozygous carriers of the wild-type allele: decreased risk of grade 3/4 gastro-intestinal toxicity in docetaxel treated OC patients in the development but not in the validation set [12].
CYP3A4	Cytochrome P450, family 3, subfamily A, polypeptide 4	Enzyme in the oxidative metabolic pathway of exogenous chemicals including taxanes and estrogens	rs2740574, g.135607G>A (CYP3A4*1B)	CYP3A4 activity determined the dominant metabolic pathway for paclitaxel [14].
				Homozygous carriers of the variant allele: decreased clearance of docetaxel [26].
				Homozygous carriers of the variant allele: increased risk of invasive OC [27].

Table 1 Overview of the 26 genotyped single nucleotide polymorphisms (SNPs) (Continued)

			rs4986910, c.1331T>C, Met444Thr (CYP3A4*3)	No correlation with pharmacokinetics, toxicity or outcome in OC patients treated with carboplatin + paclitaxel or docetaxel [9,10,12].
CYP3A5	Cytochrome P450, family 3, subfamily A, polypeptide 5	Enzyme in the oxidative metabolic pathway of exogenous chemicals including taxanes and estrogens	rs776746, c.219-237G>A	Homozygous carriers of the variant allele: increased neurotoxicity following paclitaxel treatment [25]. No correlation with pharmacokinetics, toxicity or outcome in OC patients treated with carboplatin + paclitaxel or docetaxel [9,10,12].
TP53	Tumor protein 53	Transcription factor regulating multiple cellular functions, critical for maintenance of genomic stability	rs1042522, c.215C>G, Pro72Arg	Associated with a small increase in risk of OC [29], twofold increased risk of OC in proline carriers and a longer progression-free survival in homozygous arginine allele carriers [28]. Homozygous carriers of the variant allele: increased severity of neutropenia [32].
MAPT	Microtubule-associated protein tau	Protein stimulating tubulin polymerization, stabilizing microtubules	rs11568305, c.215C>G, Pro587=	No correlation with toxicity or outcome in OC patients treated with carboplatin + paclitaxel or docetaxel [12].
GSTP1	Gluthathione S-transferase pi	Xenobiotic enzyme involved in the prevention of platinum-based DNA damage	rs1695, c.313A>G, Ile105Val	Variant allele carriers: decreased oxaliplatin-related neuropathy [30], decreased docetaxel-induced grade 2 neuropathy [31], decreased risk of hematologic toxicity [15].
			rs1138272, c.341 C>T, Ala114Val	Variant allele carriers compared to homozygous carriers of the wild-type allele: decreased PFS following cisplatin-gemcitabine [32].
				In other studies, no association with toxicity in OC patients [12,32].
ERCC1	Excision repair cross complementation group1	Enzyme involved in nucleotide excision repair of DNA	rs11615, c.354T>C, Asn118Asn	Variant allele carriers: decreased platinum resistance [34].
			rs3212961, 17677G>T	Variant allele carriers compared to homozygous carriers of the wild-type allele: increased risk on severe neutropenia and increased likelihood of overall survival following cisplatin-gemcitabine [32].
				No correlation for both genetic variants with toxicity/outcome for OC patients [12].
ERCC2	Excision repair cross complementation group2	Enzyme involved in nucleotide excision repair of DNA	rs1799793, c.934G>A, Asp312Asn	Variant allele carriers: increased severity of neutropenia in OC patients receiving cisplatin-cyclophosphamide [33].
SLC12A6	Solute carrier family 12 member 6	Integral membrane protein that lowers intracellular chloride concentrations	rs7164902,g.34551082G>A, Leu144Leu	Variant allele carriers: decreased risk on thalidomide related neuropathy grade ≥2 [36].
SERPINB2	Serpin peptidase inhibitor B member 2	Inhibitor of urokinase plasminogen activator, mediating neuro-inflammation	rs6104, 1238C>G, Ser413Cys	Variant allele carriers: decreased risk on thalidomide related neuropathy grade ≥2 [36].
PPARD	Peroxisome proliferator-activated receptor delta	Nuclear receptor protein playing a role in neuro-inflammation	rs2076169, T>C	Variant allele carriers: decreased risk on thalidomide related neuropathy grade ≥2 [36].
ICAM1	Intercellular Adhesion Molecule 1	Cell surface glycoprotein in endothelial and immune system cells	rs1799969, 241G>A	Variant allele carriers: decreased risk on thalidomide related neuropathy grade ≥2 [36].

The following 7 genetic variants failed genotyping: rs2032582 (Ser893Ala in ABCB1), rs2273697 (Val417Ile in ABCC2), rs1058930 (Ile194Met in CYP2C8), rs11572080 (Arg69Lyes in CYP2C8), rs10509681 (Lys329Arg in CYP2C8), rs12721627 (Thr185Ser in CYP3A4), rs25487 (Gln398Arg in XRCC1). Rs6103 was replaced by rs6104 because these were in full linkage disequilibrium (r^2 = 1.0). OC: ovarian cancer, NSCLS: non-small-cell lung carcinoma.

Table 2 Patient and disease characteristics, hematologic and neuro-toxicity characteristics

Patient and disease characteristics

	Total Number of patients recruited N=322	Population for hematologic analysis			Population for outcome
		All patients N=290	Paclitaxel-Carboplatin N=240	Carboplatin N=50	N=266
Age at diagnosis (years)		p=0.188*		p=0.218§	p=0.128*
Median	60	59	59	56	59
Range	(20-85)	(20-85)	(21-82)	(20-85)	(21-84)
Body mass index (BMI)		p=0.863*		p=0.063§	p=0.055*
Median	25	25	24	26	24
Range	(16-39)	(16-39)	(16-39)	(18-37)	(16-39)
Race		p=0.951*		p=0.517§	p=0.520*
Caucasian	319 (99%)	287 (99%)	238 (99%)	49 (98%)	264 (99%)
African	1 (<1%)	1 (<1%)	0 (0%)	1 (<1%)	0 (0%)
Asian	1 (<1%)	1 (<1%)	1 (<1%)	0 (0%)	1 (<1%)
Mixed: Asian-Indo-European	1 (<1%)	1 (<1%)	1 (<1%)	0 (0%)	1 (<1%)
Histologic subtype		p=0.532*		p<0.001§	p<0.001*
Serous	258 (80%)	230 (79%)	209 (87%)	21 (42%)	231 (87%)
Mucinous	20 (6%)	19 (7%)	5 (2%)	14 (28%)	6 (2%)
Endometrioid	13 (4%)	13 (4%)	5 (2%)	8 (16%)	5 (2%)
Clear cell	17 (5%)	14 (5%)	8 (3%)	6 (12%)	11 (4%)
Mixed cell	8 (3%)	8 (3%)	7 (3%)	1 (2%)	7 (3%)
Other epithelial ovarian cancer	3 (1%)	3 (1%)	3 (1%)	0 (0%)	3 (1%)
Non-epithelial	3 (1%)	3 (1%)	3 (1%)	0 (0%)	3 (1%)
FIGO stage		p=0.645*		p<0.001§	p<0.001*
I	55 (15%)	52 (18%)	11 (5%)	41 (82%)	14 (5%)
II	17 (5%)	15 (5%)	13 (5%)	2 (4%)	15 (6%)
III	196 (61%)	175 (60%)	169 (70%)	6 (12%)	184 (69%)
IV	54 (17%)	48 (17%)	47 (20%)	1 (2%)	53 (20%)
Tumor grade		p=0.235*		p<0.001§	p<0.001*
1	23 (7%)	23 (8%)	13(5%)	10 (20%)	13 (5%)
2	50 (16%)	45 (16%)	30 (12%)	15 (30%)	35 (13%)
3	249 (77%)	222 (77%)	197 (82%)	25 (50%)	218 (82%)
Residual disease		p=0.120*		p<0.001§	p=0.424*
No macroscopic disease	267 (83%)	246 (85%)	200 (83%)	46 (92%)	218 (82%)
Macroscopic disease < 1cm	7 (2%)	6 (2%)	6 (3%)	0 (0%)	7 (3%)
Macroscopic disease > 1 cm	8 (3%)	6 (2%)	6 (3%)	0 (0%)	8 (3%)
Macroscopic disease, size unknown	5 (2%)	4 (1%)	3 (1%)	1 (2%)	4 (2%)
Macroscopic disease, inoperable	35 (11%)	28 (10%)	25 (10%)	3 (6%)	29 (11%)

Hematologic toxicity characteristics

	All patients (N= 290)	Paclitaxel-Carboplatin (N=240)	Carboplatin (N=50)
Number of cycles administered			p=0.266§
<6	15 (5%)	14 (6%)	1 (2%)
6	275 (95%)	226 (94%)	49 (98%)

Table 2 Patient and disease characteristics, hematologic and neuro-toxicity characteristics *(Continued)*

Grade anemia				$p=0.118^§$
0/1	62 (21%)	51 (21%)	11 (22%)	
2	171 (59%)	136 (57%)	35 (70%)	
3	51 (18%)	48 (20%)	3 (6%)	
4	6 (2%)	5 (2%)	1 (2%)	
Use of Erythropoiesis stimulating Agent (ESA)				$p=0.073^§$
No	220 (76%)	187 (78%)	33 (66%)	
Yes	70 (24%)	53 (22%)	17 (34%)	
Grade neutropenia				$p<0.001^§$
0/1	19 (7%)	9 (4%)	10 (20%)	
2	14 (5%)	3 (1%)	11 (22%)	
3	55 (19%)	32 (13%)	23 (46%)	
4	202 (70%)	196 (82%)	6 (12%)	
Febrile neutropenia				$p=0.740^§$
0	267 (92%)	217 (90%)	50 (100%)	
3	22 (8%)	22 (9%)	0 (0%)	
4	1 (<1%)	1 (<1%)	0 (0%)	
Use of colony stimulating factor (CSF)				$p<0.001^§$
No	228 (79%)	178 (74%)	50 (100%)	
Yes	62 (21%)	62 (26%)	0 (0%)	
Grade Trombocytopenia				$p=0.089^§$
0/1	180 (62%)	156 (65%)	24 (48%)	
2	53 (18%)	41 (17%)	12 (24%)	
3	43 (15%)	31 (13%)	12 (24%)	
4	14 (5%)	12 (5%)	2 (4%)	

Neurotoxicity characteristics	Population for neurotoxicity analysis (Paclitaxel-Carboplatin) (N=265)	Population excluded for neurotoxicity (Carboplatin) (N=56)
Number of cycles administered		$p=0.596^\#$
<6	18 (7%)	2 (4%)
6	247 (93%)	54 (96%)
Grade peripheral sensory neuropathy		$p<0.001^\#$
0	109 (41%)	48 (86%)
1	108 (41%)	6 (11%)
2	39 (15%)	1 (2%)
3	9 (3%)	0 (0%)
Grade motor neuropathy		$p=0.461^\#$
0	56 (100%)	254 (96%)
1	0 (0%)	10 (4%)
2	0 (0%)	1 (<1%)
3	0 (0%)	0 (0%)
4	0 (0%)	0 (0%)

*: p-value calculated against the total population (n = 322), §: p-value calculated against the population for hematologic analysis treated with taxol-carboplatin (n = 240), $^\#$: p-value calculated against the population for neurotoxicity treated with taxol-carboplatin (n = 265).

When correlating each of the variants with grade 4 neutropenia and febrile neutropenia, we did not observe a significant association. Finally, we also correlated each of the variants to sensory neuropathy in the population that was eligible for neurotoxicity analyses, but failed to identify significant associations. None of the observed associations

Table 3 Association between genetic variants and hematologic toxicity

3A: Significant correlations with anemia

		All patients N = 290 (%)	Patients with anemia gr 3–4 N = 57 (19.6%)	Patients without anemia gr 3–4 N = 233 (80.3%)	Unadjusted OR (95%CI)	*p-value	Adjusted OR (95% CI)	**Corrected p value
ABCB1 rs1128503	CC 94 (32.4)		13 (22.8)	81 (34.8)	1.58 (1.03; 2.42)	0.035	1.71 (1.07; 2.71)	0.023
	CT 147 (50.7)		30 (52.6)	117 (50.2)				
	TT 49 (16.9)		14 (24.6)	35 (15.0)				
ABCC2 rs12762549	CC 80 (27.6)		25 (43.8)	55 (23.6)	0.55 (0.36; 0.83)	0.005	0.51 (0.33; 0.81)	0.004
	CG132 (45.5)		22 (38.6)	110 (47.2)				
	GG 76 (26.2)		10 (17.5)	66 (28.3)				
ABCA1 rs363717	AA 86 (29.6)		10 (17.5)	76 (32.6)	1.31 (1.98; 2.99)	0.001	2.08 (1.32; 3.27)	0.002
	GA 131 (45.2)		23 (40.3)	108 (33.5)				
	GG 73 (25.2)		24 (42.1)	49 (15.2)				
ERCC1 rs11615	TT 133 (45.9)		18 (31.6)	115 (49.3)	1.58 (1.06-2.35)	0.024	1.61 (1.04-2.50)	0.031
	TC 114 (39.3)		28 (49.1)	86 (36.9)				
	CC 42 (14.5)		11 (19.3)	31 (13.3)				

3B: Significant correlations with thrombocytopenia (TCP)

		All patients	Patients with TCP gr 3 – 4	Patients without TCP gr 3 – 4	Unadjusted OR	*p-value	Adjusted OR	**Corrected p value
		N = 290 (%)	N = 57 (19.6%)	N = 233 (80.3%)	(95%CI)		(95% CI)	
CYP3A4 rs4986910	TT 280 (96.5)		51(89.5)	229(98.3)	5.61 (1.46; 21.64)	0.012	4.99 (1.22; 20.31)	0.025
	CT 9 (3.1)		5(8.8)	4(1.7)				
	CC 0 (0)		0	0				

OR: Odds Ratio using wild type as reference category. *Uncorrected p values were calculated using binary logistic regression without correction for covariates. Per-allele ORs and 95% CIs are shown. There were missing genotypes for rs12762549 (n = 2), rs11615 (n = 1) and rs4986910 (n = 1). **Corrected p values were obtained using a logistic regression for the presence or absence of anemia/thrombocytopenia/febrile neutropenia while including the following covariates: genetic variant, age, BMI, AUC of carboplatin, number of administered cycles, and use of ESA for anemia or use of CSF for febrile neutropenia. In the regression for anemia, age, BMI, administered AUC of carboplatin or number of administered cycles were not identified as significant covariates (p = 0.576, p = 0.614 and p = 0.317, p = 0.481), whereas use of ESA was significant (p = 0.034). In the regression for grade 3–4 thrombocytopenia, age and AUC of administered carboplatin were a significant covariate (p = 0.023 and p = 0.014), but BMI or number of administered cycles were not (p = 0.571 and p = 0.243). In the regression for grade 4 neutropenia, BMI and age were significant covariates (p = 0.043 and p = 0.041), while administered AUC and number of administered cycles were not (p = 0.607 and p = 0.321).

with hematologic toxicity survived correction for multiple testing.

Association between genetic variants and use of growth factors

The use of ESAs or CSFs was also correlated with each of the 26 variants to examine whether they could predict the need for an ESA or CSF during treatment with chemotherapy in ovarian cancer. After correction for relevant covariates, a significant correlation for rs2074087 (*ABCC1, G > C*) and the use of ESA was noticed (p = 0.011, OR 2.09, Table 4). After correction for covariates, CSF use was significantly correlated with rs2073337 (*ABCC2, A > G*), rs1695 (*GSTP1, A > G*) and rs1799793 (*ERCC2, G > A*) (p = 0.039, OR 0.60; p = 0.017, OR 0.55; and p = 0.042, OR 0.63 respectively). None of the observed associations with use of growth factors survived correction for multiple testing.

Effects of variants on PFI and OS

The median follow-up of all patients participating to the study was 2.5 years (95% CI = 2.2-2.8 years) with 157

events for progression (59%) and 84 events for OS (31.6%). Uncorrected P-values were calculated using Cox regression analysis either adjusted for age at diagnosis only or fully adjusted for age at diagnosis, FIGO stage, tumor grade, tumor histology and residual disease after debulking surgery. Only one variant, rs1799793 (*ERCC2 G > A*), was significantly correlated with PFI in both cases (p = 0.003, HR = 0.71, 95% CI = 0.57-0.89, p = 0.016, HR = 0.75, 95% CI = 0.60-0.95). In particular, Kaplan-Meier survival analysis revealed a significant advantage in PFI for GG carriers of rs1799793 compared to AA or GA carriers (p = 0.016; Figure 1). Variants rs12762549 (*ABCC2 A > G*) and rs6104 (*SER-PINB2 C > G*) were significantly associated with PFI in the fully-adjusted model (p = 0.037 and p = 0.040, respectively), but these associations were not statistically significant in model adjusted for age only (p = 0.402 and p = 0.219, respectively). No significant correlations were found for OS.

None of the observed associations with platinum-free interval survived correction for multiple testing.

Table 4 Association between genetic variants and erythropoiesis stimulating agents (ESA) or colony stimulating factor (CSF) use

4A: Significant correlations with ESA use

	All patients	Patients with ESA use	Patients without ESA use	Unadjusted OR (95%CI)	*p-value	Adjusted OR (95% CI)	**Corrected p value
	N = 290 (%)	N = 70 (24.2%)	N = 219 (75.8%)				
ABCC1 rs2074087	GG 215 (74.4)	46 (65.7)	169 (77.2)	1.78 (1.03- 3.08)	0.054	2.09 (1.18 - 3.68)	0.011
	GC 69 (23.9)	22 (31.4)	47 (21.5)				
	CC 5 (1.7)	2 (2.8)	3 (1.4)				

4B: Significant correlations with CSF use

	All patients	Patients with CSF use	Patients without CSF use	Unadjusted OR (95%CI)	*p-value	Adjusted OR (95% CI)	**Corrected p value
	N = 290 (%)	N = 62 (21.4%)	N = 228 (78.6%)				
ABCC2 rs2073337	AA 101 (34.8)	27 (43.5)	74 (32.5)	0.61 (0.39- 0.96)	0.031	0.60 (0.37-0.99)	0.039
	AG 148 (51.0)	31 (50.0)	117 (51.3)				
	GG 41 (14.1)	4 (6.5)	37 (16.2)				
GSTP1 rs1695	AA 121 (41.7)	33 (53.2)	88 (38.6)	0.54 (0.34; 0.86)	0.010	0.55 (0.33-0.90)	0.017
	AG 137 (47.2)	27 (43.5)	110 (48.2)				
	GG 32 (11.0)	2 (3.2)	30 (13.2)				
ERCC2 Rs1799793	GG 136 (48.2)	21 (33.9)	115 (50.4)	0.67 (0.45- 1.00)	0.048	0.63 (0.41-0.98)	0.042
	GA 111 (39.4)	30 (48.4)	81 (35.5)				
	AA 35 (12.4)	9 (14.5)	26 (11.4)				

OR: Odds Ratio using wild type as reference category. *Uncorrected p values were calculated using binary logistic regression for the need for ESA/CSF use without correction for covariates. Per-allele ORs and 95% CIs are shown. There were missing genotypes for rs2074087 (n = 1), rs1799793 (n = 8). **Corrected p values were obtained using a logistic regression for the need for ESA/CSF use while including the following covariates: genetic variants, age, BMI, dosage of carboplatin (AUC) and number of administered cycles.

Discussion

We correlated paclitaxel- and carboplatin-induced toxicity with genetic variation in genes involved in pharmacokinetics of these chemotherapeutics or DNA repair, and observed various correlations supporting a role for

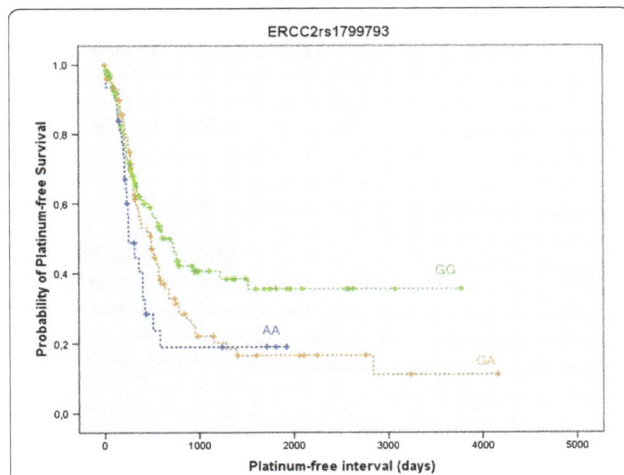

Figure 1 Kaplan-Meier curve for platinum-free interval correlated with polymorphisms of rs1799793 in ERCC2. Kaplan-Meier survival analysis reveals a significant advantage in PFI for GG cariers of rs1799793 compared to AA or GA carriers (p = 0.016).

these genes in mediating toxicity and therapy outcome. We observed that several variants correlated either with grade ≥3 anemia or thrombocytopenia, use of CSFs or ESAs, as well as the platinum-free interval (see Table 5 for an overview of all significant associations). These variants are located in genes that play an important role in transport (ABCB1, ABCC2, ABCC1, ABCA1) and hepatic metabolism (CYP3A4) of paclitaxel and base-excision repair of platinum-induced DNA damage (ERCC1, ERCC2), thus confirming a role for these genes in mediating side-effects and efficacy of paclitaxel and carboplatin. Indeed, ATP-binding cassette transporters, which are expressed on the cell-membrane surface, play an important role in the transport of taxanes [39], whereas cytochrome P450 proteins, CYP2C8, CYP3A4 and CYP3A5, catalyze the oxidative metabolism of taxanes. Furthermore, ERCC1 and ERCC2 are subunits of the endonuclease complex that plays an essential role in DNA repair by removing platinum-induced intra-strand cross-links.

Most other studies assessing similar correlations have been performed in smaller populations, and typically evaluated only few variants. Our study evaluates a more systematically-selected panel of 26 variants in a large population of ovarian cancer patients, of which 290 were evaluable for hematologic toxicity and 265 for

Table 5 Overview of all significant correlations per genetic variant

Gene	Variant allele (rs number, nucleotide)		Effect of the variant allele on toxicity or outcome	Corrected p value, adjusted OR, 95% CI	Effect of the polymorphisms according to the literature
ABCB1	rs1128503	c.1236C > T	Increased risk anemia grade 3-4	p = 0.023; OR 1.71, 1.07 – 2.71	Homozygous mutant allele carriers: decreased doctaxel clearance in 92 patients [9]
ABCC2	rs12762549	g.101620771C > G	Decreased risk anemia grade 3-4	p = 0.004; OR 0.51, 0.33-0.81	Japanese mutant allele carriers: increased risk for severe neutropenia during treatment with docetaxel in 84 patients [19]
	rs2073337	c.1668 + 148A > G	Decreased need for colony stimulating factor	p = 0.039; OR 0.60, 0.37-0.98	In vitro evidence: paclitaxel is a substrate of ABCC2 [24]
ABCC1	rs2074087	c.2284-30 G > C	Increased need for erythropoiesis stimulating agent	p = 0.011; OR 2.09, 1.18-3.68	In vitro evidence: resistance to paclitaxel with ABCC1 overexpression [23]
ABCA1	rs363717	c.1896 A > G	Increased risk anemia grade 3-4	p = 0.002; OR 2.08, 1.32-3.27	Mutant allele carriers: decreased risk to develop thalidomide related neuropathy grade ≥2 in 1495 patients [36]
CYP3A4	rs4986910	c.1331 T > C	Increased risk thrombocytopenia grade 3-4	p = 0.025; OR 4.99, 1.22-20.31	-
GSTP1	rs1695	c.313A > G	Decreased need for colony stimulating factor	p = 0.017; OR 0.55, 0.33-0.90	Mutant allele carriers: decreased oxaliplatin-related neuropathy in 90 patients [30], decreased docetaxel-induced grade 2 neuropathy in 58 patients [31], decreased risk of hematologic toxicity in 118 patients [15]
					Heterozygous mutant allele carriers compared to homozygous wildtype allele carriers: decreased PFS following cisplatin-gemcitabine in 104 patients [32]
ERCC1	rs11615	c.354 T > C	Increased risk anemia grade 3-4	p = 0.031; OR 1.61, 1.04-2.50	Mutant allele carriers: decreased platinum resistance in 60 patients [34]
					Heterozygous variant allele carriers compared to homozygous wildtype allele carriers: increased risk on severe neutropenia and increased likelihood of overall survival following cisplatin-gemcitabine in 104 patients [32]
ERCC2	rs1799793	c.934G > A	Decreased need for colony stimulating factor	p = 0.042; OR 0.63, 0.41-0.98	Heterozygous variant allele carriers compared to homozygous wildtype allele carriers: increased severity of neutropenia following cisplatin-cyclophosphamide in 104 patients [32]
			Decreased platinum free interval	p = 0.016, HR = 0.75, 0.60-0.95	

neurotoxicity. Another strength of our study is the availability of more detailed clinical toxicity data compared to previous pharmacogenetic association studies in ovarian cancer, allowing us to correlate specific entities of the hematologic toxicity spectrum, whereas other studies mostly grouped all hematologic > grade 3 toxicities into a single group [8,12,14,15] or focused on the occurrence of neutropenia alone [11,18].

Several of the previously published studies investigating the role of these variants with respect to toxicity and chemotherapy outcome confirmed the observations made in the present study. With respect to the ABC transporters, the rs1128503 (1236C > T) synonymous variant in

ABCB1 has been associated with multidrug resistance in multiple studies, and with decreased docetaxel clearance in particular, for homozygous carriers of the variant T-allele in 92 patients [9]. However, its association with severe anemia observed in our study has not been reported before. The rs1045642 (3435C > T) synonymous variant in ABCB1 increased 3′p-hydroxy-paclitaxel metabolites in 23 ovarian cancer patients carrying the T-allele [8]. *Vice versa*, in a study of 26 patients, a significant greater percent decrease in absolute neutrophil count at nadir was reported for patients homozygous for the T-allele [11], Bergmann also reported a more pronounced neutrophil decrease in patients carrying the

T-allele in 92 ovarian cancer patients carrying the T-allele. [18]. In our study, we failed to observe an association with grade ≥3 neutropenia or febrile neutropenia. Possibly, this is due to the fact that we analyzed grade ≥3 neutropenia whilst previous studies used absolute neutrophil decrease. A Japanese study demonstrated that carriers of the variant allele for rs12762549 (ABCC2,101620771 C > G) had an increased risk to develop docetaxel-induced leukopenia/ neutropenia in 84 patients [19]. In the current study, no such association was found, but we did find a significant association with anemia and PFI, thereby confirming the potential importance of this variant in mediating taxane transport. Notably, another variant in this gene, rs2073337 (1668 + 148A > G), was significantly correlated with CSF use. For rs363717 (1896 A > G) in *ABCA1*, which was selected based on its association with thalidomide-related peripheral neuropathy [36], we did not observe a significant association with sensory neurotoxicity. We observed, however, a significant association of this variant with severe anemia (p = 0.001), suggesting that ABCA1 is involved in the transport and metabolism of platinum or carboplatin, similar to its role in the transport of cholesterol [40].

With respect to the CYP genes, low CYP3A4 enzyme activity increased the conversion of paclitaxel towards its metabolite, while heterozygous patients for CYP2C8*3 had a lower clearance of paclitaxel, suggesting the role of those genes in paclitaxel pharmacokinetics in a study of 38 patients [14]. In 93 patients with ovarian cancer, Bergmann *et al.* observed an 11% reduction in paclitaxel clearance in carriers of the rs10509681 (1196A > G) variant G-allele in *CYP2C8* [16], whereas Leskelä et al. observed a correlation between neurotoxicity and these *CYP2C8* and *CYP3A5* variants in a study consisting of 118 patients [25]. In the present study, we failed however, to observe such associations. Another large study in ovarian cancer also failed to observe correlations with neurotoxicity for these variants in docetaxel or paclitaxel-treated patients [12]. We did observe, however, a significant association between rs4986910 (1331 T > C) in *CYP3A4* and thrombocytopenia. Homozygous carriers of the rs1695 (313A > G) variant G-allele in *GSTP1* have been associated with neuropathy in 90 patients receiving oxaliplatin-based chemotherapy [30]. This association was not confirmed in our study, although a correlation with febrile neutropenia and CSF use was observed.

Finally, with respect to the excision repair genes, previous studies reported a correlation between severe neutropenia and the rs1799793 (934G > A) variant A-allele in *ERCC2* in 104 ovarian cancer patients receiving a cisplatin-cyclophosphamide regimen [32]. In the current study, no correlation with severe neutropenia was described, although the rs1799793 (934G > A) variant A-allele did correlate significantly with CSF use during treatment.

Additionally, we observed an improved PFI for rs1799793 (934G > A) GG-carriers. The largest study to date exploring the association between 27 selected variants and ovarian cancer survival, which was performed by the ovarian cancer association consortium (OCAC) in >10,000 cases [41], rs1799793 (934G > A) was not tested. Nevertheless, in the high-grade serous sub-population of this large study, a significant correlation was found with another variant in *ERCC2* (rs50872 A > G) and outcome, confirming the potential importance of ERCC2 in mediating chemotherapy outcome. Unfortunately, rs50872 was not linked with rs1799793 (934G > A) ($r^2 = 0.06$), indicating that these variants represent different association signals with *ERCC2*.

In summary, we observed the strongest associations between variants in ABC-transporters and anemia. The mechanism explaining why altered transport of cytotoxic chemotherapy affects erythropoiesis rather than granulopoiesis or thrombopoiesis is not yet understood. Possibly, these variants alter intracellular concentrations of the transported cytotoxic drug in a cell type-specific manner. Another possibility is that some cell types might be more sensitive to specific changes in the concentration of certain metabolites. On the other hand, it is also possible that the effect on erythropoiesis is caused by a specific role of the affected gene during erythropoiesis. For example, a prominent role for ABCB6 during erythropoiesis as a mitochondrial porphyrin transporter essential for heme biosynthesis, has been established [42].

It is a limitation of the current study that the group for hematologic toxicity analysis included both single agent carboplatin as paclitaxel/carboplatin combination therapy although it is known that both regimens have a slightly different hematologic toxicity profile with more thrombocytopenia in carboplatin monotherapy compared to combination regimens, in our cohort the rate of grade 3–4 thrombocytopenia was 28% for carboplatin versus 18% for combination therapy. Apart from the fact that both regimens are included for hematologic analysis, this cohort is relatively homogenous including only data on first-line treatment in ovarian cancer patients with a uniform ethnicity (99% Caucasians), high number of optimal debulked patients and relatively uniform number of administered cycles of chemotherapy. To further reduce the problem of heterogeneity, pharmacogenetic research on prospective clinical trials including large populations of uniformly treated patients is warranted.

It should be noted that the candidate-gene approach employed so far selecting drug-related genes derived from platinum/taxane pharmacology only allows the analysis with candidate genes known to be involved in chemotherapy metabolism, transport or DNA repair. To discover *novel* genetic markers, other approaches such as whole-genome association studies or targeted resequencing of strong candidate genes to identify rare genetic variants, could be applied. In addition, other drug- or toxicity -related candidate genes relevant for paclitaxel-carboplatin treatment in ovarian cancer (such as GSTA-1 [32], MAD1L1 [43], OPRM1 [44], TRPV1 [44], ...) could be selected based on pharmacogenetic knowledge bases such as pharmGKB (www.pharmgkb.org).

Conclusions

The current study revealed a correlation between SNPs in genes involved in DNA repair or metabolism or transport of taxanes or platinum and toxicity or response to first-line chemotherapy in ovarian cancer, using a candidate-gene approach. Variants reported in this study may serve as biomarkers and contribute to the clinical decision-making of chemotherapy dose reductions, feasibility of chemotherapy in patients at-risk based on age and/or performance status, and use of supportive medication such as ESA or CSF. However, as none of the identified associations survived correction for multiple testing, our data are only hypothesis-generating and still need independent validation. We plan to perform such a validation by performing genome-wide screens or targeted re-sequencing of candidate genes in a large multi-centered clinical trial.

Additional files

Additional file 1: Figure S1. Study design for pharmacogenetic analyses.
Additional file 2: Table S1. Minor allele frequencies of the significant SNPs, calculated for all included patients (n = 322).

Abbreviations

SNP: Single nucleotide polymorphisms; DNA: Deoxyribonucleic acid; OR: Odds ratio; CI: Confidence interval; HR: Hazard Ratio; ATP: Adenosine 5'-triphosphate; ABCA1: ATP-binding cassette sub-family A, member 1; ABCB1: ATP-binding cassette, sub-family B, member 1; ABCC1: ATP-binding cassette, sub-family C, member 1; ABCC2: ATP-binding cassette sub-family C, member 2; ABCG2: ATP-binding cassette sub-familiy G, member 2; GSTP1: Glutathione S-transferase, pi 1; GSTT1: Glutathione S-transferase theta-1; GSTM1: Glutathione S-transferase mu-1; CYP3A4: Cytochrome P450, 3A4; CYP3A5: Cytochrome P450, 3A5; CYP2C8: Cytochrome P450, 2C8; CYP1B1: Cytochrome P450, 1B1; ERCC1: Excision repair cross-complementation group 1; ERCC2: Excision repair cross-complementation group 2; XRCC1: X-ray repair cross-complementing protein 1; SLCO1B3: Solute carrier organic anion transporter family member 1B3; SLC12A6: Solute carrier family 12 member 6; MAPT: Microtubule-associated protein tau; TUBB: Tubulin, beta class I; TP53: Tumor protein p53; SERPINB2: Serpin Peptidase Inhibitor, Clade B (Ovalbumin), Member 2; PPARD: Peroxisome Proliferator-Activated Receptor Delta; ICAM 1: Intercellular Adhesion Molecule 1; CSF: Colony stimulating factor; ESA: Erythropoiesis stimulating agent; BGOG: Belgian and Luxembourg Gynaecologic Oncology Group (BGOG); FIGO: International Federation of Gynecology and Obstetrics; CT: Computed tomography; CA 125: Cancer antigen 125; CTCAE: Common Terminology for Adverse Events; PFI: Platinum-free interval; OS: Overall survival; AUC: Area under the curve; OC: Ovarian Cancer; NSCLC: Non-small cell lung carcinoma; FDR: False discovery rate.

Competing interests

The authors declare that they have no competing interests.

Authors' contributions

SL: wrote manuscript, performed research, analyzed data; DL: designed research, performed research, analyzed data; ED: contributed new patients and data; EVN: contributed new patients and data; DS: performed research; PRD: contributed new patients and data; VR: contributed new patients and data; PV: contributed new patients and data; DL: contributed new patients and data; FA: contributed new patients and data; PN: contributed new patients and data; KL: contributed new patients and data; IV: designed research, contributed new patients and data. All authors read and approved the final manuscript.

Acknowledgements

This research project was financially supported by the Federal Public service of health, food chain safety and environment of Belgium, through the initiative 'Cancer Plan – action 29' Project KPC_29_054 (KankerPlanCancer@health.fgov.be).

Author details

[1]Division of Gynaecologic Oncology and Leuven Cancer Institute, University Hospitals Leuven, KU Leuven, Herestraat 49, 3000 Leuven, Belgium. [2]Vesalius Research Center, VIB, Leuven, Herestraat 49, Box 912, 3000 Leuven, Belgium. [3]Laboratory for Translational Genetics, Department of Oncology, KU Leuven, Herestraat 49, 3000 Leuven, Belgium. [4]Oncologisch Centrum, Algemeen Ziekenhuis Groeninge, Loofstraat 43, 8500 Kortrijk, Belgium. [5]Dienst Oncologie, Algemeen Ziekenhuis Sint Lucas, Groenebriel 1, 9000 Gent, Belgium. [6]Dienst Medische Oncologie, Onze-Lieve-Vrouwziekenhuis, Moorselbaan 164, 9300 Aalst, Belgium. [7]Dienst Medische Oncologie, Jessa Ziekenhuis, Stadsomvaart 11, 3500 Hasselt, Belgium.

References

1. Ferlay J, Parkin DM, Steliarova-Foucher E. Estimates of cancer incidence and mortality in Europe in 2008. Eur J Cancer. 2010;46:765–81.
2. Cannistra SA. Cancer of the ovary. N Engl J Med. 2004;351:2519–29.
3. du Bois A, Luck HJ, Meier W, Adams HP, Mobus V, Costa S, et al. A randomized clinical trial of cisplatin/paclitaxel versus carboplatin/paclitaxel as first-line treatment of ovarian cancer. J Natl Cancer Inst. 2003;95:1320–9.
4. du Bois A, Herrstedt J, Hardy-Bessard AC, Muller HH, Harter P, Kristensen G, et al. Phase III trial of carboplatin plus paclitaxel with or without gemcitabine in first-line treatment of epithelial ovarian cancer. J Clin Oncol. 2010;28:4162–9.
5. Pfisterer J, Weber B, Reuss A, Kimmig R, du Bois A, Wagner U, et al. Randomized phase III trial of topotecan following carboplatin and paclitaxel in first-line treatment of advanced ovarian cancer: a gynecologic cancer intergroup trial of the AGO-OVAR and GINECO. J Natl Cancer Inst. 2006;98:1036–45.
6. Ozols RF, Bundy BN, Greer BE, Fowler JM, Clarke-Pearson D, Burger RA, et al. Phase III trial of carboplatin and paclitaxel compared with cisplatin and paclitaxel in patients with optimally resected stage III ovarian cancer: a Gynecologic Oncology Group study. J Clin Oncol. 2003;21:3194–200.
7. Aapro MS, Cameron DA, Pettengell R, Bohlius J, Crawford J, Ellis M, et al. EORTC guidelines for the use of granulocyte-colony stimulating factor to reduce the incidence of chemotherapy-induced febrile neutropenia in adult patients with lymphomas and solid tumours. Eur J Cancer. 2006;42:2433–53.
8. Nakajima M, Fujiki Y, Kyo S, Kanaya T, Nakamura M, Maida Y, et al. Pharmacokinetics of paclitaxel in ovarian cancer patients and genetic polymorphisms of CYP2C8, CYP3A4, and MDR1. J Clin Pharmacol. 2005;45:674–82.
9. Bosch TM, Huitema AD, Doodeman VD, Jansen R, Witteveen E, Smit WM, et al. Pharmacogenetic screening of CYP3A and ABCB1 in relation to population pharmacokinetics of docetaxel. Clin Cancer Res. 2006;12:5786–93.
10. Henningsson A, Marsh S, Loos WJ, Karlsson MO, Garsa A, Mross K, et al. Association of CYP2C8, CYP3A4, CYP3A5, and ABCB1 polymorphisms with the pharmacokinetics of paclitaxel. Clin Cancer Res. 2005;11:8097–104.
11. Sissung TM, Mross K, Steinberg SM, Behringer D, Figg WD, Sparreboom A, et al. Association of ABCB1 genotypes with paclitaxel-mediated peripheral neuropathy and neutropenia. Eur J Cancer. 2006;42:2893–6.

12. Marsh S, Paul J, King CR, Gifford G, McLeod HL, Brown R. Pharmacogenetic assessment of toxicity and outcome after platinum plus taxane chemotherapy in ovarian cancer: the Scottish Randomised Trial in Ovarian Cancer. J Clin Oncol. 2007;25:4528–35.

13. Johnatty SE, Beesley J, Paul J, Fereday S, Spurdle AB, Webb PM, et al. ABCB1 (MDR 1) polymorphisms and progression-free survival among women with ovarian cancer following paclitaxel/carboplatin chemotherapy. Clin Cancer Res. 2008;14:5594–601.

14. Green H, Soderkvist P, Rosenberg P, Mirghani RA, Rymark P, Lundqvist EA, et al. Pharmacogenetic studies of Paclitaxel in the treatment of ovarian cancer. Basic Clin Pharmacol Toxicol. 2009;104:130–7.

15. Kim HS, Kim MK, Chung HH, Kim JW, Park NH, Song YS, et al. Genetic polymorphisms affecting clinical outcomes in epithelial ovarian cancer patients treated with taxanes and platinum compounds: a Korean population-based study. Gynecol Oncol. 2009;113:264–9.

16. Bergmann TK, Brasch-Andersen C, Green H, Mirza M, Pedersen RS, Nielsen F, et al. Impact of CYP2C8*3 on paclitaxel clearance: a population pharmacokinetic and pharmacogenomic study in 93 patients with ovarian cancer. Pharmacogenomics J. 2011;11:113–20.

17. Tian C, Ambrosone CB, Darcy KM, Krivak TC, Armstrong DK, Bookman MA, et al. Common variants in ABCB1, ABCC2 and ABCG2 genes and clinical outcomes among women with advanced stage ovarian cancer treated with platinum and taxane-based chemotherapy: a Gynecologic Oncology Group study. Gynecol Oncol. 2012;124:575–81.

18. Bergmann TK, Brasch-Andersen C, Green H, Mirza MR, Skougaard K, Wihl J, et al. Impact of ABCB1 variants on neutrophil depression: a pharmacogenomic study of paclitaxel in 92 women with ovarian cancer. Basic Clin Pharmacol Toxico. 2012;110(2):199–204.

19. Kiyotani K, Mushiroda T, Kubo M, Zembutsu H, Sugiyama Y, Nakamura Y. Association of genetic polymorphisms in SLCO1B3 and ABCC2 with docetaxel-induced leukopenia. Cancer Sci. 2008;99:967–72.

20. Smith NF, Acharya MR, Desai N, Figg WD, Sparreboom A. Identification of OATP1B3 as a high-affinity hepatocellular transporter of paclitaxel. Cancer Biol Ther. 2005;4:815–8.

21. Chew H, Sandanaraj E, Singh O, Chen X, Tan EH, Lim WT, et al. Influence of SLCO1B3 haplotype-tag SNPs on docetaxel disposition in Chinese nasopharyngeal cancer patients. Br J Clin Pharmacol. 2012;73:606–18.

22. Crouthamel MH, Wu D, Yang Z, Ho RJ. A novel MDR1 G1199T variant alters drug resistance and efflux transport activity of P-glycoprotein in recombinant Hek cells. J Pharm Sci. 2006;95:2767–77.

23. Vanhoefer U, Cao S, Minderman H, Toth K, Scheper RJ, Slovak ML, et al. PAK-104P, a pyridine analogue, reverses paclitaxel and doxorubicin resistance in cell lines and nude mice bearing xenografts that overexpress the multidrug resistance protein. Clin Cancer Res. 1996;2:369–77.

24. Huisman MT, Chhatta AA, van Tellingen O, Beijnen JH, Schinkel AH. MRP2 (ABCC2) transports taxanes and confers paclitaxel resistance and both processes are stimulated by probenecid. Int J Cancer. 2005;116:824–9.

25. Leskela S, Jara C, Leandro-Garcia LJ, Martinez A, Garcia-Donas J, Hernando S, et al. Polymorphisms in cytochromes P450 2C8 and 3A5 are associated with paclitaxel neurotoxicity. Pharmacogenomics J. 2011;11:121–9.

26. Baker SD, Verweij J, Cusatis GA, van Schaik RH, Marsh S, Orwick SJ, et al. Pharmacogenetic pathway analysis of docetaxel elimination. Clin Pharmacol Ther. 2009;85:155–63.

27. Pearce CL, Near AM, Van Den Berg DJ, Ramus SJ, Gentry-Maharaj A, Menon U, et al. Validating genetic risk associations for ovarian cancer through the international Ovarian Cancer Association Consortium. Br J Cancer. 2009;100:412–20.

28. Gadducci A, Di Cristofano C, Zavaglia M, Giusti L, Menicagli M, Cosio S, et al. P53 gene status in patients with advanced serous epithelial ovarian cancer in relation to response to paclitaxel- plus platinum-based chemotherapy and long-term clinical outcome. Anticancer Res. 2006;26:687–93.

29. Schildkraut JM, Goode EL, Clyde MA, Iversen ES, Moorman PG, Berchuck A, et al. Single nucleotide polymorphisms in the TP53 region and susceptibility to invasive epithelial ovarian cancer. Cancer Res. 2009;69:2349–57.

30. Lecomte T, Landi B, Beaune P, Laurent-Puig P, Loriot MA. Glutathione S-transferase P1 polymorphism (Ile105Val) predicts cumulative neuropathy in patients receiving oxaliplatin-based chemotherapy. Clin Cancer Res. 2006;12:3050–6.

31. Mir O, Alexandre J, Tran A, Durand JP, Pons G, Treluyer JM, et al. Relationship between GSTP1 Ile(105)Val polymorphism and docetaxel-induced peripheral neuropathy: clinical evidence of a role of oxidative stress in taxane toxicity. Ann Oncol. 2009;20:736–40.

32. Khrunin AV, Moisseev A, Gorbunova V, Limborska S. Genetic polymorphisms and the efficacy and toxicity of cisplatin-based chemotherapy in ovarian cancer patients. Pharmacogenomics J. 2010;10:54–61.

33. Khrunin A, Ivanova F, Moisseev A, Khokhrin D, Sleptsova Y, Gorbunova V, et al. Pharmacogenomics of cisplatin-based chemotherapy in ovarian cancer patients of different ethnic origins. Pharmacogenomics. 2012;13:171–8.

34. Kang S, Ju W, Kim JW, Park NH, Song YS, Kim SC, et al. Association between excision repair cross-complementation group 1 polymorphism and clinical outcome of platinum-based chemotherapy in patients with epithelial ovarian cancer. Exp Mol Med. 2006;38:320–4.

35. Krivak TC, Darcy KM, Tian C, Bookman M, Gallion H, Ambrosone CB, et al. Single nucleotide polypmorphisms in ERCC1 are associated with disease progression, and survival in patients with advanced stage ovarian and primary peritoneal carcinoma; a Gynecologic Oncology Group study. Gynecol Oncol. 2011;122:121–6.

36. Johnson DC, Corthals SL, Walker BA, Ross FM, Gregory WM, Dickens NJ, et al. Genetic factors underlying the risk of thalidomide-related neuropathy in patients with multiple myeloma. J Clin Oncol. 2011;29:797–804.

37. Eisenhauer EA, Therasse P, Bogaerts J, Schwartz LH, Sargent D, Ford R, et al. New response evaluation criteria in solid tumours: revised RECIST guideline (version 1.1). Eur J Cancer. 2009;45:228–47.

38. Reumers J, De Rijk P, Zhao H, Liekens A, Smeets D, Cleary J, et al. Optimized filtering reduces the error rate in detecting genomic variants by short-read sequencing. Nat Biotechnol. 2012;30:61–8.

39. Marsh S. Pharmacogenomics of taxane/platinum therapy in ovarian cancer. Int J Gynecol Cancer. 2009;19 Suppl 2:S30–4.

40. Brooks-Wilson A, Marcil M, Clee SM, Zhang LH, Roomp K, van Dam M, et al. Mutations in ABC1 in Tangier disease and familial high-density lipoprotein deficiency. Nat Genet. 1999;22:336–45.

41. White KL, Vierkant RA, Fogarty ZC, Charbonneau B, Block MS, Pharoah PD, et al. Analysis of Over 10,000 Cases Finds No Association between Previously Reported Candidate Polymorphisms and Ovarian Cancer Outcome. Cancer Epidemiol Biomarkers Prev. 2013;22:987–92.

42. Krishnamurthy PC, Du G, Fukuda Y, Sun D, Sampath J, Mercer KE, et al. Identification of a mammalian mitochondrial porphyrin transporter. Nature. 2006;443:586–9.

43. Santibanez M, Gallardo D, Morales F, Lopez A, Prada D, Mendoza J, et al. The MAD1 1673 G. A polymorphism alters the function of the mitotic spindle assembly checkpoint and is associated with a worse response to induction chemotherapy and sensitivity to treatment in patients with advanced epithelial ovarian cancer. Pharmacogenet Genomics. 2013;23:190–9.

44. McWhinney-Glass S, Winham SJ, Hertz DL, Yen Revollo J, Paul J, He Y, et al. Cumulative genetic risk predicts platinum/taxane-induced neurotoxicity. Clin Cancer Res. 2013;19:5769–76.

14

Effects of simvastatin on cell viability and proinflammatory pathways in lung adenocarcinoma cells exposed to hydrogen peroxide

Luca Gallelli[1], Daniela Falcone[1], Monica Scaramuzzino[1], Girolamo Pelaia[2], Bruno D'Agostino[4]*, Maria Mesuraca[3], Rosa Terracciano[1], Giuseppe Spaziano[4], Rosario Maselli[2], Michele Navarra[5] and Rocco Savino[1]

Abstract

Lung cancer is characterized by a high mortality rate probably attributable to early metastasis. Oxidative stress is involved in development and progression of lung cancer, through cellular and molecular mechanisms which at least in part overlap with proinflammatory pathways. Simvastatin is a statin with pleiotropic effects that can also act as an anti-oxidant agent, and these pharmacologic properties may contribute to its potential anti-cancer activity. Therefore, the aim of this study was to evaluate, in the human lung adenocarcinoma cell line GLC-82, the effects of a 24-hour treatment with simvastatin on hydrogen peroxide (H_2O_2)-induced changes in cell viability, ERK phosphorylation, matrix metalloproteinase (MMP) expression, innate immunity signaling, NF-κB activation and IL-8 secretion. Cell counting was performed after trypan blue staining, cell proliferation was assessed using MTT assay, and apoptosis was evaluated through caspase-3 activation and Tunel assay. Western blotting was used to analyze protein extracts, and IL-8 release into cell culture supernatants was assessed by ELISA. Our results show that simvastatin (30 μM) significantly (P <0.01) inhibited the proliferative effect of H_2O_2 (0.5 mM) and its stimulatory actions on ERK1/2 phosphorylation, NF-κB activation and IL-8 production. Furthermore, simvastatin decreased H_2O_2-mediated induction of the cellular expression of MMP-2 and MMP-9, as well as of several components of the signaling complex activated by innate immune responses, including MyD88, TRAF2, TRAF6 and TRADD. In conclusion, these findings suggest that simvastatin could play a role in prevention and treatment of lung cancer via modulation of important proinflammatory and tumorigenic events promoted by oxidative stress.

Keywords: Lung cancer, NF-κB, Matrix metalloproteinases, Innate immunity, IL-8, Simvastatin

Background

The respiratory system is remarkably susceptible to oxidative stress because of its peculiar anatomical and functional properties, mainly related to the large area exposed to the external environment. Therefore, the cellular/tissue injury triggered by the oxidant burden generated by air pollutants in association with cigarette smoking plays a pivotal role in the pathogenesis of several inflammatory and proliferative lung disorders, including chronic obstructive pulmonary disease (COPD), asthma, acute respiratory distress syndrome (ARDS), idiopathic pulmonary fibrosis (IPF), cystic fibrosis, and also lung cancer.

In particular, inhaled oxidants such as ozone and nitrogen dioxide cause sequestration of inflammatory cells into the pulmonary microcirculation, thus leading to their accumulation within air spaces. Cigarette smoke, which contains many oxidants and free radicals in both its gaseous and particulate phases [1], significantly contributes to recruit macrophages into the airways, as well as to increase neutrophil numbers within lung microvessels. Once recruited and activated, macrophages, neutrophils and eosinophils produce and release reactive oxygen

* Correspondence: bruno.dagostino@unina2.it
[4]Department of Experimental Medicine-Section of Pharmacology, School of Medicine, Second University of Naples, via Costantinopoli 16, 80136 Naples, Italy
Full list of author information is available at the end of the article

species (ROS) such as hydroxyl radicals and superoxide anion ($O_2.^-$), the latter being rapidly converted to hydrogen peroxide (H_2O_2) by superoxide dismutase (SOD) [2]. ROS may interfere with signal transduction pathways regulating the functions of transcription factors such as nuclear factor κB (NF-κB) and activator protein-1 (AP-1) [3]. NF-κB and AP-1 are responsible for the coordinated expression of several genes that control inflammation, cell proliferation and apoptosis. Within this context a key role is played by mitogen-activated protein kinases (MAPK), whose targets are mainly represented by nuclear transcription factors, also including those involved in oxidative stress. In particular, the ERK1/2 subgroup of MAPK is activated by a MAPK kinase kinase named Raf (most commonly Raf-1), whose activation in turn requires the GTP-bound form of Ras family proteins [4]. Once activated, Raf-1 phosphorylates the MAPK kinases MEK1 and MEK2, that finally stimulate ERK1 and ERK2.

Airborne pollutants and cigarette smoke can induce the bronchial epithelium to acquire a proinflammatory phenotype, characterized by an increased production of autacoids, cytokines, and chemokines [5]. Oxidant-induced phenotypic changes may thus significantly contribute to the key pathogenic role played by bronchial epithelial cells in inflammatory airway disorders such as asthma and COPD. Moreover, ROS may also contribute via several different signalling pathways, including MAPK activation, to development and progression of lung cancer [6].

Lung cancer is the leading cause of neoplastic death worldwide. More than 80% of lung cancer cases belong to the non small cell lung cancer (NSCLC) type, which can be further subdivided into adenocarcinoma (approximately 40% of all NSCLCs), squamous cell carcinoma and large cell carcinoma [7]. The metastatic potential of NSCLC strongly correlates with the cellular expression of matrix metalloproteinases (MMPs), which are regulated by NF-κB and by the metastasis suppressor RECK (reversion-inducing-cysteine-rich protein with kazal motif) [8,9]. Moreover, the complex cellular and molecular mechanisms underlying the development and progression of NSCLC are also significantly affected by the innate immune system [6]. Indeed, the latter represents the first line of defense against noxious agents such as ROS, which can damage the airway epithelium.

The poor survival rate of patients with NSCLC is mostly due to its high metastatic potential and also to a relative drug resistance [7]. Therefore, new and more effective pharmacological treatments for NSCLC are strongly needed. In this regard, increasing attention is currently being paid to statins because of their capability of inhibiting 3-hydroxy-3-methylglutaryl coenzyme A (HMG-CoA) reductase, which is the rate limiting enzyme within the mevalonate pathway. Hence, by blocking the synthesis of mevalonate and its isoprenoid derivatives farnesyl pyrophosphate (FPP) and geranyl geranyl pyrophosphate (GGPP), statins also prevent prenylation-dependent activation of oncogenic Ras proteins [10]. Indeed, statins may have a cytostatic effect on cancer cells, and can prolong the survival of cancer patients [11]. They also act as anti-oxidant, anti-inflammatory and anti-angiogenic factors, and could therefore prevent or inhibit cancer cell growth [12]. Furthermore, we have recently shown that simvastatin is able to induce a decrease in cell proliferation and a significant increase of apoptosis in human NSCLC cell cultures [13], as well as to modulate Ras, MMP-2/9 and NF-κB activity in pulmonary neoplastic tissues obtained from patients undergoing therapeutic surgery for lung cancer [14].

On the basis of the above mentioned considerations, the aim of our present study has been to investigate, in the human lung adenocarcinoma cell line GLC-82 exposed to H_2O_2, the effects of simvastatin on cell viability and apoptosis, ERK phosphorylation, MMP2/9 and RECK protein expression, NF-κB nuclear content and interleukin-8 (IL-8) secretion. Moreover, we also assessed the effects of simvastatin on H_2O_2-induced changes in the expression of some important proteins of the signaling network underlying innate immune responses, including MyD88, tumor necrosis factor (TNF) receptor-associated factors (TRAF)2/6, and TNF receptor type 1-associated death domain protein (TRADD).

Methods

Reagents

The anti-caspase-3 monoclonal antibody E83-77 was purchased from Abcam (Cambridge, UK). Trypan blue was purchased from Sigma (St. Louis, MO, USA). Anti-phospho-ERK1/2, anti-NF-κB-p65, anti-RECK, anti-MyD88, anti-TRAF2, anti-TRADD, anti-TRAF6, anti-MMP2 and anti-MMP9 monoclonal antibodies were purchased from New England Biolabs (Beverly, MA, USA); an anti-(total)-ERK1/2 polyclonal antibody was commercially provided by Santa Cruz Biotechnology, Inc. (Santa Cruz, CA, USA). Purified crystalline powders of simvastatin were commercially obtained from Sigma (St. Louis, MO, USA), and then dissolved into refrigerated and light-protected DMSO stock solution.

Culture and treatment of human lung cancer cells

GLC-82, a human lung adenocarcinoma cell line [13], was cultured at 37°C, 5% CO_2, in Dulbecco's modified Eagle's medium (DMEM) supplemented with 10% FCS, penicillin 100 U/ml, streptomycin 100 μg/ml, and amphotericin B 25 μg/ml in a humidified 5% CO_2 atmosphere. For each treatment, cells were plated in a 100-mm polystyrene dish (Falcon, Becton-Dickinson, Lincoln Park, NJ, USA) and ten ml of supplemented DMEM were then added. When GLC-82 cells grew to about 70% confluence, they were exposed for 2 hours to H_2O_2 (0.5 mM) and then cells were or not exposed for 24 hour to simvastatin (30 μM). The medium was not changed after treatment. The solvent employed to dissolve this drug was used as a control. After this period, the medium was removed for IL-8 assessment (see later), and cells were processed for protein extraction and immunoblotting.

Cell viability and proliferation

Cell viability was assessed by light microscopy and dye exclusion, using Trypan blue. Cell numbers were evaluated by direct counting using a hemocytometer, in agreement with our previous reports [15-17]. Cell proliferation was investigated by 3-[4,5-dimethylthiazol-2-yl]-2,5 diphenyl tetrazolium bromide (MTT) assay, based on the conversion by mitochondrial dehydrogenases of the substrate containing a tetrazolium ring into blue formazan, detectable spectrophotometrically. The level of blue formazan was then used as an indirect index of cell density. Briefly, after treatment with either H_2O_2 and/or simvastatin, cells were exposed to MTT (5 μg/mL) for 150 min at 37°C. The medium was then removed and cells were solubilized with acidified isopropanol and 2% sodium dodecyl sulfate (SDS). After complete solubilization, presence of blue formazan was evaluated spectrophotometrically at a reference wavelength of 650 nm. All experiments were carried out in triplicate.

Protein extraction and immunoblot analysis

Following treatment with simvastatin, cells were lysed for Western blotting in radioimmunoprecipitation assay (RIPA) buffer, as previously described [18]. Moreover, nuclear extracts were obtained using the NE-PER cell fractionation kit (Thermo Scientific, Rockford, IL, USA). Briefly, whole cell lysates or nuclear proteins were then separated on a 12.5% sodium dodecyl sulfate-polyacrylamide gel electrophoresis (SDS-PAGE) and transferred onto polyvinylidene difluoride (PVDF) membranes (Amersham Pharmacia, Little Chalfont, UK). Immunoblotting was performed using the above mentioned monoclonal antibodies. After being "stripped", membranes were re-probed with a polyclonal antibody against total (phosphorylated and unphosphorylated) ERK1/2 proteins. Antibody binding was visualized by enhanced chemiluminescence (ECL-Plus; Amersham Pharmacia); intensities of experimental bands were analyzed by computer-assisted densitometry and expressed as arbitrary units, as previously described [19]. These experiments were performed in triplicate.

TUNEL assay

TdT (terminal deoxynucleotidyl transferase)-mediated dUTP nick-end labeling (TUNEL) assay was performed

in agreement with our previous reports [13]. Briefly, cells were plated on 24 9 24 mm cover slips (Carlo Erba Reagenti, Milan, Italy) and placed in six-well microtitre plates (Corning Incorporated, Corning, NY, USA) in DMEM supplemented with 10% FCS, penicillin 100 U/ml, streptomycin 100 mg/ml, and fungizone 25 mg/ml; 24 h after plating, when cells had reached 50–60% confluence, they were treated or not with H_2O_2 (0.5 mM) for 2 hours, and then were exposed or not to simvastatin (30 μM) for 24 hours; the incubation medium was not changed. Following treatment, TUNEL assay was performed using MEBSTAIN Apoptosis TUNEL Kit Direct (MBL, Woburn, MA, USA), strictly following instructions provided by the manufacturer. Photographs were acquired using a Leica GRDM confocal microscope (Leica, Wetzlar, Germany).

IL-8 secretion

Culture supernatants were collected and assayed for IL-8 by ELISA using a commercially available kit (Peli-Kine kit; Eurogenetics, Hampton, UK; sensitivity limit, 1 pg/ml), according to manufacturer's protocol. These experiments were performed in triplicate.

Statistical analysis

All data are expressed as mean ± standard error (SEM). Statistical evaluation of the results was performed by analysis of variance (ANOVA). Differences identified by ANOVA were pinpointed by unpaired Student's t test. The threshold of statistical significance was set at P <0.05.

Results
Cell viability

MTT assay detected an increase in cell number in cells pretreated with H_2O_2 (0.5 mM). In contrast, a 24 hours treatment with simvastatin (30 μM) was able to significantly decrease (P < 0.01) the cell number with respect to both control and pretreatment with H_2O_2. Therefore, simvastatin was able to modify normal growth cell, as well as to change the effect of H_2O_2 on cell proliferation (Figure 1).

Caspase-3 activation

Human GLC-82 cells were characterized by relatively low levels of caspase-3 activation, detected at baseline conditions as well as after exposure to H_2O_2 (0.5 mM) and after simvastatin treatment. Simvastatin (30 μM) significantly increased (P <0.01) the expression of active caspase-3 (Figure 2).

TUNEL assay

H_2O_2 (0.5 mM) did not modify the number of TUNEL-positive cells, with respect to untreated cells (control). By contrast, in the presence of H_2O_2, simvastatin (30 μM) significantly (P < 0.01) increased (of about 30%) the number of TUNEL-positive cells (Figure 3).

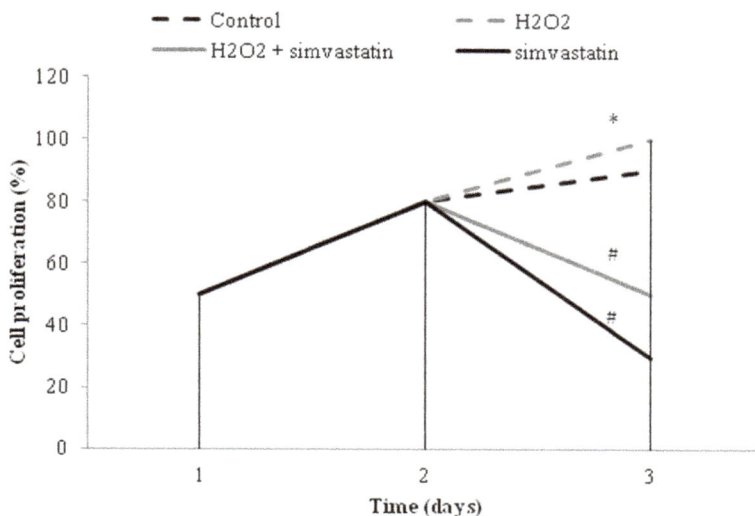

Figure 1 Cell viability. Effects of hydrogen peroxide (H_2O_2) on GLC-82 cell proliferation in the presence or absence of a 24 hours treatment with simvastatin (30 µM). Cell proliferation was assessed by MTT assay. *P < 0.01 (H_2O_2 vs control); #P <0.01 (H_2O_2 + simvastatin and simvastatin vs H_2O_2). Data represent the mean of three experiments.

ERK phosphorylation

Exposure of GLC-82 cells for 2 hours to H_2O_2 caused a significant (P < 0.01) increase in ERK1/2 phosphorylation; this effect was significantly inhibited in presence of a 24 hours treatment with simvastatin (P < 0.01) (Figure 4). Simvastatin (30 µM) induced a significant decrease (P < 0.01) of p-ERK expression. Both H_2O_2 and simvastatin exerted their effects uniquely on phosphorylation-dependent activation of ERK1/2, without affecting its total expression, as demonstrated by the unchanged binding patterns of the anti-(total)ERK polyclonal antibody (data not shown).

Matrix metalloproteinase expression

H_2O_2 induced a significant (P <0.01) increase in MMP-2 and MMP-9 expression. These effects were reverted by treatment with simvastatin (Figure 5). Moreover, simvastatin induced a significant decrease of both MMP-2 and MMP-9 baseline expression.

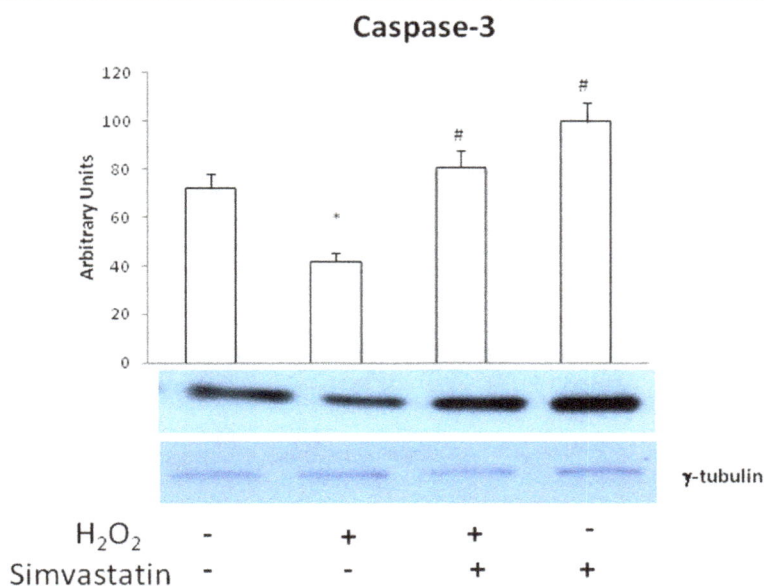

Figure 2 Caspase-3 activation. Western blot evaluation of caspase-3 expression with and without H_2O_2, in the presence or absence of a 24 hours treatment with simvastatin. Data represent the mean ± SEM of three experiments. **P <0.01. #P <0.01 (H_2O_2 + simvastatin and simvastatin vs H_2O_2).

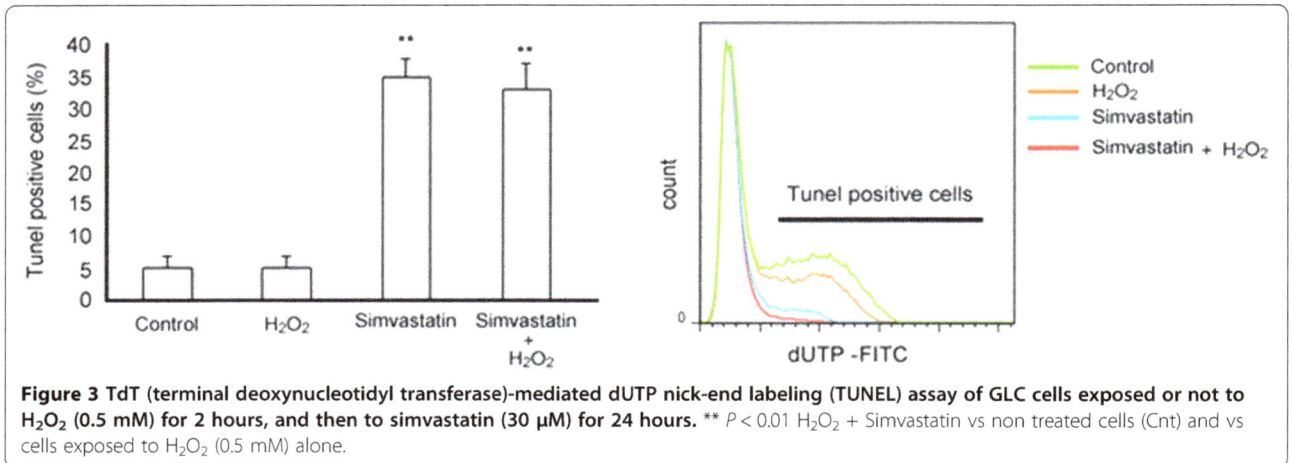

Figure 3 TdT (terminal deoxynucleotidyl transferase)-mediated dUTP nick-end labeling (TUNEL) assay of GLC cells exposed or not to H_2O_2 (0.5 mM) for 2 hours, and then to simvastatin (30 μM) for 24 hours. ** $P < 0.01$ H_2O_2 + Simvastatin vs non treated cells (Cnt) and vs cells exposed to H_2O_2 (0.5 mM) alone.

RECK expression

H_2O_2 induced a significant (P <0.01) decrease in RECK expression, whereas treatment with simvastatin significantly (P <0.01) enhanced RECK cellular content (Figure 6).

NF-κB nuclear content

H_2O_2 elicited a significant (P <0.01) increase in NF-κB nuclear levels, and this effect was significantly inhibited by treatment with simvastatin (P <0.01) (Figure 7).

MyD88 and TRAF6 expression

H_2O_2 induced a significant (P < 0.01) increase in MyD88 and TRAF6 expression, and these effects were significantly (P <0.01) inhibited by treatment with simvastatin (Figure 8).

TRADD and TRAF2 expression

H_2O_2 caused a significant (P <0.01) increase in TRADD and TRAF2 expression. These effects were significantly (P <0.01) inhibited by treatment with simvastatin (Figure 9).

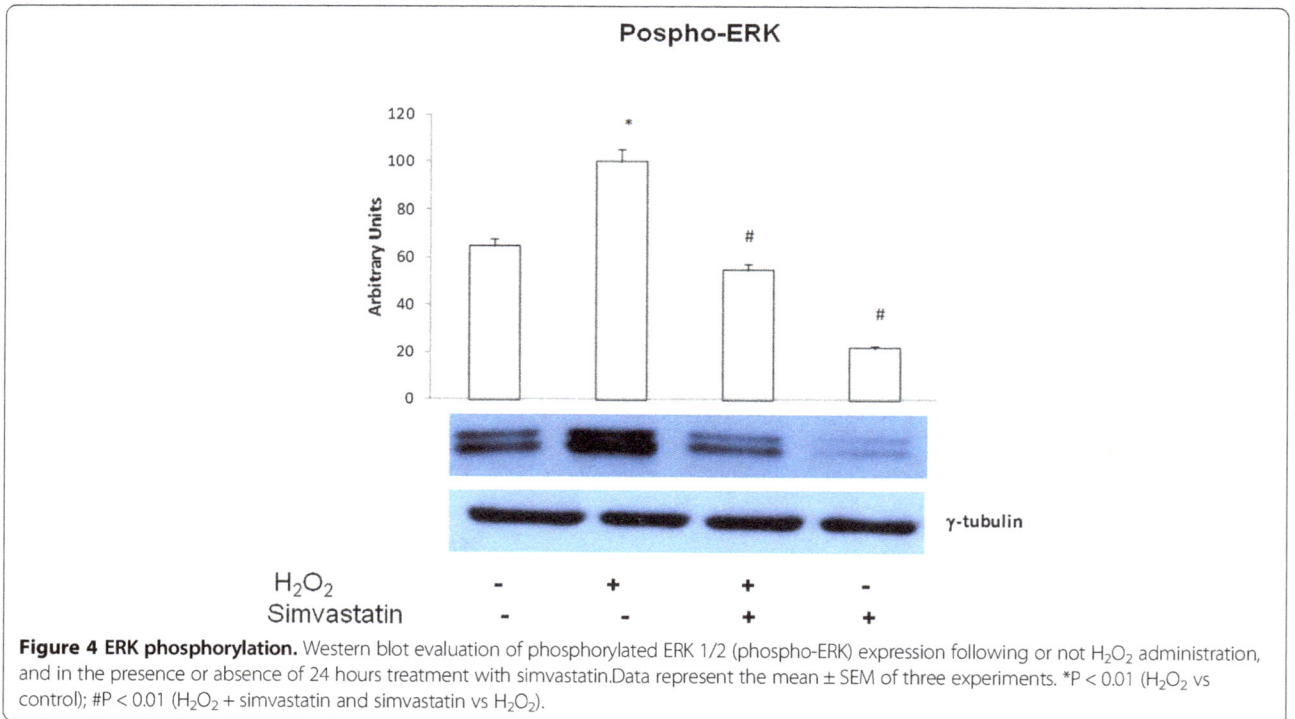

Figure 4 ERK phosphorylation. Western blot evaluation of phosphorylated ERK 1/2 (phospho-ERK) expression following or not H_2O_2 administration, and in the presence or absence of 24 hours treatment with simvastatin.Data represent the mean ± SEM of three experiments. *P < 0.01 (H_2O_2 vs control); #P < 0.01 (H_2O_2 + simvastatin and simvastatin vs H_2O_2).

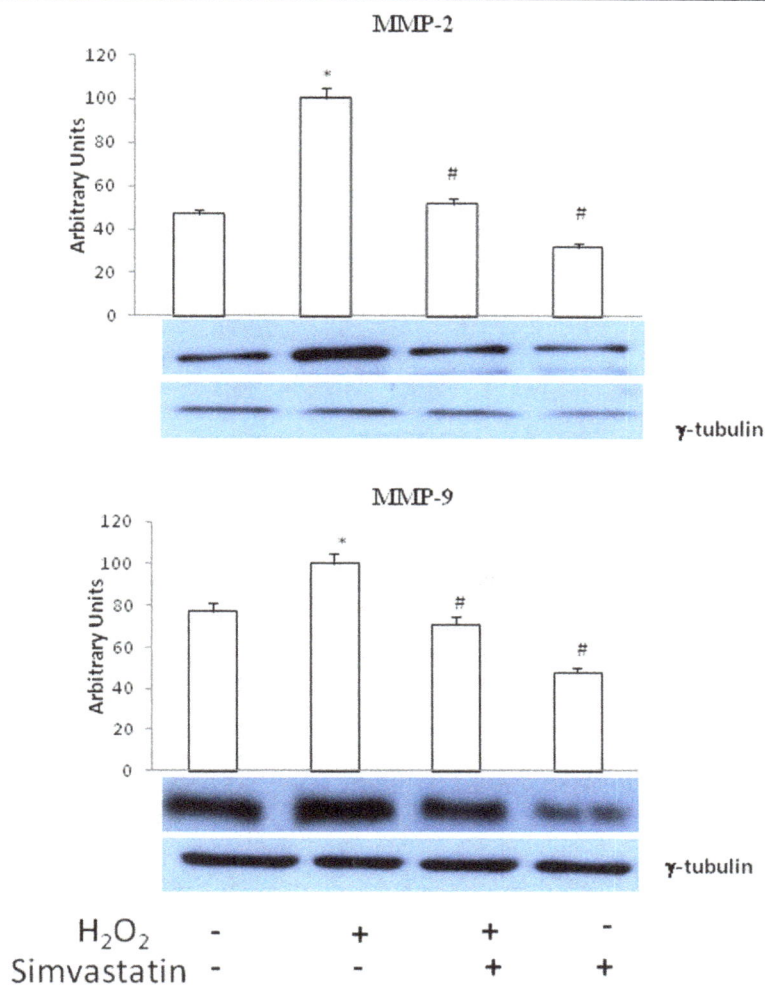

Figure 5 Matrix metalloproteinase expression. Western blot evaluation of MMP-2 (upper panel) and MMP-9 (lower panel) expression following or not H_2O_2 administration, and in the presence or absence of 24 hours treatment with simvastatin. Data represent the mean ± SEM of three experiments *P < 0.01 (H_2O_2 vs control); #P < 0.01 (H_2O_2 + simvastatin and simvastatin vs H_2O_2).

IL-8 secretion

H_2O_2 elicited a significant (P <0.01) increase in IL-8 secretion, which was significantly (P <0.01) prevented by pretreatment with simvastatin (Figure 10).

Discussion

In this study we evaluated the effects of simvastatin on lung adenocarcinoma GLC-82 cells, exposed to hydrogen peroxide (H_2O_2). Interestingly, oxidants are capable of exerting a tumorigenic action via molecular mechanisms which at least in part are also activated by proinflammatory pathways [20,21], and several authors have shown that both oxidative stress and inflammation are involved in the development and progression of cancer [22].

Therefore, we focused our attention on several cellular events triggered by oxidative stress. Within such a research context, it is noteworthy to point out that simvastatin was able to induce a comprehensive inhibition of many phenomena related to lung cancer.

In this regard, Manfredini et al. have previously reported that simvastatin is able to modulate oxidative DNA damage [23], and we also showed that simvastatin significantly decreased H_2O_2-induced cell proliferation rate, probably through inhibition of Ras-dependent phosphorylative activation of the ERK1/2 subgroup of MAPKs [13]. In fact, H_2O_2 dramatically enhanced ERK phosphorylation, and such a stimulatory action was markedly reduced by simvastatin. This implies that simvastatin affects ERK function by inhibiting mevalonate-dependent post-translational prenylation of Ras, thus impairing the sequential activation of the Ras/Raf/MEK/ERK signalling cascade [24]. Therefore, this mechanism may be also involved in the observed pro-apoptotic action of simvastatin, documented by the increased expression of active caspase-3 [25].

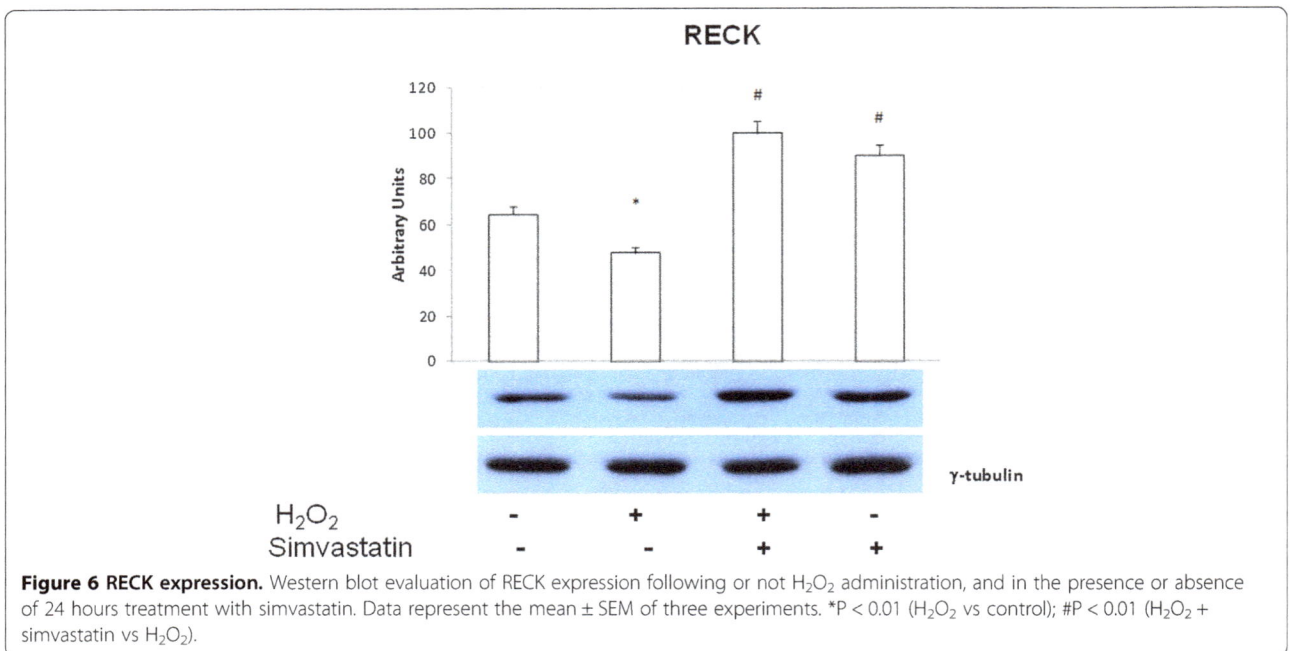

Figure 6 RECK expression. Western blot evaluation of RECK expression following or not H_2O_2 administration, and in the presence or absence of 24 hours treatment with simvastatin. Data represent the mean ± SEM of three experiments. *P < 0.01 (H_2O_2 vs control); #P < 0.01 (H_2O_2 + simvastatin vs H_2O_2).

Interestingly, in our present study the anti-proliferative and pro-apoptotic effects of simvastatin were also paralleled by a drug-induced up-regulation of RECK protein, which plays a pivotal role in inhibiting matrix metalloproteinases. MMP-2 and MMP-9 are responsible for extracellular matrix degradation, and for the consequent neo-angiogenesis, vascular invasion and metastatic potential that characterize malignant tumours [26-28]. Indeed, in many cancers RECK down-regulation is associated with high levels of MMP-9 [9]. Otherwise, preservation of RECK expression in some neoplasms correlates with a relatively low microvascular density as well as with a better prognosis, due to a decreased tendency to metastatic invasion [29]. Consistently with these considerations, our results show that H_2O_2 down-regulated RECK in GLC-82 cells, whereas simvastatin restored its expression. Moreover, H_2O_2 enhanced MMP-2 and MMP-9

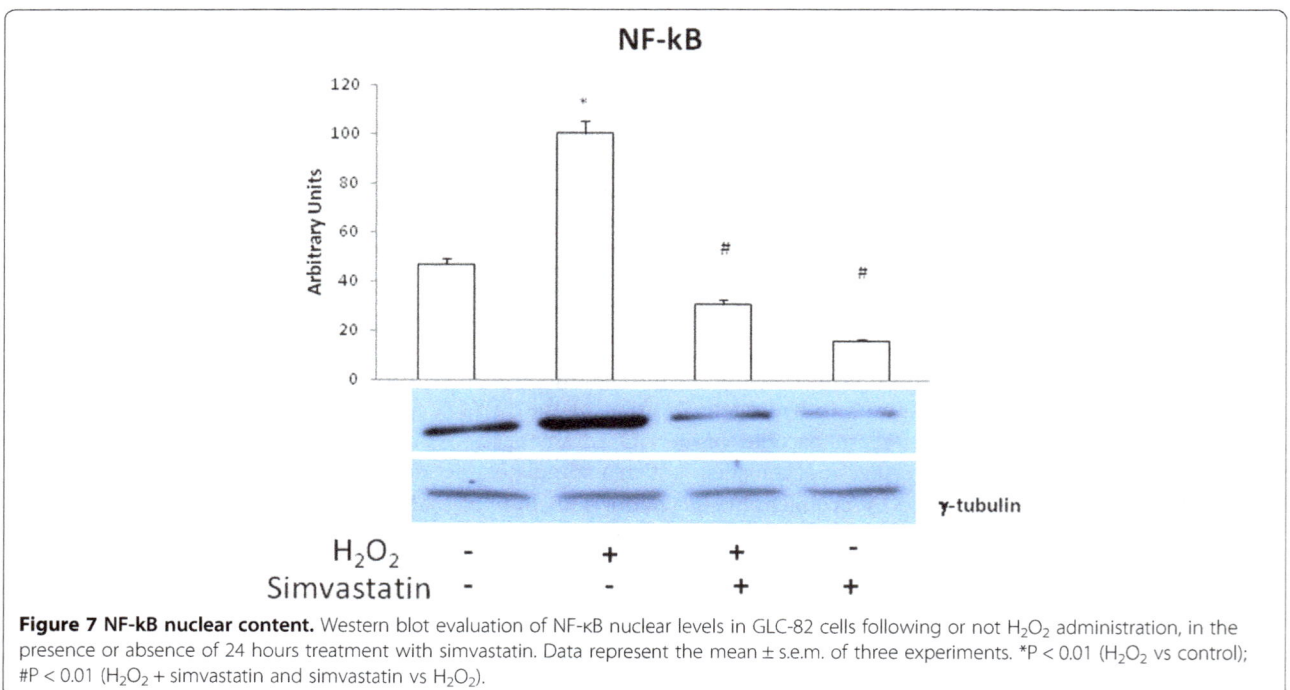

Figure 7 NF-kB nuclear content. Western blot evaluation of NF-κB nuclear levels in GLC-82 cells following or not H_2O_2 administration, in the presence or absence of 24 hours treatment with simvastatin. Data represent the mean ± s.e.m. of three experiments. *P < 0.01 (H_2O_2 vs control); #P < 0.01 (H_2O_2 + simvastatin and simvastatin vs H_2O_2).

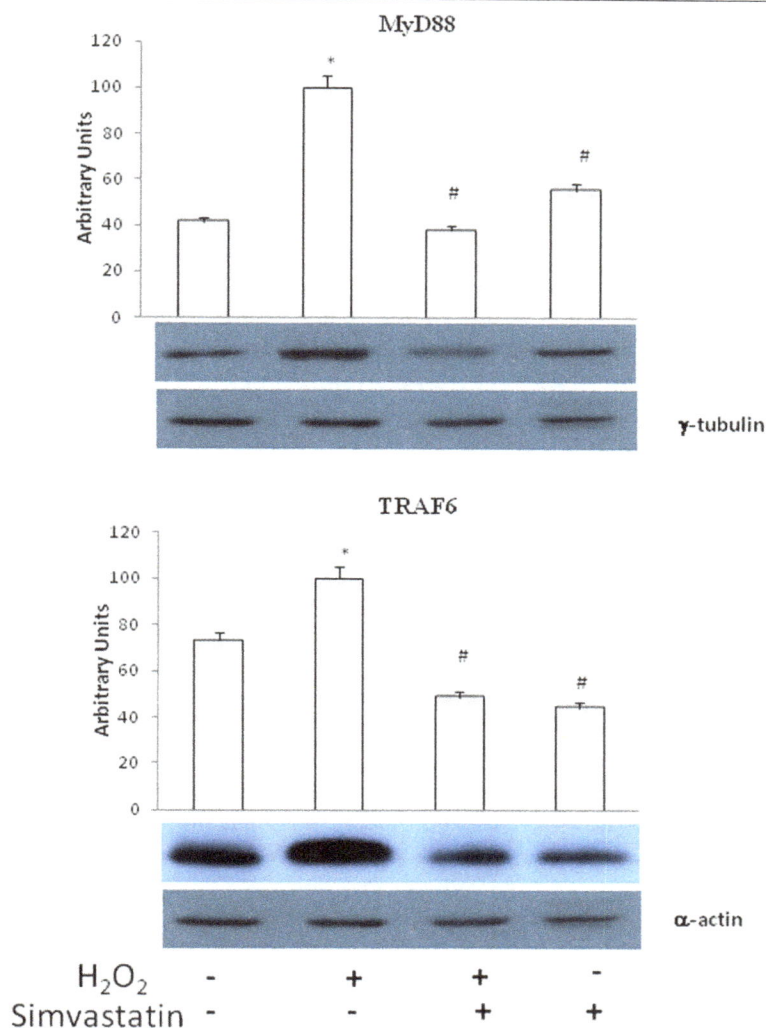

Figure 8 MyD88 and TRAF6 expression. Western blot evaluation of MyD88 (upper panel) and TRAF6 (lower panel) expression following H_2O_2 administration, in the presence or absence of 24 hours treatment with simvastatin. Data represent the mean ± SEM of three experiments. *P <0.01 (H_2O_2 vs control); #P <0.01 (H_2O_2 + simvastatin vs H_2O_2).

cellular expression, and these effects of oxidative stress were prevented by simvastatin.

Other important observations reported in the present study refer to further aspects of signal transduction. In particular, our data demonstrate that the noxious effects of oxidative stress on human lung adenocarcinoma cell lines, as well as the potential anti-cancer activity of statins, are also attributable to interferences with the signalling pathways linked to innate immunity [30]. In this regard, it is remarkable that H_2O_2 induced the expression of MyD88, a key molecular component of the intracellular signalling machinery activated by Toll-like receptors (TLRs), and once again simvastatin abrogated such effect. MyD88 associates with TLRs; upon stimulation, MyD88 recruits IL-1 receptor-associated kinase (IRAK) to TLRs via interaction of the death domains of

both molecules [31]. IRAK is activated by phosphorylation and then associates with tumor necrosis factor (TNF) receptor-associated factor 6 (TRAF6). Similarly to MyD88, the opposite actions of H_2O_2 and simvastatin translated into significant increases and decreases in TRAF6 expression, respectively. Therefore, on the basis of this experimental work, we canspeculate that oxidative stress triggers a particular type of tissue injury which is sensed by the surveillance network of innate immunity via TLR stimulation. In fact, it has been demonstrated that H_2O_2 can prime the responsiveness of the innate immune system through a recruitment of TLRs to cell plasma membrane [32]. However, this chain of molecular events, including the essential step of MyD88 activation, ultimately culminates in the downstream involvement of the transcription factor NF-κB,

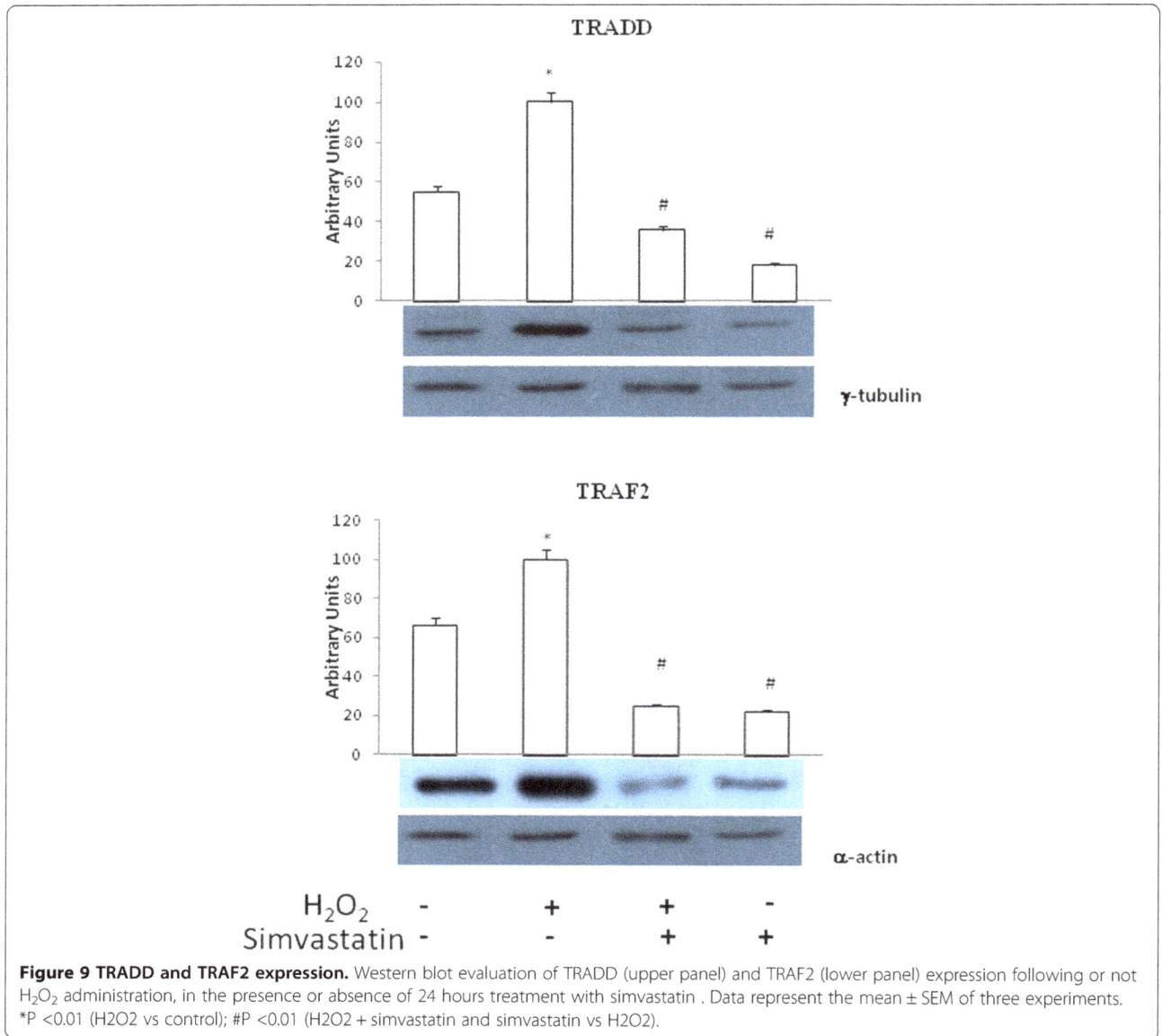

Figure 9 TRADD and TRAF2 expression. Western blot evaluation of TRADD (upper panel) and TRAF2 (lower panel) expression following or not H_2O_2 administration, in the presence or absence of 24 hours treatment with simvastatin . Data represent the mean ± SEM of three experiments. *P <0.01 (H2O2 vs control); #P <0.01 (H2O2 + simvastatin and simvastatin vs H2O2).

which is a key effector of the carcinogenic and proinflammatory attitudes of oxidative stress. It can thus be argued that, by interrupting such complex molecular cascades, statins can have relevant anti-cancer and anti-inflammatory properties.

Other important components of the macromolecular complex associated with TNF receptor superfamily, whose stimulation leads to NF-κB activation, include TRADD and TRAF2 proteins [33]. Here it is shown that both TRADD and TRAF2 were susceptible to up-regulation induced by H_2O_2, and this effect was prevented by simvastatin. Because the above mentioned signaling pathways converge towards NF-κB activation, it was not surprising to detect in GCL-82 cells, as a result of their exposure to H_2O_2, an increased nuclear content of NF-κB. Indeed,

nuclear translocation of this transcription factor is the essential step underlying its activation. Consistently with the overall experimental design of this study, it was well expected to find the observed decrease of NF-κB nuclear levels elicited by simvastatin.

Moreover, a further evidence of the opposite actions of H_2O_2 and simvastatin was found by analyzing, in GLC-82 cell culture supernatants, the changes referring to the concentrations of IL-8, which acts as a powerful chemoattractant for neutrophils [34]. In particular, IL-8 secretion was up-regulated and down-regulated by H_2O_2 and simvastatin, respectively. Indeed, this proinflammatory chemokine is encoded by a gene targeted by the transcriptional stimulatory activity of NF-κB [35].

IL-8

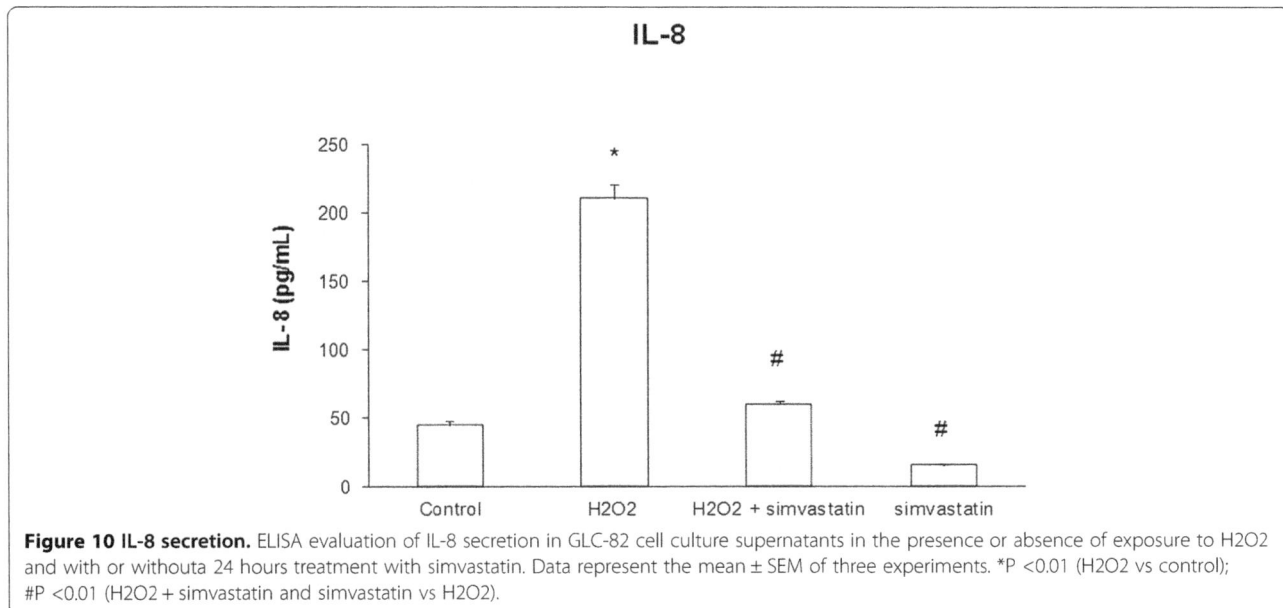

Figure 10 IL-8 secretion. ELISA evaluation of IL-8 secretion in GLC-82 cell culture supernatants in the presence or absence of exposure to H2O2 and with or without a 24 hours treatment with simvastatin. Data represent the mean ± SEM of three experiments. *P <0.01 (H2O2 vs control); #P <0.01 (H2O2 + simvastatin and simvastatin vs H2O2).

Therefore, taken together these results strongly suggest the existence of a tight cross-talk involving the proliferative, metastatic and proinflammatory mechanisms activated by oxidative stress in GLC-82 cells. Moreover, our data clearly demonstrate that in this lung adenocarcinoma cell line simvastatin can effectively interfere with the complex signal transduction networks underlying such mechanisms. These findings confirm and further extend our previous data obtained in the same GLC-82 cell line, showing that simvastatin was able to significantly decrease cell proliferation and increase apoptosis via inhibition of the ERK1/2 subgroup of MAPKs [13].

With regard to MMP-2 and MMP-9, it is well known that these enzymes promote cancer progression through extracellular matrix and basement membrane degradation, resulting in the exposure of cryptic locations linked to invasion, metastasis and angiogenesis. The 5′ flanking regions of the MMP-2 and MMP-9 genes contain several functional regulatory motifs that bind transcription factors such as NF-κB [36,37]. Through the interactions between NF-κB and its DNA binding sites, various agents including growth factors and cytokines are able to regulate MMP expression. Hence, the coordinated inhibitory effects of simvastatin on MMP2/9 expression and NF-κB activation imply the involvement of HMG-CoA reductase pathway in the process of metastatic invasion related to NF-κB and MMP activity. In fact, cancer cells usually express high levels of HMG-CoA reductase, which appear to be required by NSCLC cells to satisfy their increased need for isoprenoids and lipids.

Thus, by blocking Ras prenylation, simvastatin could interfere with NF-κB-dependent signaling networks responsible not only for MMP expression, but also for IL-8 synthesis. Indeed, it is reasonable to infer that, by inhibiting Ras/Raf-induced phosphorylative activation of MAPKs, simvastatin may be able to prevent IL-8 production elicited in GLC-82 cells by NF-κB activation due to oxidative stress.

Conclusion

In conclusion, our results show that simvastatin is able to inhibit the effects of H_2O_2 on lung cancer cells, suggesting that simvastatin is able to induce an antiproliferative, pro-apoptotic and antinflammatory effects in presence of a pro-inflammatory mediator. These data could support the role of simvastatin in the prevention of cancer and lung inflammatory disease (i.e. chronic obstructive pulmonary diseases). In fact to date no definitive reports have been published regarding these diseases [38,39]. However, in order to validate these preliminary observations further studies are needed, especially including controlled clinical trials.

Competing interests
The authors declare that they have no competing interests.

Authors' contributions
GL is the guarantor of the paper, taking responsibility for the integrity of the work as a whole, from inception to published article. D'AB made substantial contributions to the final version to be published. SG made substantial contributions to drafting the article. FD contributed to study conception and design, data acquisition, analysis and interpretation and drafting the article. SM contributed to study conception and design, data acquisition, analysis and interpretation and drafting the article. PG contributed to study conception and design, data acquisition, analysis and interpretation and drafting the article. MM contributed to study conception and design, data acquisition, analysis and interpretation and drafting the article. TR contributed to study conception and design, data acquisition, analysis and interpretation and drafting the article. MR contributed to study conception and design, data acquisition, analysis and interpretation and drafting the

article. NM contributed to study conception and design, data acquisition, analysis and interpretation and drafting the article. SR contributed to study conception and design, data acquisition, analysis and interpretation and drafting the article. All authors read and approved the final manuscript.

Acknowledgments

Daniela Falcone and Monica Scaramuzzino" were supported by a fellowship of the PhD Programme in Molecular Oncology, Experimental Immunology and Development of Innovative Therapies. This research was supported in part by a grant from Sicily Region (PO FESR Sicilia 2007/2013, CUP G73F11000050004 to MN, project "MEPRA", N. 133 of Linea d'Intervento 4.1.1.1).

Author details

[1]Department of Health Science, University of Catanzaro, Catanzaro, Italy. [2]Department of Medical and Surgical Sciences, University of Catanzaro, Catanzaro, Italy. [3]Department of Experimental Medicine, University of Catanzaro, Catanzaro, Italy. [4]Department of Experimental Medicine-Section of Pharmacology, School of Medicine, Second University of Naples, via Costantinopoli 16, 80136 Naples, Italy. [5]Department of Drug Sciences and Health Products, University of Messina, IRCCS centro neurolesi "Bonino-Pulejo", Messina, Italy.

References

1. Pryor WA, Prier DG, Church DF: Electron-spin resonance study of mainstream and sidestream cigarette smoke: nature of the free radicals in gasphase smoke and in cigarette tar. *Environ Health Perspect* 1983, 47:345–355.
2. Thannickal VJ, Fanburg BL: Reactive oxygen species in cell signaling. *Am J Physiol Lung Cell Mol Physiol* 2000, 279:L1005–L1028.
3. Chung KF, Adcock IM: Multifaceted mechanisms in COPD: inflammation, immunity, and tissue repair and destruction. *Eur Respir J* 2008, 31:1334–1356.
4. Chang L, Karin M: Mammalian MAP kinase signalling cascades. *Nature* 2001, 410:37–40.
5. Holgate ST: The sentinel role of the airway epithelium in asthma pathogenesis. *Immunol Rev* 2011, 242:205–219.
6. Milara J, Cortijo J: Tobacco, inflammation, and respiratory tract cancer. *Curr Pharm Des* 2012, 18:3901–3938.
7. Zalcman G, Bergot E, Lechapt E: Update on nonsmall cell lung cancer. *Eur Respir Rev* 2010, 19:173–185.
8. Deryugina EI, Quigley JP: Matrix metalloproteinases and tumor metastasis. *Cancer Metastasis Rev* 2006, 25:9–34.
9. Takahashi C, Sheng Z, Horan TP, Kitayama H, Maki M, Hitomi K, Kitaura Y, Takai S, Sasahara RM, Horimoto A, Ikawa Y, Ratzkin BJ, Arakawa T, Noda M: Regulation of matrix metalloproteinase-9 and inhibition of tumor invasion by the membrane-anchored glycoprotein RECK. *Proc Natl Acad Sci U S A* 1998, 95:13221–13226.
10. Kostantinopolous PA, Karamouzis MV, Papavassiliou AG: Post-translational modifications and regulation of the RAS superfamily of GTPases as anticancer targets. *Nat Rev Drug Discov* 2007, 6:541–555.
11. Nielsen SF, Nordestgaard BG, Bojesen SE: Statin use and reduced cancer-related mortality. *N Engl J Med* 2012, 367:1792–1802.
12. Beri A, Sural N, Mahajan SB: Non-atheroprotective effects of statins: a systematic review. *Am J Cardiovasc Drugs* 2009, 9:361–370.
13. Pelaia G, Gallelli L, Renda T, Fratto D, Falcone D, Caraglia M, Busceti MT, Terracciano R, Vatrella A, Maselli R, Savino R: Effects of statins and farnesyl transferase inhibitors on ERK phosphorylation, apoptosis and cell viability in non-small lung cancer cells. *Cell Prolif* 2012, 45:557–565.
14. Falcone D, Gallelli L, Di Virgilio A, Tucci L, Scaramuzzino M, Terracciano R, Pelaia G, Savino R: Effects of simvastatin and rosuvastatin on RAS protein, matrix metalloproteinases and NF-κB in lung cancer and in normal pulmonary tissues. *Cell Prolif* 2013, 46:172–182.
15. Pelaia G, Gallelli L, D'Agostino B, Vatrella A, Cuda G, Fratto D, Renda T, Galderisi U, Piegari E, Crimi N, Rossi F, Caputi M, Costanzo FS, Vancheri C, Maselli R, Marsico SA: Effects of TGF-beta and glucocorticoids on map kinase phosphorylation, IL-6/IL-11 secretion and cell proliferation in primary cultures of human lung fibroblasts. *J Cell Physiol* 2007, 210:489–497.
16. Gallelli L, Pelaia G, D'Agostino B, Cuda G, Vatrella A, Fratto D, Gioffrè V, Galderisi U, De Nardo M, Mastruzzo C, Salinaro ET, Maniscalco M, Sofia M, Crimi N, Rossi F, Caputi M, Costanzo FS, Maselli R, Marsico SA, Vancheri C: Endothelin-1 induces proliferation of human lung fibroblasts and IL-11 secretion through an ET(A) receptor-dependent activation of MAP kinases. *J Cell Biochem* 2005, 96:858–868.
17. Pelaia G, Cuda G, Vatrella A, Gallelli L, Fratto D, Gioffrè V, D'Agostino B, Caputi M, Maselli R, Rossi F, Costanzo FS, Marsico SA: Effects of hydrogen peroxide on MAPK activation, IL-8 production and cell viability in primary cultures of human bronchial epithelial cells. *J Cell Biochem* 2004, 93:142–152.
18. Gallelli L, Pelaia G, Fratto D, Muto V, Falcone D, Vatrella A, Curto LS, Renda T, Busceti MT, Liberto MC, Savino R, Cazzola M, Marsico SA, Maselli R: Effects of budesonide on p38 MAPK activation, apoptosis and IL-8 secretion, induced by TNF-α and *Haemophilus influenzae* in human bronchial epithelial cells. *Int J Immunopathol Pharmacol* 2010, 23:471–479.
19. Gallelli L, Falcone D, Pelaia G, Renda T, Terracciano R, Malara N, Vatrella A, Sanduzzi A, D'Agostino B, Rossi F, Vancheri C, Maselli R, Marsico SA, Savino R: IL-6 receptor superantagonist SANT7 inhibits TGF-β-induced proliferation of human lung fibroblasts. *Cell Prolif* 2008, 41:393–407.
20. Valko M, Izakovic M, Mazur M, Rhodes CJ, Telser J: Role of oxygen radicals in DNA damage and cancer incidence. *Mol Cell Biochem* 2004, 266:37–56.
21. Franco R, Schoneveld O, Georgakilas AG, Panayiotidis MI: Oxidative stress, DNA methylation and carcinogenesis. *Cancer Lett* 2008, 266:6–11.
22. Nowsheen S, Aziz K, Kryston TB, Ferguson NF, Georgakilas A: The interplay between inflammation and oxidative stress in carcinogenesis. *Curr Mol Med* 2012, 12:672–680.
23. Manfredini V, Biancini GB, Vanzin CS, Dal Vesco AM, Cipriani F, Biasi L, Treméa R, Deon M, Peralba Mdo C, Wajner M, Vargas CR: Simvastatin treatment prevents oxidative damage to DNA in whole blood leukocytes of dyslipidemic type 2 diabetic patients. *Cell Biochem Funct* 2010, 28:360–366.
24. Khanzada UK, Pardo OE, Meier C, Downward J, Seckl MJ, Arcaro A: Potent inhibition of small-cell lung cancer cell growth by simvastatin reveals selective functions of Ras isoforms in growth factor signaling. *Oncogene* 2006, 25:877–887.
25. Nicholson DW, Thornberry NA: Caspases: killer proteases. *Trends Biochem Sci* 1997, 22:299–306.
26. Egeblad M, Werb Z: New functions for the matrix metalloproteinases in cancer progression. *Nat Rev Cancer* 2002, 2:161–174.
27. Duffy MJ, Maguire TM, Hill A, McDermott E, O'Higgins N: Metalloproteinases: role in breast carcinogenesis, invasion and metastasis. *Breast Cancer Res* 2000, 2:252–257.
28. Curran S, Murray GI: Matrix metalloproteinases: molecular aspects of their roles in tumour invasion and metastasis. *Eur J Cancer* 2000, 36:1621–1630.
29. Chen Y, Tseng SH: The potential of RECK inducers as antitumor agents for glioma. *Anticancer Res* 2012, 32:2991–2998.
30. Pinto A, Morello S, Sorrentino R: Lung cancer and Toll-like receptors. *Cancer Immunol Immunother* 2011, 60:1211–1220.
31. Lin SC, Lo YC, Wu H: Helical assembly in the MyD88-IRAK4-IRAK2 complex in TLR/IL-1R signalling. *Nature* 2010, 465:885–890.
32. Powers KA, Szaszi K, Khadaroo RG, Tawadros PS, Marshall JC, Kapus A, Rotstein OD: Oxidative stress generated by hemorrhagic shock recruits Toll-like receptor 4 to the plasma membrane in macrophages. *J Exp Med* 2006, 203:1951–1961.
33. Jackson-Bernitsas DG, Ichikawa H, Takada Y, Myers JN, Lin XL, Darnay BG, Chaturvedi MM, Aggarwal BB: Evidence that TNF-TNFR1-TRADD-TRAF2-RIP-TAK1-IKK pathway mediates constitutive NF-κB activation and proliferation in human head and neck squamous cell carcinoma. *Oncogene* 2007, 26:1385–1397.
34. Biggioni M, Dewald B, Moser B: Interleukin-8 and related chemotactic cytokines-CXC and CC chemokines. *Adv Immunol* 1984, 55:97–179.
35. Hoffmann E, Dittrich-Breiholz O, Holtmann H, Kracht M: Multiple control of interleukin-8 gene expression. *J Leukoc Biol* 2002, 72:847–855.
36. Sato H, Seiki M: Regulatory mechanism of 92-kDa type IV collagenase gene expression which is associated with invasiveness of tumor cells. *Oncogene* 1993, 8:395–405.
37. Takahra T, Smart DE, Oakley F, Mann DA: Induction of myofibroblast MMP-9 transcription in three-dimensional collagen I gel cultures: regulation by NF-kappaB, AP-1 and Sp1. *Int J Biochem Cell Biol* 2004, 36:353–363.

38. Wang J, Li C, Tao H, Cheng Y, Han L, Li X, Hu Y: **Statin use and risk of lung cancer: a meta-analysis of observational studies and randomized controlled trials.** *PLoS One* 2013, **25**:e77950.
39. Horita N, Miyazawa N, Kojima R, Inoue M, Ishigatsubo Y, Ueda A, Kaneko T: **Statins reduce all-cause mortality in chronic obstructive pulmonary disease: a systematic review and meta-analysis of observational studies.** *Respir Res* 2014, **15**:80.

15

Anti-malarial prescribing practices in Sudan eight years after introduction of artemisinin-based combination therapies and implications for development of drug resistance

Abeer Abuzeid Atta Elmannan[1*], Khalid Abdelmutalab Elmardi[2], Yassir Ali Idris[3], Jonathan M Spector[4], Nahid Abdelgadir Ali[2] and Elfatih Mohamed Malik[3]

Abstract

Background: The World Health Organization (WHO) recommends artemisinin-based combination therapies (ACTs) as first-line treatment for uncomplicated malaria. Sudan revised its malaria treatment policy accordingly in 2004. However, eight years after ACTs were introduced in Sudan the patterns of ACT prescribing practices among health care providers remain unclear. We systematically analyzed use of ACTs in a large number of primary health facilities and we discuss the public health implications of our findings.

Methods: This cross-sectional study was based on WHO's guidance for investigating drug use in health facilities. Data were collected from 40 randomly selected primary health centers in five localities in Gezira State, Sudan. The primary outcome of the study was the proportion of patients who were adequately managed according to Sudan's recommended malaria treatment guidelines. Twelve drug-use indicators were used to assess key ACT prescribing practices.

Results: One thousand and two hundred patients diagnosed with uncomplicated malaria were recruited into the study. ACT was prescribed for 88.6%patients and artemether injections were (incorrectly) prescribed in 9.5% of cases. Only 40.9% of patients in the study were correctly diagnosed and 26.9% were adequately managed according to the nationally recommended treatment guidelines. Incorrect prescribing activities included failure to use generic medicine names (88.2%), incorrect dosage (27.7%), and unexplained antibiotic co-prescription (24.2%). Dispensing practices were also poor, with labeling practices inadequate (97.1%) and insufficient information given to patients about their prescribed treatment (50.5%).

Conclusion: Irrational malaria treatment practices are common in Sudan. This has important public health implications since failure to adhere to nationally recommended guidelines could play a role in the future development of drug resistance. As such, identifying ways to improve the anti-malarial prescribing practices of heath workers in Sudan may be a priority.

Keywords: Malaria, Artemisinin-based combination therapy, Drug resistance, Sudan, Sub-Saharan Africa

* Correspondence: abeeratta@gmail.com
[1]Al Neelain University, Steen Street, P.O. Box 7294, Code: 11123 Khartoum, Sudan
Full list of author information is available at the end of the article

Background

The World Health Organization (WHO) recommends artemisinin-based combination therapies (ACTs) as first-line treatment for uncomplicated malaria [1,2]. ACTs consist of two anti-malarial compounds: an artemisinin derivative, which induces rapid reduction of parasite load in blood over a period of days, and a partner drug, which eradicates remaining parasites [3].

Recently, artemisinin resistance has been observed in four Southeast Asian countries (Cambodia, Myanmar, Thailand, and Viet Nam) [4-6]. This has been attributed to factors including irrational prescribing practices, poor patient compliance with prescribed regimens, improper use of artemisinin monotherapies, and inadequate access to quality assured forms of the drug [7-9]. Fortunately, ACTs remain effective as long as resistance to the partner drug has not developed [10]. But while resistance to ACTs has not yet been observed, concern exists that poor treatment practices may promote ACT resistance in the future, a situation similar to the global spread of chloroquine resistance that has occured [11].

In 2011, WHO encouraged the scale-up of interventions to protect the efficacy of ACTs, which was supported by the release of the Global Plan for Artemisinin Resistance Containment [8]. Currently, WHO recommends five forms of ACTs: artemether-lumefantrine (AL), artesunate-sulfadoxine/pyrimethamine (ASP), artesunate-amodiaquine (ASAQ), artesunate-mefloquine (ASMQ), and dihydroartemisinin-piperaquine (DHAPQ) [12]. Malaria-endemic countries in Sub-Saharan Africa have adopted several of these different formulations of ACTs in their national strategies for malaria control and elimination [13].

In 2004 Sudan revised its Malaria treatment policy in favor of use of ACTs. The nationally recommended first- and second-line treatments are ASP and AL, respectively [14,15], both of which are provided free of charge at primary health care facilities in Sudan. According to national treatment guidelines in Sudan, peripheral blood smears should be obtained on febrile patients that are suspected of having malaria in order to confirm the diagnosis before treatment (presumptive diagnosis of malaria is no longer accepted for prescribing treatment, except in the increasingly rare event that no laboratory facility or rapid diagnostic testing capability are available). However, some data suggest that the malaria guidelines in Sudan are far from universally adhered to. A cluster-sample survey conducted in 15 states in Sudan five years following ACT introduction found that only 35% of febrile patients were treated according to test results [16]. Another survey revealed that the nationally recommended first-line treatment (ASP) was prescribed in only 44% of prescriptions [17]. Eight years after introduction of public policy aimed at harmonizing effective and appropriate anti-malarial treatment across the country, the patterns of ACT use in Sudan remain largely unclear.

In this study we aimed to systematically explore patterns of ACT use among health care providers in primary health care units in Sudan, and to assess the significance of the findings in the context of risks for drug resistance. We suspected that the results of this investigation could provide a useful quantitative analysis of specific ACT prescribing problems that are common in Sudan, and could potentially help to inform strategies for promoting rational use of ACT nationally.

Methods

Study setting

This was a cross-sectional study conducted in Gezira State, which is located in the east-central region of the Sudan. Gezira is a large state with a total area of 27,549 km [18]. Administratively, it is divided into eight localities, containing 65 hospitals and greater than 800 primary health care facilities.

Study population

The study population consisted of patients that sought medical care at primary health care facilities throughout Gezira State and who were diagnosed with uncomplicated malaria. Uncomplicated malaria was confirmed by the demonstration of asexual forms of the parasite in the thick or thin peripheral blood smear or by rapid diagnostic test in the presence of fever. We based our sampling method and sample size calculation on guidelines published by WHO ("How to Investigate Drug Use in Health Facilities") [19]. Patients were recruited through a three-step sampling methodology in which we took advantage of existing administrative divisions of the state and clustering at the level of primary health centers. Firstly, five of Gezira State's 8 localities were randomly selected for participation in the study. Second, 40 "clusters" (i.e., primary health centers) within those five states were randomly selected. Finally, 30 patients were recruited from each primary health center included in the study in order to arrive at the sample size of 1,200 patients. The study took place over a 5 month period (July-November 2011). During the study period, study teams visited each primary health center and recruited the first 30 consecutive patients who were diagnosed with uncomplicated malaria and who verbally consented to be in the study. In health facilities with high patient volume, only 2–3 days were required to recruit the necessary number of patients. In other health facilities with lower patient volumes, up to 12 days were needed to recruit 30 patients diagnosed with uncomplicated malaria.

Data collection and analyses

Data were collected prospectively. The primary outcome of this study was the proportion of patients who were adequately managed according to the nationally recommended treatment guidelines. Adequate management was defined by patient history of fever, positive blood smear for malaria, and first-line anti-malarial treatment prescribed in the correct dose.

Seven core drug use indicators drawn from WHO's prescribing and patient-care indicators [19] were used to assess key practices of health care providers. The prescribing indicators were: anti-malarial prescribed in generic name, antibiotic co-prescribed, analgesic co-prescribed, and anti-malarial dosage form correctly written. The patient-care indicators were: anti-malarial prescribed was fully dispensed, anti-malarial adequately labeled, and patient adequately informed about the prescribed anti-malarial. We also measured an additional 5 indicators that were developed for the purpose of this study in order to evaluate essential components of the nationally recommended protocol for diagnosing and treating malaria correctly in Sudan. These supplementary indicators were: patient history of fever, whether or not a clinical examination was performed, blood smear evaluation, positive blood smear, and correct diagnosis (as defined by patient history of fever and positive blood smear).

Study staff reviewed patients' prescriptions to collect data relating to prescribing indicators. Exit interviews with patients were conducted to explore patient-care practices. Data collectors attended an intensive training workshop prior to the start of the study to help ensure standardized data collection. Training components included familiarization with drug use indicators, how to properly extract information from anti-malarial drug-containing prescriptions, how to interview patients, and how to record and code indicators. At study sites, data collectors recruited patients at the pharmacy when patients came to collect their medicines following clinical encounters. Through a verbal consent process, data collectors explained the purpose and risks of the study to patients. Those who consented to participate were interviewed and their prescriptions were reviewed. Data were recorded on standardized forms and coded.

Statistics
Chi-squared test was utilized to compare frequencies of prescription, patient-care, and supplementary indicators between types of anti-malarial medications prescribed. Data were analyzed using SPSS 22.0 (IMB SPSS Inc., Chicago, IL, USA).

Ethical considerations
Ethical approvals for this study were obtained from Al Neelain University Institutional Review Board, the Sudan National Fund for Promoting Medical Services, and Gezira State Ministry of Health. Verbal-only consent was approved

by the three boards, as it was not practical to obtain written informed consent from all patients.

Results
The five localities within Gezira State that were randomly selected for this study were Greater Medani, Gezira South, Gezira East, Hasahisa, and Kamleen. The names of the 40 primary health centers within these five localities that were randomly selected for participation are being kept anonymous to maintain confidentiality of patients and health providers.

Of the 1,200 prescriptions reviewed, 88.6% included ACT (Table 1). Of these, virtually all were ASP; only two ACT prescriptions contained AL. One hundred and fourteen (114) patients were prescribed artemether injections, comprising 9.5% of the prescriptions. As the main focus of this was ACT prescribing practices, we restricted subsequent data analysis to the 1,175 patients (98%) who were prescribed either ASP or artemether injections.

Just fewer than 41% percent of the 1,200 patients in the study were correctly diagnosed with uncomplicated malaria, and 26.9% of patients were adequately managed for uncomplicated malaria according to the nationally recommended treatment guidelines.

The frequencies of prescribing, patient-care, and supplementary indicators stratified by anti-malarial medicine prescribed are presented in Tables 2, 3 and 4. Only 11.8% of prescriptions contained the generic name, and strong evidence of association existed between prescribing in generic name and the type of anti-malarial prescribed (p <0.000). Although ASP was prescribed in greater than 90% of prescriptions, it was written generically in only 6.7% of prescriptions. It was observed that many prescribers tended to write the informal name for ASP ("Rajimat" which translates to "missiles" in English). Conversely, artemether, while incorrectly prescribed, was written generically in 58.5% of prescriptions. Nearly 25% of prescriptions contained an antibiotic without a clear indication for its use.

Regarding dispensing practices, the prescribed anti-malarial was fully dispensed in the vast majority of cases,

Table 1 Anti-malarial treatment formulations prescribed in 40 primary health centers in Gezira State, Sudan

	n	%
Artesunate-sulfadoxine/pyrimethaminetablets	1,061	88.4
Artemether injection	114	9.5%
Quinine injection	14	1.2%
Quinine tablets	5	0.4%
Sulfadoxine/pyrimethamine tablets	4	0.3%
Artemether-lumefantrine tablets	2	0.2%
Total	1,200	100.0%

Table 2 Prescribing indicators stratified by anti-malarial medication prescribed

	ASP n (%) N = 1,061	ART* n (%) N = 114	All prescriptions n (%) N = 1,175	95% CI	Chi-squared p value
Anti-malarial prescribed in generic name	71 (6.7%)	67 (58.8%)	138 (11.8%)	10-13.6	0.000
Antibiotic co-prescribed	248 (23.4%)	36 (31.6%)	284 (24.2%)	21.8-26.7	0.000
Analgesic co-prescribed	342 (32.2%)	84 (73.7%)	426 (36.3%)	33.6-39.1	0.065
Anti-malarial dosage form correctly written	769 (72.5%)	80 (70.2%)	849 (72.3%)	69.7-74.9	0.584

*Artemether injection.

signifying a high availability of anti-malarial medications at the study sites. However, labeling practices were adequate in only 2.9% of dispensed treatment packages. More than half of patients were inadequately informed about their anti-malarial treatment.

Discussion

More than eight years have elapsed since the introduction of ACT for malaria in Sudan. However, proper case management for patients with malaria remains a challenge. In this large study of prescribing practices among healthcare workers in Gezira State, the recommended first-line drug was prescribed in most patients, which would seem to indicate confidence among heath care providers in this approach to treatment. Nevertheless, misuse of ACTs was widespread. Artemether injections were prescribed inappropriately, patients were not diagnosed according to standard guidelines, patients received inadequate education regarding their therapy, and treatment packages were poorly labeled. Overall, a minority of patients were diagnosed and treated according to the nationally recommended guidelines. A previous study in Ghana showed similar results [20].

A variety of factors may explain the findings in this study. For instance, poor supervision of health care providers, coupled with inadequate training and few opportunities for continuing education, could be a contributing cause of irrational ACT prescribing. Patient-related factors may also play a large role. Self-treatment of malaria is a common practice in Sudan [21], as well as in other countries [22]. Patient demand for treatment may influence the prescribing behaviors of health care providers. This may be especially true at the primary health care level where-working conditions are sometimes unfavorable due to

heavy workloads and low salaries. Additionally, it is not infrequent that such facilities encounter medication stock outs, which can lead by necessity to haphazard prescribing of other anti-malarial drugs (e.g., prescribing artemether injections for uncomplicated malaria despite the fact that this is not recommended therapy).

The majority of health care providers in this study requested a laboratory confirmation for malaria before prescribing treatment. However, among those who were prescribed ASP, only half were smear positive. Higher rates were reported in a Kenyan study where nearly 80% of patients with negative blood smears were prescribed malaria treatment [23]. This may raise concerns about Sudanese healthcare worker's acceptance of laboratory results. Lack of trust of health care providers in laboratory diagnosis could be a factor in overreliance on clinical diagnosis of malaria. In the past, when laboratory facilities were largely unavailable in rural and remote areas, presumptive treatment of malaria was widely accepted. In recent years, however, with the expansion of health services across the country including the introduction of rapid diagnostic tests, presumptive treatment is no longer recommended as long as laboratory facilities are available. Moreover, requesting a laboratory investigation without utilizing its result is a waste of resources and poses unnecessary cost for patients. Most importantly, prescribing ACT for malaria negative patients increases the risk of developing drug resistance in the future, and should therefore be restricted. Unless all efforts come together to ensure accurate and safe diagnosis of malaria patients, barriers to effective clinical practices are likely to remain.

According to the national malaria treatment policy, the first-line treatment is made available free of charge

Table 3 Patient-care indicators stratified by anti-malarial medication prescribed

	ASP n (%) N = 1061	ART* n (%) N = 114	All prescriptions n (%) N = 1175	95% CI	Chi-squared p value
Anti-malarial prescribed was fully dispensed	1,028 (96.9%)	104 (91.2%)	1,132 (96.3%)	95.1-97.3	0.006
Anti-malarial adequately labeled	34 (3.2%)	0 (0.0%)	34 (2.9%)	2-3.9	0.069
Patient adequately informed about the prescribed anti-malarial	510 (48.1%)	64 (56.1%)	574 (48.9%)	46-51.8	0.115

*Artemether injection.

Table 4 Supplementary indicators stratified by anti-malarial medication prescribed

	ASP n (%) N = 1,061	ART* n (%) N = 114	All prescriptions n (%) N = 1,175	95% CI	Chi-squared p value
Patient presented with history of fever	891 (84.0%)	90 (78.9%)	981 (83.5%)	81.4-85.6	0.184
Patient clinically examined	221 (20.8%)	28 (24.6%)	249 (21.2%)	18.9-23.5	0.338
Peripheral blood smear for malarial obtained	1,029 (97.0%)	105 (92.1%)	1,134 (96.5%)	95.5-97.6	0.013
Peripheral blood smear positive for malaria	516 (50.1%)	73 (69.5%)	589 (51.9%)	49-54.8	0.000
Patient correctly diagnosed with uncomplicated malaria	425 (40.1%)	56 (49.1%)	481 (40.9%)	38.1-43.7	0.071

*Artemether injection.

in primary health care facilities. Overall, prescribing ACT using the generic name was widely neglected. Prescribers tend to use the term "Rajimat" to refer to the first–line therapy instead of prescribing it generically. It appears that the system for reviewing written prescriptions is either lacking or ineffective. Furthermore, the rate of antibiotic co-prescribing is evidently high. In some cases the healthcare provider may be uncertain about the diagnosis and therefore prescribe an antibiotic along with the anti-malarial. Haphazard antibiotic prescribing promotes the development of drug resistance and puts patients at risk of adverse drug effects. Our investigation also showed that the ACT dosage form was incorrectly written in the majority of prescriptions. For a prescription to be considered correctly written it should at minimum contain the medication's dose (written in milligrams), quantity, and schedule. That information was incorrect, incomplete, or not written in the vast majority of prescriptions reviewed in our study. This practice has serious implications related to patient safety, including increasing the potential for treatment failure, promoting drug resistance, and increasing the risk of complications either due to the disease itself or to the administering of an inappropriate dose.

Interestingly, the availability of ACT in the study sites was high during the study period. Most ACT prescriptions were fully dispensed. This is a positive finding, since reliable availability of first-line therapies at primary health facilities would be expected to promote their rational use. However, labeling of dispensed drug packages was grossly inadequate. Moreover, information given to patients about their prescribed treatment was insufficient in most cases. Patient education and information enhance their adherence to prescribed therapies, leading to better treatment outcomes [24-26]. Heavy patient load in primary health facilities could be a main contributory factor.

Given that a multifactorial etiology is likely the cause for poor ACT prescribing patterns among health workers in Sudan, it would seem difficult to significantly improve the situation unless collaborative efforts take place by many different stakeholders. Examples of potentially important interventions include targeted training programmes for health workers, strategies for providing clear ACT information to patients and to the general public, strict policies focused on ACT deployment, and continuous monitoring of existing practices. Clear regulations relating to ACT use should be institutionalized, and more support is needed to encourage health care providers to adhere to the recommended guidelines. Evidence-based interventions such as implementing a self-administered checklist have proven to be effective for improving the performance of health care providers in disciplines such as surgery and childbirth [27,28]. Perhaps similar checklist-based interventions could promote the rational use of ACTs in Sudan.

This study has a several limitations. Prescribing data in this study were collected prospectively over a limited period of time and the fact that healthcare providers were aware that their practices were being observed could be a source of bias via the Hawthorne effect. However, retrospective collection of information was not feasible in this setting since records in most health facilities are severely incomplete. Interruptions in the anti-malarial drug supply chain or seasonality were also possible sources of bias. Another limitation of this study is the cluster sampling method used. While it is a well-accepted statistical method for increasing efficiency of data capture, similarities between individuals within clusters could result in the study sample being less representative of the study population. Nevertheless, Gezira state covers a huge geographical area and random sampling was impractical.

Conclusion

The results of this study suggest that poor anti-malarial prescribing practices are prevalent in Sudan. This has important public health implications since failure to adhere to nationally recommended guidelines could play a role in the development of drug resistance. As such, there may be urgent need for identifying ways to improve the anti-malarial prescribing practices of heath workers in Sudan. Understanding the specific behaviors of health workers, such as those highlighted in this investigation, may help to provide a blueprint for how to tailor quality improvement interventions that will be successful.

Abbreviations

ACT: Artemsinin-based combination therapy; AL: Artemether-lumefantrine; ART: Injectable artemisinin; ASAQ: Artesunate-amodiaquine; ASMQ: Artesunate-mefloquine; ASP: Artesunate-sulfadoxine/pyrimethamine; DHAPQ: Dihydroartemisinin-piperaquine; WHO: World Health Organization.

Competing interests

The authors declare that they have no competing interests.

Authors' contributions

AM, EM and KE contributed to the study concept, design and interpretation of results. YI contributed to planning fieldwork and training of data collectors. NA contributed to data analysis and interpretation of results. JS provided advice and critically reviewed study results. All authors read and approved the final manuscript.

Acknowledgments

We wish to acknowledge the financial support provided by the National Fund for Promoting Medical Services, the National Malaria Control Programme, and Al Neelain University in Sudan. We are also grateful to Dr. Sakhr Omer, the Coordinator of the malaria programme in Gezira State for facilitating field visits, the field teams who participated in data collection, and to all patients and health care providers that participated in this study.

Author details

[1]Al Neelain University, Steen Street, P.O. Box 7294, Code: 11123 Khartoum, Sudan. [2]Federal Ministry of Health, Khartoum, Sudan. [3]Gezira State Ministry of Health, Wad Medani, Sudan. [4]Harvard School of Public Health, 677 Huntington Avenue, Boston, MA 02115, USA.

References

1. World Health Organization. Anti-malarial drug combination therapy: report of a WHO technical consultation. Geneva, Switzerland: World Health Organization; 2001.
2. World Health Organization. Guidelines for the treatment of malaria. Geneva. 2006. ISBN 92-4-154694-8.
3. White NJ. Anti-malarial drug resistance. J Clin Invest. 2004;113:1084–92.
4. Noedl H, Se Y, Schaecher K, Smith BL, Socheat D, Fukuda MM. Evidence of artemisinin-resistant malaria in western Cambodia. N Engl J Med. 2008;359:2619–20.
5. Phyo AP, Nkhoma S, Stepniewska K, Ashley EA, Nair S, McGready R, et al. Emergence of artemisinin-resistant malaria on the Western border of Thailand: a longitudinal study. Lancet. 2012;379:1960–6.
6. Ashley EA, Dhorda M, Fairhurst RM, Amaratunga C, Lim P, Suon S, et al. Spread of artemisinin resistance in plasmodium falciparum malaria. New Eng J Med. 2014;371:411–23.
7. World Health Organization. Malaria rapid diagnostic test performance, Results of WHO product testing of malaria RDTs. Geneva: World Health Organization; 2010.
8. World Health Organization. Global plan for artemisinin resistance. [http://www.who.int/malaria/publications/atoz/artemisininresistance%20containment%202011.pdf]
9. Meremikwu M, Okomo U, Nwachukwu C, Oyo-Ita A, Eke-Njoku J, Okebe J, et al. Anti-malarial drug prescribing practice in private and public facilities in south-east Nigeria: a descriptive study. Malar J. 2007;6:55.
10. Global malaria programme. Update on artemisinin resistance. (WHO, April 2012).
11. WHO. The world medicines situation. Geneva: World Health Organization; 2004. http://apps.who.int/medicinedocs/pdf/s6160e/s6160e.pdf.
12. World Health Organization. Guidelines for the treatment of malaria. 2nd ed. Geneva: World Health Organization; 2010.
13. Nyunt MM, Plowe CV. Pharmacologic advances in the global control and treatment of malaria: combination therapy and resistance. Clin Pharmacol Ther. 2007;82:601–5.
14. Elamin SB, Malik EM, Abdelgadir T, Khamiss AH, Mohammed MM, Ahmed ES, et al. Artesunate plus sulfadoxine-pyrimethamine for treatment of uncomplicated Plasmodium falciparum malaria in Sudan. Malar J. 2005;4:41.
15. Malik EM, Mohamed TA, Elmardi KA, Mowien RM, Elhassan AH, Elamin SB, et al. From chloroquine to artemisinin-based combination therapy: the Sudanese experience. Malar J. 2006;5:65.
16. Abdelgader TM, Ibrahim AM, Elmardi KA, Githinji S, Zurovac D, Snow RW, et al. Progress towards implementation of ACT malaria case-management in public health facilities in the Republic of Sudan: a cluster-sample survey. BMC Public Health. 2012;12:11.
17. Elmardi KA, Noor AM, Githinji S, Abdelgadir TM, Malik EM, Snow RW. Self-reported fever, treatment actions and malaria infection prevalence in the northern states of Sudan. Malar J. 2011;10:128.
18. "Home – Al-Gezira State". Sudan Tribune. 2003–2013. Retrieved March 19, 2013.
19. WHO. How to investigate drug use in health facilities. Selected Drug Use Indicators - EDM Research Series No. 007. (1993).
20. Dodoo A, Fogg C, Asiimwe A, Nartey E, Kodua A, Tenkorang O, et al. Pattern of drug utilization for treatment of uncomplicated malaria in urban Ghana following national treatment policy change to artemisinin-combination therapy. Malar J. 2009;8:2.
21. Malik EM, Hanafi K, Ali SH, Ahmed ES, Mohamed KA. Treatment-seeking behaviour for malaria in children under five years of age: implication for home management in rural areas with high seasonal transmission in Sudan. Malar J. 2006;5:60. Malar J. 2006 Jul 22;5:60.
22. Cot M, Hesran JY, Miailes P, Esveld M, Etya'ale D, Breart G. Increase in birth weight following chloroquine chemoprophylaxis during the first pregnancy: results of a randomized trial in Cameroon. Am J Trop Med Hyg. 1995;53:581–5.
23. Zurovac D, Midia B, Ochola SA, English M, Snow RW. Microscopy and outpatient malaria case management among older children and adults in Kenya. Trop Med Int Health. 2006;11:432–40.
24. Fogg C, Bajunirwe F, Piola P, Biraro S, Grandesso F, Ruzagira E, et al. Adherence to a six-dose regimen of artemether-Lumefantrine for treatment of uncomplicated Plasmodium falciparum malaria in Uganda. Am J Trop Med Hyg. 2004;5:525–35.
25. Piola P, Fogg C, Bajunirwe F, Biraro S, Grandesso F, Ruzagira E, et al. Supervised versus unsupervised intake of six-dose artemether-lumefantrine for treatment of acute, uncomplicated Plasmodium falciparum malaria in Mbarara, Uganda: a randomised trial. Lancet. 2005;365:1467–73.
26. Mutabingwa TK, Anthony D, Heller A, Hallett R, Ahmed J, Drakeley C, et al. Amodiaquine alone, amodiaquine + sulfadoxine-pyrimethamine, amodiaquine + artesunate, and artemether-lumefantrine for outpatient treatment of malaria in Tanzanian children: a four-arm randomised effectiveness trial. Lancet. 2005;365:1474–80.
27. Spector JM, Agrawal P, Kodkany B, Lipsitz S, Lashoher A, Dziekan G, et al. Improving quality of care for maternal and newborn health: prospective pilot study of the WHO safe childbirth checklist program. PLoS One. 2012;7(5):e35151.
28. Haynes AB, Weiser TG, Berry WR, Lipsitz SR, Breizat AH, et al. A surgical safety checklist to reduce morbidity and mortality in a global population. N Engl J Med. 2009;360:491–9.

16

Psychotropic drug use among people with dementia – a six-month follow-up study

Maria Gustafsson[1*], Stig Karlsson[2], Yngve Gustafson[3] and Hugo Lövheim[3]

Abstract

Background: Psychotropic drugs are widely used among old people with dementia but few studies have described long-term treatment in this group of patients. The purpose of this study was to explore the long-term use of psychotropic drugs in old people with dementia.

Methods: Data on psychotropic drug use, functioning in the activities of daily living (ADL), cognitive function and behavioral and psychological symptoms were collected at baseline and six months later, using the Multi-Dimensional Dementia Assessment Scale (MDDAS). The data were collected in 2005–2006. Detailed data about the prescribing of psychotropic drugs were collected from prescription records. This study was conducted in 40 specialized care units in northern Sweden, with a study population of 278 people with dementia.

Results: At the start of the study, 229 of the participants (82%) were prescribed at least one psychotropic drug; 150 (54%) used antidepressants, 43 (16%) used anxiolytics, 107 (38%) used hypnotics and sedatives, and 111 (40%) used antipsychotics. Among the baseline users of antidepressants, anxiolytics, hypnotics and sedatives and antipsychotics, 67%, 44%, 57% and 57% respectively, still used the same dose of the same psychotropic drug after six months. Associations were found between behavioral and psychological symptoms and different psychotropic drugs.

Conclusion: Psychotropic drug use was high among people with dementia living in specialized care units and in many cases the drugs were used for extended periods. It is very important to monitor the effects and adverse effects of the prescribed drug in this frail group of people.

Keywords: Psychotropic drugs, Dementia, BPSD, Psychotropic prescribing

Background

The prescribing of drugs for old people is extensive and often inappropriate [1]. A Swedish study of people living in nursing homes shows that over 70% of the residents had one or more potentially inappropriate prescription according to quality indicators published by the Swedish National Board of Health and Welfare [2].

The inappropriate use of drugs has been associated with an increased risk of hospitalization among old people [3] and studies show that up to 30% of hospital admissions are directly connected to drug-related problems [4,5]. Older people are at increased risk of adverse drug reactions, and older people with dementia are especially vulnerable [6].

Of particular concern is the high risk of adverse effects among old people treated with psychotropic drugs. These drugs are widely used among people with dementia [7,8] despite the fact that this group is particularly at risk of the adverse cognitive effects of drugs with anticholinergic properties, such as antipsychotics and certain antihistamines [8,9]. In addition, serious events such as hospital admission or death are frequent following even short-term use of antipsychotics among people with dementia [10]. Many older people with dementia and neuropsychiatric symptoms can be withdrawn from chronic antipsychotic treatment without deterioration, however, some people could benefit from continuing their antipsychotic medication [11]. Benzodiazepines can cause problems with impaired cognition [12], incident mobility and ADL disability among old people [13]. Benzodiazepines and other hypnotics and sedatives might also worsen sleep apnea syndrome [14] and are therefore contraindicated

* Correspondence: maria.gustafsson@pharm.umu.se

[1]Department of Pharmacology and Clinical Neurosciences, Division of Clinical Pharmacology and Department of Community Medicine and Rehabilitation, Geriatric Medicine, Umeå University, Umeå, Sweden

Full list of author information is available at the end of the article

among people with this condition. Sleep apnea syndrome is common among people with dementia, with reported prevalence's of around 50% and higher [15,16]. Antidepressants also have several side-effects in individuals with dementia, such as falls [17] and hyponatraemia [18]. Taken together, many psychotropic drugs are considered inappropriate, or should be used for a limited period only, or with caution among older people [19].

Behavioral and psychological symptoms are common among people with dementia [20]. Psychotropic drugs are frequently used in nursing homes to treat these symptoms, [21] despite their limited efficacy in this patient group [22,23]. Only a few studies have described long-term psychotropic treatment among people with dementia [21,24]. The aim of one of these studies was to track changes in the prescribing patterns of antidepressants, antipsychotics, anxiolytics and hypnotics over six months among nursing homes residents in Australia [24]. It was found that treatment with psychotropic drugs was, in most cases, not adjusted over time.

We have previously reported data showing that the use of antipsychotic drugs among people with dementia living in specialized care units was high and the treatment in many cases remained unchanged after six months [25]. The study also showed that people who exhibited aggressive behavior or passiveness, or had mild cognitive impairment were at increased risk of being prescribed antipsychotics [25]. The purpose of the present study was to explore the prevalence, associated factors, including behavioral and psychological symptoms, and long-term use of all psychotropic drugs in old people with dementia living in specialized care units. Previously reported analyses of antipsychotic drugs in particular [25] are not included.

Methods
Subjects and settings
Data for this study were taken from a research study concerning the use of physical restraint [26]. This was an intervention study conducted in 2005–2006, which included 40 specialized care units for persons with dementia in nine municipalities in northern Sweden. All specialized care units in these areas were inventoried, i.e. 99 units were contacted - and those units with the highest prevalence of physical restraint use ($\geq$ 20%) were selected for inclusion in the study. Our study population comprised 353 people with dementia, and complete data from baseline and a six-month follow up were obtained for 278 persons. Among these 278 people, the mean age was 82 years and 75% were women. All had a dementia diagnosis, and 23% were prescribed an anti-dementia drug. Records were incomplete for 75 out of the 353 people because of incomplete data (16), death (47) or dropout (12). The study was approved by the Regional Ethical Review Board in Umeå (registration number 02–105).

Procedures
The assessments were made using the Multi-Dimensional Dementia Assessment Scale (MDDAS) [27]. The member of staff who knew each resident best and were most involved in their care performed the assessments based on observations made over the preceding 7 days.

The scale measures, for example, functioning in the activities of daily living (ADL), cognition, and behavior and psychological symptoms. MDDAS also includes a registration of current drug prescription. The MDDAS has good intra- and inter-rater reliability [27]. The ADL function score ranges from 4–24, where a higher score indicates greater ADL independence. This score is based on the patient's ability to cope with hygiene, dressing, eating and bladder and bowel control. Cognitive impairment was measured using an assessment scale developed by Gottfries and Gottfries [28]. The scale comprises 27 items that measure a person's cognitive function. Scores of less than 24 are considered to indicate cognitive impairment, correlating with a sensitivity of 90% and a specificity of 91% [28] to the usual cut-off point, 24/30, of the Mini-mental State Examination (MMSE) [29]. The scale is further subdivided into three groups, mild cognitive impairment (16–23), moderate cognitive impairment (8–15) and severe cognitive impairment (0–7). The MDDAS contains 25 behavioral items and 14 psychological symptom items. Each item is rated on a three-point scale indicating whether the symptom was present at least once a day, once a week, or never during the one-week observation period. These variables are dichotomized between at least once a week and less than once a week in the present study.

The prescription records were collected at the start of the study and six months later. The majority used an automated multidose dispensing service where the person's drugs are dispensed in one-dose-unit bags for each dose occasion.

In this present study, the prescription records collected earlier were searched in order to identify those patients from the study population who were treated with psychotropic drugs. All patients were listed according to age, sex, and treatment with antidepressants (N06A), anxiolytics (N05B), hypnotics and sedatives (N05C), and antipsychotics (N05A). The WHO ATC (Anatomical Therapeutic Chemical Index) classification system was used. Information about dose and type of antidepressant, anxiolytics, hypnotics and sedatives drugs was collected. Pro re nata (PRN) drugs were not included, as information was lacking about the actual use of these drugs.

Statistics and calculations
PASW Statistics 18 was used for data handling and statistical calculations. A p-value of < 0.05 was considered

statistically significant. A multiple logistic regression model was constructed to find factors independently associated with psychotropic drug use. The behavioral and the psychological symptom items of the MDDAS were grouped and weighted (in each group every symptom was multiplied by the calculated factor loading and then added to the next symptom) according to a factor analysis previously described by Lövheim et al. [30]. The factors were then normalized and included in a logistic regression model that also included background variables (age, sex and level of cognitive impairment). As many of the behavioral and psychological symptoms correlated strongly, the behaviors and symptoms were tested in the regression model in a stepwise procedure, where the behavior that had the strongest bivariate correlation was included first, and all other behaviors and symptoms were included subsequently one by one to see if any of them contributed independently. The behavior and symptom factors were: aggressive behavior, wandering behavior, restless behavior, verbally disruptive/attention-seeking behavior, passiveness, hallucinatory symptoms, depressive symptoms, disoriented symptoms and regressive/inappropriate behavior. Ultimately, all significant behaviors and symptoms were included in a final model, one for each drug group.

McNemars test without Yates correction was used to compare the prevalence of symptoms at baseline and follow-up, among people receiving various psychotropic treatments.

Results

The characteristics of the study population and the prevalence of psychotropic drug use at the start of the study are presented in Table 1. Two hundred and twenty-nine (82%) of the people were prescribed at least one psychotropic drug. One hundred and fifty (54%) used antidepressants, 131 (47%) used anxiolytics, hypnotics and sedatives, and

Table 1 Characteristics of study population and prevalence of psychotropic drug use at baseline

Cases, n	278
Women, n (%)	209 (75.2)
Mean age ± SD	82.0 ± 8.0
ADL score (4–24) mean ± SD	12.6 ± 5.4
Cognitive score (0–27) mean ± SD	10.7 ± 7.3
Antidepressant (N06A) use, n (%)	150 (54.0)
Anxiolytics, hypnotics and sedatives (N05B&C) use, n (%)	131 (47.1)
Anxiolytics drug (N05B) use, n (%)	43 (15.5)
Hypnotic and sedative drug (N05C) use, n (%)	107 (38.5)
Antipsychotic drug (N05A) use, n (%)	111 (39.9)
Any psychotropic drug use, n (%)	229 (82.4)

SD = Standard deviation, ADL = Activities of daily living.

111 (40%) used antipsychotics. In addition, 74 people in the study population (27%) were prescribed anxiolytics/hypnotics/sedatives and an antidepressant drug simultaneously. Sixty-two people (22%) were prescribed anxiolytics/hypnotics/sedatives and an antipsychotic drug simultaneously and 61 people (22%) an antidepressant drug and an antipsychotic drug simultaneously. There were 61 people (22%) who used three or more psychotropic drugs concomitantly.

Furthermore, among antipsychotics (N05A), antidepressants (N06A), anxiolytics (N05B) and hypnotics and sedatives (N05C), 64 people (23%) were prescribed inappropriate drugs, according to the National Board of Health and Welfare (levomepromazine, clozapine, clomipramine, hydroxyzine, diazepam, flunitrazepam and propiomazine) [19]. Eight people used two inappropriate drugs concomitantly.

Multiple logistic regression analyses

Multiple logistic regression analyses were performed for three psychotropic drug classes: antidepressants (N06A), anxiolytics (N05B) and hypnotics and sedatives (N05C) (Table 2). Younger participants or people with moderate cognitive impairment (compared to severe cognitive impairment) were at increased risk of being prescribed an antidepressant drug. There was no association between antidepressant drug use and depressive symptoms or any other BPSD factor.

Those who exhibited verbally disruptive/attention-seeking behavior (a factor consisting of the following symptoms: shrieks and shouts continuously, constantly seeks attention of the staff, interrupted night's sleep, seeks help, disturbed and restless, complains) were at increased risk of being prescribed an anxiolytic drug.

Three variables were associated with hypnotic and sedative drug use: younger age, mild cognitive impairment (compared to severe cognitive impairment) and disoriented symptoms (a factor consisting of the following symptoms: lies in other patients' beds, take things from other patients' boxes and closets and undresses in the dayroom).

A multiple regression analysis was also performed including the symptom interrupted night's sleep and background variables. No association was found between this symptom and the prescribing of hypnotic and sedative drugs (data not shown).

An earlier study explored the associations between antipsychotics (N05A) and behavioral and psychological symptoms in this study population [25].

Antidepressant drugs

Selective serotonin reuptake inhibitors (SSRI) were the drugs mainly prescribed among the 150 persons who used antidepressant drugs (Table 3). Citalopram accounted for

Table 2 Multiple logistic regression regarding different psychotropic drug use

	Odds ratio	95% confidence interval	p-value
Antidepressants (N06A)			
Male sex	0.727	0.381-1.385	0.332
Higher age	0.932	0.897-0.969	0.000
Moderate cognitive impairment[a]	1.971	1.072-3.622	0.029
Mild cognitive impairment[a]	0.933	0.460-1.894	0.848
Anxiolytics (N05B)			
Male sex	0.522	0.181-1.505	0.229
Higher age	0.985	0.939-1.032	0.521
Moderate cognitive impairment[a]	0.606	0.242-1.514	0.283
Mild cognitive impairment[a]	1.331	0.509-3.481	0.560
Verbally disruptive/attention-seeking behavior	2.193	1.389-3.462	0.001
Hypnotics and sedatives (N05C)			
Male sex	1.769	0.917-3.413	0.089
Higher age	0.932	0.896-0.971	0.001
Moderate cognitive impairment[a]	1.401	0.725-2.705	0.316
Mild cognitive impairment[a]	3.627	1.685-7.810	0.001
Disoriented symptoms	1.545	1.169-2.041	0.002

Model Cox and Snell R^2: 0.078, concordance between observed and predicted value: 65.4% (antidepressants): 0.070/85.5% (anxiolytics): 0.138/69.9% (hypnotics and sedatives). [a]Cognitive score ranges from 0–27 points and a score of less than 24 is considered to indicate cognitive impairment. The scale is subdivided into three groups, 0–7 (severe cognitive impairment), 8–15 (moderate cognitive impairment) and 16–23 (mild cognitive impairment). Severe cognitive impairment is reference category.

52% of the antidepressants prescribed followed by sertraline (20%) and mirtazapine (16%). At the start of the study, 150 persons (54%) were prescribed antidepressant drugs (Figure 1). After six months, 100 out of these 150 (67%) were still being treated with the same antidepressant drug in the same dose. Seventeen of these 150 patients showed changes in their prescriptions indicating an escalation of treatment during the six-month period: four people had another antidepressant added, six people had changed to another antidepressant drug and seven had received an increased dose. In total, 33 people had reduced their antidepressant treatment in various ways; 12 had a lower dose or fewer antidepressant drugs, 21 had finished their antidepressant medication completely. This means that 86% (129/150) were still being treated with antidepressant drugs after 6 months. Among the 128 taking no antidepressant drug at the start of the study; eight people were prescribed an antidepressant drug after six months. There was a significant decrease in the proportion of people with at least one of the three depressive symptoms (sad, crying and anxious and fearful) from baseline to the six-month

follow-up among people who were treated with antidepressants on both occasions (from 88/120 (73.3%) to 72/120 (60.0%), p = 0.008).

Anxiolytic drugs

Concerning anxiolytics, 43 patients (15%) were prescribed such a drug at the start of the study (Figure 2). Oxazepam accounted for 70% of the anxiolytic prescriptions followed by hydroxyzine (16%). After six months, 19/43 patients (44%) were still being treated with the same drug and in the same dose. Five people showed changes in their prescriptions indicating an escalation of treatment during the six-month period, while 19 people had reduced their anxiolytic treatment; 5 were on a lower dose and 14 had ended their anxiolytic treatment, meaning that 67% (29/43) were still being treated with anxiolytic drugs after 6 months. After six months an additional ten people were prescribed an anxiolytic drug. There was no significant change from baseline to follow-up in the proportion of people judged to be anxious and fearful among those treated with anxiolytics on both occasions (data not shown).

Hypnotic and sedative drugs

A total of 107 persons (38%) in the study population used hypnotic and sedative drugs at the start of the study (Figure 3). Propiomazine (28%) accounted for the largest share of the hypnotic and sedative prescriptions. After six months, 61 of these 107 (57%) were still being treated with the same drug at the same dose. Of these 107 patients, there were changes in the prescriptions of 15 indicating an escalation in treatment during the six-month period. Of these fifteen people, eight had another hypnotic and sedative drug added, three changed to another hypnotic and sedative drug and four were given an increased dose. In total 31 people reduced their treatment; eight had a lower dose or fewer hypnotic and sedative drugs, 23 finished their treatment. In other words, 78% (84/107) were still being treated with hypnotics and sedatives after 6 months. After six months an additional four people were also prescribed a hypnotic and sedative drug. There was no significant change from baseline to follow-up in the proportion of people with interrupted night's sleep among those treated with hypnotics and sedatives on both occasions (data not shown).

Discussion

The prevalence of psychotropic drug use (82%) in the study population is in line with or somewhat higher than that reported previously among people with dementia [21,31]. The use of more than one psychotropic drug also seems to be common. This study reveals that many people with dementia who live in specialized care units appear to be on stable doses of psychotropic drugs for

Table 3 Characteristics of psychotropic drugs at the start of the study

Drug	n (%)	Dose, mean (mg) ± SD	Range (mg)	Dose, median (mg)
Antidepressants (N06A)				
Citalopram	84 (52.5)	19.6 ± 6.1	10-40	20.0
Clomipramine	1 (0.6)	175.0		175.0
Escitalopram	1 (0.6)	10.0		10.0
Sertraline	32 (20.0)	68.0 ± 31.3	25-150	50.0
Mianserine	8 (5.0)	27.5 ± 10.3	10-40	30.0
Mirtazapine	26 (16.3)	30.6 ± 7.9	15-60	30.0
Venlafaxine	8 (5.0)	112.5 ± 56.7	75-225	75.0
Anxiolytics (N05B)				
Hydroxyzine	7 (15.9)	32.9 ± 22.1	10-75	25.0
Diazepam	1 (2.3)	3.3		3.3
Oxazepam	31 (70.5)	24.0 ± 26.8	5-135	15.0
Alprazolam	4 (9.0)	2.6 ± 2.5	0.5-6	2.0
Buspirone	1 (2.3)	15.0		15.0
Hypnotics and sedatives (N05C)				
Clometiazol	35 (26.3)	651.4 ± 273.7	300-1500	600.0
Flunitrazepam	15 (11.3)	0.7 ± 0.3	0.5-1	0.5
Propiomazine	37 (27.8)	33.4 ± 12.5	12-50	25.0
Zolpidem	19 (14.3)	6.4 ± 2.5	2.5-10	5.0
Zopiclone	27 (20.3)	6.9 ± 2.2	5-15	7.5

n = number of prescriptions, percent is calculated within each drug group.

six months or possibly longer; after six months, 67%, 44% and 57% were being treated with the same dose of the same antidepressant, anxiolytic or hypnotic/sedative drug respectively. Also, 57% of the study population were being treated with the same dose of the same antipsychotic drug after six months [25].

We found in the present study that more than every second person was prescribed an antidepressant drug (54%) and 67% of those who were prescribed antidepressants were still being treated with the same drug in the same dose after six months. Put another way, for at least 33% changes were made concerning their antidepressant treatment. These results differ from those reported by O'Connor et al. where antidepressants in particular were not adjusted over time. For example in only one out of 59 cases treated in that study was antidepressant medication stopped over the six-month period [24].

We found no association between antidepressant treatment and depressive symptoms. This result also differs from those reported in other studies [7]. The rather

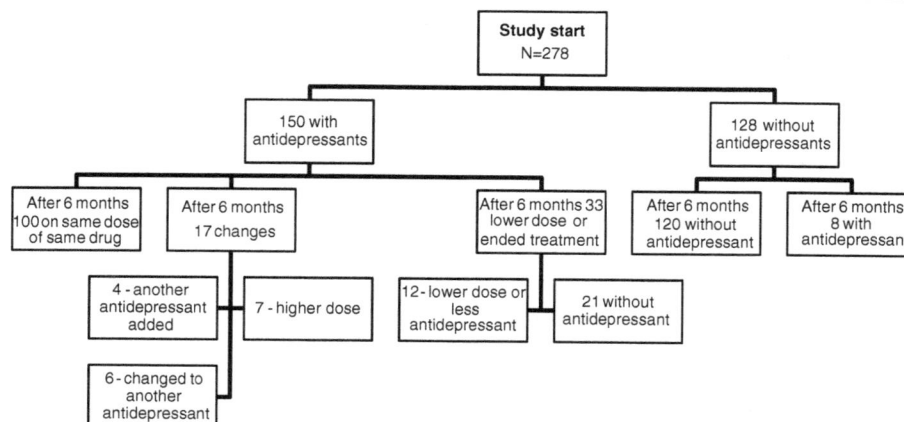

Figure 1 Antidepressants (N06A) – flow chart of participants from baseline to six-month follow-up.

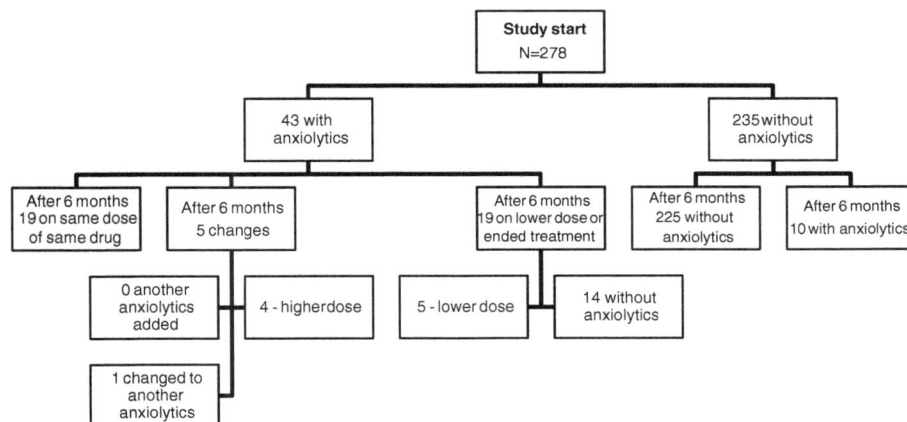

Figure 2 Anxiolytics (N05B) - flow chart of participants from baseline to six-month follow-up.

small study population might explain this finding, or possibly, these drugs were used also for other indications besides depression – which the high prevalence of antidepressant drugs might indicate. In Sweden, SSRI is recommended as a first-line treatment for irritability, agitation and anxiety among people with dementia [32]. It may also be that people taking an antidepressant drug have no current depressive symptoms because the drug treatment had been successful, therefore few conclusions can be drawn from a lack of association between depressive symptoms and antidepressants. It is much more worrying if persons taking antidepressants are still depressed.

Unlike the situation for all other psychotropic classes, properly monitored, long-term treatment with antidepressants might be appropriate among people with dementia. However, the very high prevalence of antidepressant drug use in this study raises concern. Recent results show that antidepressants have no antidepressant effects among people with dementia, but they do entail an increased risk of adverse events [33]. Nevertheless, we saw a significant

decrease in the prevalence of depressive symptoms from baseline to follow-up among people who were treated with antidepressants. However, considering the observational nature of the data, these results have to be interpreted very cautiously. True treatment effects cannot be differentiated from any natural variation in symptoms over time.

Regarding anxiolytics, almost half the patients (44%) were being treated with the same drug and in the same dose after six months. This group includes some of the benzodiazepines (diazepam, oxazepam and alprazolam). These results are in agreement with an earlier study where it was found that benzodiazepines were prescribed with no clear indication for their use and were continued long-term in spite of the risks [34]. Benzodiazepines should not be used for longer than 2–4 weeks by elderly people because of their adverse effects, inducement of dependency and limited efficacy when used continuously [35]. Apart from the long-term use seen in this study, it seems that in most cases a proper benzodiazepine (short-acting) was prescribed.

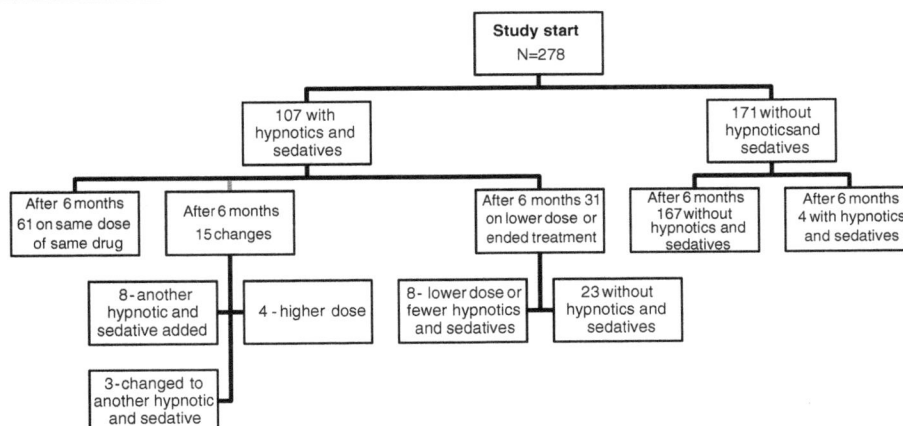

Figure 3 Hypnotics and sedatives (N05C) - flow chart of participants from baseline to six-month follow-up.

The high prevalence and long-term use of hypnotic and sedative drugs (38%) in this study warrants concern. More than half the patients (57%) were being treated with the same hypnotic and sedative drug in the same dose after six months. Hypnotic and sedative drugs administered regularly, every night for more than a month, without re-examination are considered as an inappropriate regimen among the elderly according to the Swedish National Board of Health and Welfare [19]. The usefulness and safety of the long-term treatment of elderly people with sleeping pills is not documented. A significant tolerance can be developed to the hypnotic/sedative effect, while the negative effect on psychomotor skills and cognition remains. Intermittent treatment is therefore recommended. Flunitrazepam (long-acting benzodiazepine) should be avoided unless there are special circumstances because of the high risk of side effects in the elderly [19]. Also, given the high prevalence of people with dementia who suffer from sleep apnea syndrome [15,16], treatment with benzodiazepines in this population is in many cases contraindicated. Propiomazine and clometiazol were two commonly used drugs in this study. They were previously manufactured and sold by Swedish pharmaceutical companies and there is a strong tradition of using these drugs in treatment in Sweden. The use of propiomazine among older people, especially those with dementia, is considered inappropriate because of the risk of side effects such as extra pyramidal symptoms. Clometiazol may be used for a short time when urgent sedation is needed and if the patient is adequately monitored [19].

No association was found between the symptom interrupted night's sleep and the prescribing of hypnotic and sedative drugs, nor did we find any change in the prevalence of interrupted night's sleep from baseline to six-month follow-up among patients who were treated with hypnotics/sedatives, or in the proportion of people who were anxious and fearful among those taking anxiolytics. This might possibly be a consequence of a tolerance of benzodiazepines and similar drugs already developed at baseline.

The regression analysis shows an association between hypnotics/sedatives and the factor disoriented symptoms and also an association between verbally disruptive/attention-seeking behavior and anxiolytic drugs. The earlier regression analysis with antipsychotics showed that people who exhibited aggressive behavior or passiveness, or had mild cognitive impairment were at increased risk of being prescribed antipsychotics [25]. In another recently published study we found that verbally disruptive/attention-seeking behavior was associated with all psychotropic drug classes, including antipsychotics [7]. Disoriented symptoms and passiveness were also associated with the use of antipsychotics in that study [7]. Taking

these findings together might indicate that psychotropic drugs are being used for the wrong reasons in some cases. For example, continuous shouting can be very stressful for the staff. A Dutch study investigated associations between the use of psychotropic drugs and staff distress, aspects of the physical environment and the patient's neuropsychiatric symptoms, and found an association between staff distress at patient's agitation and the use of antipsychotic and anxiolytic drugs [36]. Another study from Taiwan found a correlation between the use of psychotropic drugs and the severity of the caregiver's burden [37]. Concerning aggressive behavior, antipsychotics have been shown to have some efficacy [38], however, evidence of the efficacy of psychotropic drugs for treating patients with verbally disruptive/attention-seeking behavior is limited [23]. Psychotropic drugs with their risk of potentially severe side effects should, however, only be used for the benefit of the person taking them, taking into account both positive and negative effects. Staff distress cannot be regarded as a valid reason for initiating such treatment.

In this study we have been able to describe the long-term use of psychotropic drugs among people with dementia at a detailed level. We found that many people were treated with the same psychotropic drug in the same dose after six months, which indicates long-term treatment among this group of people. Given the significant risk of adverse effects among people with dementia, it is important that proper monitoring of drug therapy is implemented to ensure the appropriate and safe use of medication.

This study has some advantages. The pharmaceutical registration was of high quality since the prescription records were searched in detail. We can also assume that compliance was high since the vast majority of those taking the drugs used an automated dose dispensing system and the staff delivered the drugs.

The study also has some limitations that should be considered. The data were collected in 2005–2006. We cannot know if the prescribing has changed since then, but there is no reason to believe that long-term treatment with psychotropic drugs among people with dementia has changed considerably.

The rather small number of people in the study population may have meant that we did not discover some associations between the psychotropics and behavioral and psychological symptoms. Data were registered at the start of the study and six months later, but we know nothing about what happened between those two dates, for example whether dose reductions were tried and reversed because of aggravated symptoms. We do not know the duration of psychotropic treatment at the time of recruitment into the study, and we do not know the background of the participants or if they had other diseases. Some people might have bipolar disorder or other chronic psychiatric illnesses where long-term treatment of some psychotropic drugs might be appropriate when properly monitored.

Also, the selection of specialized care units was not random but based on the prevalence of the use of physical restraint. It could be that people in these homes have severe problems with BPSD and, therefore, receive long-term treatment of psychotropic drugs to a greater extent. However, comparing this population with an unselected material of persons living in specialized care units for people with dementia (a subset of the material presented in Lövheim et al. 2006) [39], also assessed with the MDDAS, there were no differences concerning the prevalence of aggressive behavior and verbally disruptive/attention-seeking behavior (data not shown). We believe that the selection of participants does not affect the main results of the study, but it should be borne in mind when interpreting the results.

Conclusion

Psychotropic drug use among people with dementia living in specialized care units was high and in many cases the drugs seemed to be used for extended periods. It is very important to monitor the effects and adverse effects of the prescribed drug in this frail group of people.

Competing interests
The authors declare that they have no competing interests.

Authors' contributions
SK and YG were responsible for the study concept, design and acquisition of subjects. MG reviewed the data a second time and MG and HL made the statistical analysis. MG and HL analyzed and interpreted the data and prepared the manuscript. All authors critically revised the manuscript, added their comments and approved the final version.

Acknowledgements
This study was supported financially by a grant from the Lions Research Foundation for Age-related Diseases, the Swedish Dementia Association, the County Council of Västerbotten, King Gustaf V's and Queen Victoria's Freemason Foundation, the Field Research Center for the Elderly in Västerbotten and the Swedish Research Council, Grant K2005-27-VX-15357-01A.

Author details
[1]Department of Pharmacology and Clinical Neurosciences, Division of Clinical Pharmacology and Department of Community Medicine and Rehabilitation, Geriatric Medicine, Umeå University, Umeå, Sweden. [2]Department of Nursing, Umeå University, Umeå, Sweden. [3]Department of Community Medicine and Rehabilitation, Geriatric Medicine, Umeå University, Umeå, Sweden.

References
1. Olsson J, Bergman A, Carlsten A, Oké T, Bernsten C, Schmidt IK, Fastbom J: Quality of drug prescribing in elderly people in nursing homes and special care units for dementia: a cross-sectional computerized pharmacy register analysis. Clin Drug Investig 2010, 30:289–300.
2. Bergman A, Olsson J, Carlsten A, Waern M, Fastbom J: Evaluation of the quality of drug therapy among elderly patients in nursing homes. Scand J Prim Health Care 2007, 25:9–14.
3. Lau DT, Kasper JD, Potter DEB, Lyles A, Bennett RG: Hospitalization and death associated with potentially inappropriate medication prescriptions among elderly nursing home residents. Arch Intern Med 2005, 165:68–74.
4. Col N, Fanale JE, Kronholm P: The role of medication noncompliance and adverse drug reactions in hospitalizations of the elderly. Arch Intern Med 1990, 150:841–845.
5. Mannesse CK, Derkx FH, de Ridder MA, Man in 't Veld AJ, van der Cammen TJ: Contribution of adverse drug reactions to hospital admission of older patients. Age Ageing 2000, 29:35–39.
6. Hajjar ER, Hanlon JT, Artz MB, Lindblad CI, Pieper CF, Sloane RJ, Ruby CM, Schmader KE: Adverse drug reaction risk factors in older outpatients. Am J Geriatr Pharmacother 2003, 1:82–89.
7. Gustafsson M, Sandman P-O, Karlsson S, Gustafson Y, Lövheim H: Association between behavioral and psychological symptoms and psychotropic drug use among old people with cognitive impairment living in geriatric care settings. Int Psychogeriatr 2013, 25:1415–1423.
8. Moore AR, O'Keeffe ST: Drug-induced cognitive impairment in the elderly. Drugs Aging 1999, 15:15–28.
9. Cancelli I, Beltrame M, Gigli GL, Valente M: Drugs with anticholinergic properties: cognitive and neuropsychiatric side-effects in elderly patients. Neurol Sci 2009, 30:87–92.
10. Rochon PA, Normand S-L, Gomes T, Gill SS, Anderson GM, Melo M, Sykora K, Lipscombe L, Bell CM, Gurwitz JH: Antipsychotic therapy and short-term serious events in older adults with dementia. Arch Intern Med 2008, 168:1090–1096.
11. Declercq T, Petrovic M, Azermai M, Vander Stichele R, De Sutter AIM, van Driel ML, Christiaens T: Withdrawal versus continuation of chronic antipsychotic drugs for behavioural and psychological symptoms in older people with dementia. Cochrane Database Syst Rev 2013, 28:CD007726.
12. Hanlon JT, Horner RD, Schmader KE, Fillenbaum GG, Lewis IK, Wall WE Jr, Landerman LR, Pieper CF, Blazer DG, Cohen HJ: Benzodiazepine use and cognitive function among community-dwelling elderly. Clin Pharmacol Ther 1998, 64:684–692.
13. Gray SL, LaCroix AZ, Hanlon JT, Penninx BWJH, Blough DK, Leveille SG, Artz MB, Guralnik JM, Buchner DM: Benzodiazepine use and physical disability in community-dwelling older adults. J Am Geriatr Soc 2006, 54:224–230.
14. Hetta J, Schwan A: Läkemedelsboken 2011–2012, Sömnstörningar [In English: Sleep Disturbances]. Uppsala: Läkemedelsverket; 2011:1005–1015.
15. Gehrman PR, Martin JL, Shochat T, Nolan S, Corey-Bloom J, Ancoli-Israel S: Sleep-disordered breathing and agitation in institutionalized adults with Alzheimer disease. Am J Geriatr Psychiatry 2003, 11:426–433.
16. Ancoli-Israel S, Klauber MR, Butters N, Parker L, Kripke DF: Dementia in institutionalized elderly: relation to sleep apnea. J Am Geriatr Soc 1991, 39:258–263.
17. Richards JB, Papaioannou A, Adachi JD, Joseph L, Whitson HE, Prior JC, Goltzman D, Canadian Multicentre Osteoporosis Study Research Group: Effect of selective serotonin reuptake inhibitors on the risk of fracture. Arch Intern Med 2007, 167:188–194.
18. Coupland CAC, Dhiman P, Barton G, Morriss R, Arthur A, Sach T, Hippisley-Cox J: A study of the safety and harms of antidepressant drugs for older people: a cohort study using a large primary care database. Health Technol Assess 2011, 15:1–202. iii–iv.
19. Socialstyrelsen: Indikatorer för god läkemedelsterapi hos äldre [In English: Indicators of good drug therapy in old people. Information from the National Board of Health and Welfare]. Retrieved April 10, 2013 from http://www.socialstyrelsen.se/Lists/Artikelkatalog/Attachments/18085/2010-6-29.pdf.
20. Zuidema SU, Derksen E, Verhey FRJ, Koopmans RTCM: Prevalence of neuropsychiatric symptoms in a large sample of Dutch nursing home patients with dementia. Int J Geriatr Psychiatry 2007, 22:632–638.
21. Selbaek G, Kirkevold Ø, Engedal K: The course of psychiatric and behavioral symptoms and the use of psychotropic medication in patients with dementia in Norwegian nursing homes–a 12-month follow-up study. Am J Geriatr Psychiatry 2008, 16:528–536.
22. Gauthier S, Cummings J, Ballard C, Brodaty H, Grossberg G, Robert P, Lyketsos C: Management of behavioral problems in Alzheimer's disease. Int Psychogeriatr 2010, 22:346–372.
23. Cerejeira J, Lagarto L, Mukaetova-Ladinska EB: Behavioral and psychological symptoms of dementia. Front Neurol 2012, 3:73.
24. O'Connor DW, Griffith J, McSweeney K: Changes to psychotropic medications in the six months after admission to nursing homes in Melbourne, Australia. Int Psychogeriatr 2010, 22:1149–1153.

25. Gustafsson M, Karlsson S, Lövheim H: **Inappropriate long-term use of antipsychotic drugs is common among people with dementia living in specialized care units.** *BMC Pharmacol Toxicol* 2013, **14**:10.

26. Pellfolk TJ-E, Gustafson Y, Bucht G, Karlsson S: **Effects of a restraint minimization program on staff knowledge, attitudes, and practice: a cluster randomized trial.** *J Am Geriatr Soc* 2010, **58**:62–69.

27. Sandman PO, Adolfsson R, Norberg A, Nyström L, Winblad B: **Long-term care of the elderly. A descriptive study of 3600 institutionalized patients in the county of Västerbotten, Sweden.** *Compr Gerontol A* 1988, **2**:120–132.

28. Adolfsson R, Gottfries CG, Nyström L, Winblad B: **Prevalence of dementia disorders in institutionalized Swedish old people. The work load imposed by caring for these patients.** *Acta Psychiatr Scand* 1981, **63**:225–244.

29. Folstein MF, Folstein SE, McHugh PR: **"Mini-mental state". A practical method for grading the cognitive state of patients for the clinician.** *J Psychiatr Res* 1975, **12**:189–198.

30. Lövheim H, Sandman P-O, Karlsson S, Gustafson Y: **Behavioral and psychological symptoms of dementia in relation to level of cognitive impairment.** *Int Psychogeriatr* 2008, **20**:777–789.

31. Zuidema SU, de Jonghe JFM, Verhey FRJ, Koopmans RTCM: **Psychotropic drug prescription in nursing home patients with dementia: influence of environmental correlates and staff distress on physicians' prescription behavior.** *Int Psychogeriatr* 2011, **23**:1632–1639.

32. Läkemedelsverket: *Läkemedelsbehandling och bemötande vid Beteendemässiga och Psykiska Symtom vid Demenssjukdom - BPSD. [In English: Drug therapy and treatment for Behavioral and Psychological Symptoms of dementia - BPSD. Information from the Medical Products Agency].* Retrieved April 10, 2013 from http://www.lakemedelsverket.se/malgrupp/Halso—sjukvard/Behandlings-rekommendationer/Behandlingsrekommendation—listan/Beteendemassiga-och-psykiska-symtom-vid-demenssjukdom–BPSD/.

33. Banerjee S, Hellier J, Dewey M, Romeo R, Ballard C, Baldwin R, Bentham P, Fox C, Holmes C, Katona C, Knapp M, Lawton C, Lindesay J, Livingston G, McCrae N, Moniz-Cook E, Murray J, Nurock S, Orrell M, O'Brien J, Poppe M, Thomas A, Walwyn R, Wilson K, Burns A: **Sertraline or mirtazapine for depression in dementia (HTA-SADD): a randomised, multicentre, double-blind, placebo-controlled trial.** *Lancet* 2011, **378**:403–411.

34. Simon GE, Ludman EJ: **Outcome of new benzodiazepine prescriptions to older adults in primary care.** *Gen Hosp Psychiatry* 2006, **28**:374–378.

35. Ashton H: **The diagnosis and management of benzodiazepine dependence.** *Curr Opin Psychiatry* 2005, **18**:249–255.

36. Nijk RM, Zuidema SU, Koopmans RTCM: **Prevalence and correlates of psychotropic drug use in Dutch nursing-home patients with dementia.** *Int Psychogeriatr* 2009, **21**:485–493.

37. Chiu M-J, Chen T-F, Yip P-K, Hua M-S, Tang L-Y: **Behavioral and psychologic symptoms in different types of dementia.** *J Formos Med Assoc* 2006, **105**:556–562.

38. Ballard C, Waite J: **The effectiveness of atypical antipsychotics for the treatment of aggression and psychosis in Alzheimer's disease.** *Cochrane Database Syst Rev* 2006, **25**:CD003476.

39. Lövheim H, Sandman PO, Kallin K, Karlsson S, Gustafson Y: **Relationship between antipsychotic drug use and behavioral and psychological symptoms of dementia in old people with cognitive impairment living in geriatric care.** *Int Psychogeriatr* 2006, **18**:713–726.

17

Pharmacokinetics of piperacillin/tazobactam in cancer patients with hematological malignancies and febrile neutropenia after chemotherapy

José C Álvarez[1†], Sonia I Cuervo[1,2,3†], Javier R Garzón[2], Julio C Gómez[2,3], Jorge Augusto Díaz[2,4†], Edelberto Silva[2,4,5*†], Ricardo Sánchez[1,2,3†] and Jorge A Cortés[1†]

Abstract

Introduction: Patients with febrile neutropenia (FN) exhibit changes in extracellular fluid that may alter the plasma concentrations of beta-lactams and result in therapeutic failure or toxicity. We evaluated the pharmacokinetics of piperacillin/tazobactam in patients with hematological malignancies and FN after receiving chemotherapy at a primary public cancer center.

Methods: This was an open, nonrandomized, observational, descriptive, and prospective study. Samples from 15 patients with hematological malignancies and FN were evaluated after the administration of chemotherapy. Five blood samples were taken from each patient when the antibiotic level was at steady-state 10, 60, 120, 180, and 350 min after each dose. Antibiotic concentrations were measured using gel diffusion with *Bacillus subtilis*. All study participants provided written informed consent.

Results: We investigated the pharmacokinetics of piperacillin in 14 patients between the ages of 18 years and 59 years and with a mean absolute neutrophil count of 208 cells per mm^3 (standard deviation (SD) ± 603.2). The following pharmacokinetic measurements were obtained: maximum concentration, 94.1–1133 mg/L; minimum concentration, 0.47–37.65 mg/L; volume of distribution, 0.08–0.65 L/kg (mean, 0.34 L/kg); drug clearance (CL), 4.42–27.25 L/h (mean, 9.93 L/h); half-life ($t_{1/2}$), 0.55–2.65 h (mean, 1.38 h); and area under the curve, 115.12–827.16 mg·h/L.

Conclusion: Patients with FN after receiving chemotherapy exhibited significant variations in the pharmacokinetic parameters of piperacillin compared with healthy individuals; specifically, FN patients demonstrated an increase in $t_{1/2}$ and decreased CL.

Keywords: Pharmacokinetics, Piperacillin/tazobactam, Beta-lactam antibiotics, Neutropenia, Fever, Chemotherapy, Hematological malignancies

Background

Variations in the pharmacokinetic (PK) and pharmacodynamic (PD) parameters of hydrophilic antimicrobial agents have been described previously in different pathological conditions (e.g., sepsis, trauma, burns, hypoalbuminemia), in animal models and in clinical trials evaluating febrile neutropenia (FN). These variations were identified because the extracellular fluid (ECF) levels in these patients were different than in healthy patients. Changes in ECF levels affect the plasma concentrations of antibiotics [1,2].

Beta-lactams are the first-choice antibiotics for the treatment of FN after chemotherapy, and inadequate serum levels of these antibiotics may lead to therapeutic failure. Cefepime, piperacillin/tazobactam, imipenem/cilastatin, and meropenem are beta-lactam antibiotics that exhibit activity against *Pseudomonas aeruginosa*, and these

* Correspondence: esilvag@unal.edu.co
†Equal contributors
[2](GREICAH): Grupo de Investigación en Enfermedades Infecciosas en Cáncer y alteraciones hematológicas, Bogotá, Colombia
[4]Departamento de Farmacia, Facultad de Ciencias, Universidad Nacional de Colombia, Bogotá, Colombia
Full list of author information is available at the end of the article

antibiotics are recommended as monotherapy for the empirical treatment of FN after chemotherapy [3].

Little information is available on the kinetic behavior of piperacillin or the piperacillin/tazobactam combination in cancer patients. However, addition of piperacillin or amikacin to moxalactam administration in FN patients has been shown to alter PK parameters compared with healthy individuals [4], and a randomized clinical trial evaluating PK parameters demonstrated a decrease in the volume of distribution (Vd) and drug clearance (CL) and an increase in half-life (t½) [5].

We investigated the PK parameters of piperacillin in Latin American patients with hematological malignancies and FN after receiving chemotherapy.

Methods

We conducted an open, nonrandomized, observational, descriptive, and prospective study in the Hematology Department of the National Cancer Institute (NCI) in Bogota, Colombia. The Ethics Committees of the National University of Colombia and NCI approved the protocol. All study participants provided written informed consent.

Patients

The inclusion criteria were patients: aged >18 years with a *de novo* diagnosis or recent diagnosis of hematological malignancy; currently undergoing chemotherapy; who had FN after receiving chemotherapy; did not have renal or liver failure; being treated with piperacillin/tazobactam (4.5 g, i.v.) every 6 h in the event of FN. Pregnancy tests were negative for women of reproductive age.

The exclusion criteria were patients: with chronic kidney disease defined as a estimated glomerular filtration rate (eGFR) <60 mL/min/1.73 m^2 [6]; with liver failure defined as Child–Turcotte–Pugh classes B or C [7]; who received combined antimicrobial therapy due to a polymicrobial bloodstream infection.

Definitions

Neutropenia was defined as an absolute neutrophil count <1,000 cells per mm^3 or in cases where a count <1,000 cells per mm^3 was anticipated 3–5 days after chemotherapy. Neutropenia was also declared in cases of acute leukemia with a neutrophil count with a blast percentage >90%.

Fever was defined as a temperature of 38°C for 1 h or one temperature measurement >38.3°C. FN was secondary to intensive antineoplastic induction, re-induction, or maintenance chemotherapy.

Laboratory tests

Five samples were taken from each of the 15 patients 10, 60, 120, 180, and 350 min after the dose of piperacillin/tazobactam attained a steady state. Piperacillin/tazobactam

was administered as a generic product (Vitalis®) purchased by the institution for use in all patients. The piperacillin content in samples from different batches and patient sera was measured using a biological gel diffusion assay with *Bacillus subtilis* ATCC 6633. The following PK parameters were calculated from the concentration–time plots: maximum concentration (C$_{max}$), minimum concentration (C$_{min}$), Vd, CL, t½, and the area under the curve (AUC$_{0-\infty}$).

Statistical analyses

STATA IC® ver11.1 software was used for analyses. Two-tailed Student's *t*-tests were used to compare independent samples at a significance defined as p < 0.05. PK parameters were compared between group of patients with albumin levels >3 g/dL*vs.* those with <3 g/dL, those who received a piperacillin/tazobactam in bolus dose, and those who received chemotherapy with Hyper-CVAD *vs.* another chemotherapy regimen (for Hyper-CVAD chemotherapy, course A comprised cyclophosphamide, vincristine, doxorubicin and dexamethasone, and course B consisted of methotrexate and cytarabine).

Results

Originally, the study cohort was 15 patients. However, 1 patient (patient 003) was excluded because the inhibition zone was not clearly visible due to serum hyperviscosity and the white blood cell (WBC) count was 262,400 cells per mm^3. The ages of the 14 studied patients ranged from 18 years to 59 years (mean, 31.9 years; standard deviation (SD), 15.4), and 8 of the patients were women. The albumin values recorded were between 2.1 g/dL and 4 g/dL (mean, 3.04 g/dL; SD, 0.56), and the neutrophil count was 0–2,380 cells per mm^3 (mean, 208 cells/mm^3; SD, 603.2). In 71.4% of patients, the Hyper-CVAD chemotherapy regimen was used alone or in combination with rituximab or imatinib (Table 1).

Concentrations (μg/mL) *versus* time were plotted for each patient to generate an exponential curve, which was used to calculate PK parameters. Visual inspection revealed one-compartment model behavior of piperacillin/tazobactam. Table 2 presents the PK parameters for each patient.

Statistically significant differences in PK parameters were evaluated by comparing the albumin values (Table 3) in patients with levels <3 g/dL and >3 g/dL and the use of Hyper-CVAD chemotherapy against other regimens.

Discussion

The present study confirmed previous observations of differences in the PK parameters of piperacillin/tazobactam in patients with FN and cancer. Patients with cancer and FN after chemotherapy are prone to cachexia, hypoalbuminemia, and the development of a third space

Table 1 General characteristics of patients

Parameter	Number (%)
Age (years)	
18– 24	7 (50.0)
25 - 31	3 (21,4)
40 - 60	4 (28.6)
Sex	
Female	8 (57.1)
Male	6 (42.9)
Weight (kg)	
40 - 50	5 (35.7)
51 – 60	6 (42.9)
61 - 80	3 (21.4)
Mean ± SD = 56.4 ± 11.2	
Height (cm)	
150 – 160	9 (64.3)
161 – 170	4 (28.6)
171 – 180	1 (7.1)
BMI kg/m^2	
17.0 – 22.0	8 (57.2)
22.1 – 27.0	5 (35.7)
27.1 – 32.0	1 (7.1)
Mean ± SD = 21.9 ± 4.0	
Creatinine clearance (mg/mL)	
80 - 110	3 (21.4)
111 - 140	6 (42.9)
141 - 170	5 (35.7)
Albumin g/dL	
2.0 – 2.6	3 (21.4)
2.7 – 3.3	7 (50.0)
3.4 – 4.0	4 (28.6)
Mean ± SD = 3.0 ± 0.6	
Antibiotic given in the previous month?	
Yes	5 (35.7)
No	9 (64.3)
Malignancy	
Lymphoma	2 (14.3)
Lymphoid leukemia	9 (64.3)
Myeloid leukemia	3 (21.4)
Number of neutrophils/mm^3	
Range	0–2380
Mean ± SD	208(603.2)
Therapy cycles	
1 – 2	6 (42.9)
3 – 5	3(21.4)
6 - 8	5 (35.7)

Table 1 General characteristics of patients *(Continued)*

FN-associated chemotherapy	
Hyper-CVAD	10 (71.4)
No Hyper-CVAD	4 (28.6)

BMI, body mass index; FN, febrile neutropenia; GFR, glomerular filtration rate. For Hyper-CVAD chemotherapy, course A comprised cyclophosphamide, vincristine, doxorubicin and dexamethasone, and course B consisted of methotrexate and cytarabine.
Mentioned on page 6.

[2]. Furthermore, the high protein content in exudates favors drug binding to proteins, which slows distribution of the drug in the systemic circulation, decreases C_{max} and increases $t_{1/2}$.

The current study, in which piperacillin/tazobactam was administered as a bolus dose every 6 h, confirmed that the C_{min}, elimination rate (Ke), and $t_{1/2}$ parameters of piperacillin/tazobactam were modified in patients whose albumin levels were <3 g/dL. However, patients with an albumin level <3 g/dL would be expected to exhibit a higher free faction of antibiotic and a higher CL because these two parameters are directly related (renal CL = unbound drug × eGFR) [8]. Indeed, a difference in GFR was observed between subgroups because this rate increased in patients with albumin levels > 3 g/dL. However, other statistically significant differences between these groups were not observed. Organ function can be diminished in patients with lower albumin levels. For example, kidney function may increase tumor progression or decrease functional reserve, and non-renal CL or other non-quantified clinical variables may also be altered.

Table 4 summarizes the values of the means and SD for the calculated PK parameters and other patient characteristics in comparison with the work of Drusano et al. [4], Drusano et al. [5] and Mattoes et al. [9].

Analyses of the piperacillin/tazobactam concentration against time plots revealed a one-compartment model, as described previously in an *in vitro* study by Strayer et al. [10]. The PK parameters of piperacillin alone at 3 g every 6 h were compared with those of 3 g piperacillin every 6 h or 4 g every 8 h in combination with 0.375 g or 0.5 g tazobactam, respectively (Table 3). The PK parameters in our FN patients were related directly to higher Vd and CL values, which explains the similar $t_{1/2}$ value as that observed by Strayer et al. (Table 4) [10].

A one-compartment model of behavior was observed previously when piperacillin/tazobactam was administered as a prolonged infusion to 13 patients who were hospitalized for the treatment of an infectious process [11]. Of these patients, 6 were noncritical and 7 were critical, and they received 4.5 g of piperacillin/tazobactam as a 4-h intravenous infusion every 8 h. These previous results by Shea et al. [11] suggested that the lower $t_{1/2}$ value was due

Table 2 PK parameters for each patient

Patient	C_{max} (µg/mL)	C_{min} (µg/mL)	VD (L/kg)	Ke (h^{-1})	CL (L/h)	$t_{1/2}$ (h)	AUC [0-inf]	Dose in mg/kg
1	283.97	13.29	0.26	0.53	7.45	1.31	398.78	54.05
2	200.56	16.87	0.35	0.44	8.70	1.59	419.14	52.63
4	337.21	6.36	0.22	0.69	8.15	1.01	232.15	70.18
5	211.53	18.76	0.35	0.43	8.19	1.60	446.61	46.51
6	153.13	18.74	0.61	0.36	9.30	1.95	311.08	85.11
7	97.37	3.88	0.52	0.57	23.54	1.21	163.28	63.49
8	94.10	2.22	0.65	0.64	27.25	1.08	115.12	58.82
10	465.78	13.64	0.15	0.57	4.93	1.21	607.15	86.96
11	162.34	5.18	0.42	0.53	13.13	1.30	317.32	66.67
12	179.52	37.65	0.45	0.26	5.84	2.65	418.48	60.61
13	318.81	28.34	0.26	0.44	5.48	1.59	667.45	62.50
14	319.55	19.07	0.30	0.50	6.20	1.40	477.15	78.43
15	513.74	4.52	0.10	0.82	6.38	0.85	678.99	86.96
16	1133	0.47	0.08	1.25	4.42	0.55	827.16	66.67
Mean	319.33	13.50	0.34	0.57	9.93	1.38	434.28	67.11
σ(n-1)	266.08	10.71	0.18	0.24	6.95	0.51	205.17	13.01

Mentioned on page 6.

to an increase in CL, despite a similar Vd, for PK parameters (Table 4) [11].

Piperacillin doses between 8 g per day and 18 g per day were administered with tazobactam to four groups of healthy patients. Auclair et al. found that one-compartment model behavior was determined by visual inspection of the logarithmic relationship of plasma and urinary concentrations against time [12]. Piperacillin elimination is accomplished primarily *via* active tubular secretion by the kidney, but elimination is assisted by glomerular filtration and biliary excretion. Saturation of these mechanisms at plasma concentrations of piperacillin/tazobactam is unlikely. A nonlinear elimination, as explained by the Michaelis–Menten equation, would occur in the event of saturation, which would require a different PK analysis (Table 4) [12]. The filtration rate of a drug and the subsequent elimination rate are dependent upon the volume of the glomerular filtrate and free drug concentrations in the plasma (Table 4) [13].

One limitation of this study was the lack of a standardized method for administration of piperacillin/tazobactam by nurses with regard to the reconstitution of the powder

forms of the drugs, solvent volume, or rate of infusion of the diluted antibiotic. This variability underlies representation of the concentration–time plots for antibiotic administration as an infusion in some patients and a bolus in others. Therefore, calculations of PK parameters were undertaken using interpretations of these two modes of drug administration. Mattoes et al. [10] investigated 12 healthy adults who received piperacillin/tazobactam (4.5 g, i.v.) every 6 h and demonstrated that patients with FN exhibited higher values of Vd and lower values of CL. These results may explain the lower values of Ke and higher values of $t_{1/2}$ as compared with healthy individuals. PK parameters were investigated in patients in the intensive care unit (ICU) after administration of a 4-g bolus of piperacillin every 8 h or a 4-g bolus with subsequent continuous 8-g infusion for 24 h. PK parameters in patients who received a bolus administration compared with patients with FN in our study exhibited a similar value of CL and lower value of Vd, which would explain the lower $t_{1/2}$ value compared with ICU patients. Langgartner et al. found that PK parameters often differed in healthy subjects because a previous study found that

Table 3 PK parameters in patients with albumin >3 g/dL and <3 g/dL with statistically significant differences

PK parameter	Albumin <3 g/dL	Albumin >3 g/dL	Student's *t*-test	P
C_{min} (µg/mL)	8.3	20.4	4.5135	0.0305
Ke (h^{-1})	0.7	0.4	−2.4515	0.0486
$t_{1/2}$ (h)	1.1	1.7	−2.5709	0.0245

Mentioned on pages 6 and 8.

Table 4 Summary of PK parameters for piperacillin/tazobactam as compared with other studies

Parameter	Present study	Strayer et al.	Shea et al.	Auclair et al.	Mattoes et al.	Langaartner et al.	Drusano et al. 1985	Drusano et al. 1989
C_{max} (μg/mL)	319.3 ± 266.08	366.7	108.2 ± 31.7	SD	282.2 ± 57.7	231 ± 66	152	SD
C_{min} (μg/mL)	13.5 ± 10.71	SD	27.6 ± 26.3	SD	SD	11.5 ± 14.8	12	SD
VD (L/kg)	0.34 ± 0.18	SD	0.28 ± 0.07	0.12	0.2	34.6*	0.21 ± 0.14	0.13 ± 0.03
Ke (h^{-1})	0.57 ± 0.24	SD	SD	SD	0.86 ± 0.09	SD	SD	SD
CL (L/h)	9.93 ± 6.45	SD	8.6 ± 3.0	7.8	10.9 ± 2.5	10.23	8.31 ± 3.39	6.1 ± 2.54
$t_{1/2}$ (h)	1.38 ± 0.51	1.3	2.1 ± 1.2	0.9	0.81 ± 0.08	2.4 ± 1.2	1.47 ± 0.95	1.54 ± 0.42
$AUC_{[0-\infty)}$ mg·h/L	434.28 ± 205.17	488.9	527.5 ± 216.1	290	380.4 ± 72.6	391 ± 183	635.3 ± 253.2	SD
Weight (kg)	56.4 ± 26.78	In vitro	79.6 ± 13.8	SD	69.8 ± 15.7	60 - 86	69.5	70.2 ± 29.05

*Data shown in L.
Mentioned on pages 7, 8 and 9.

an increase in $t_{1/2}$ and decrease in CL were due to decreased clearance of creatinine (Table 4) [14].

In another study, moxalactam was administered to FN patients and piperacillin or amikacin were included randomly. Drusano et al. measured the following PK parameters for piperacillin: Vd = 0.21 (SD = 0.14) L/kg; CL = 8.31 (SD 3.39) L/h/1.73 m^2; and $t_{1/2}$ = 1.47 (SD = 0.95) h (Table 4) [4]. Furthermore, Drusano et al. conducted a randomized, double-blind clinical trial in which one group received piperacillin and amikacin and the other group received imipenem/cilastatin. PK parameters were measured and decreases were found in Vd (0.13 (SD = 0.03) L/kg) and CL (6.1 (SD = 2.54) L/h/1.73 m^2) and an increase in $t_{1/2}$ (1.54 (SD = 0.42) h) noted [5].

Conclusions

We found that piperacillin/tazobactam exhibited a one-compartment model of PK behavior in neutropenic patients. These data are in accordance with those of previous reports.

FN patients after chemotherapy exhibited important variations in PK parameters compared with healthy individuals. FN patients exhibited an increase in $t_{1/2}$ and a decrease in CL.

FN patients should receive piperacillin/tazobactam doses based on weight (75 mg/kg) due to the low weight of these FN patients and the observed variations in plasma concentrations.

Study limitations

One important limitation of this study was the inability to standardize the infusion rate or the amount of piperacillin/tazobactam diluent. This variation caused the values of plasma concentrations of antibiotics to differ from the expected values over time in some patients. This problem necessitated evaluation of the exponential curves from which the PK parameters were calculated with fewer samples than were taken. Serum sample measurements for piperacillin/tazobactam corresponded to those for

different batches from the same drug company, but the piperacillin content in one sample from a different batch was not significantly different (results to be published).

Abbreviations
ECF: Extracellular fluid; FN: Febrile neutropenia; ICU: Intensive care unit; NCI: National cancer institute; PD: Pharmacodynamic; PK: Pharmacokinetic.

Competing interests
The authors declare that they have no competing interest.

Authors' contribution
JCA collaborated on data collection, PK calculations, and drafting of the manuscript. SIC participated in the design and preparation of the manuscript and coordinated the research at the research site. JRG presented the research idea and designed the research protocol. JCG collaborated on the selection and enrolment of patients, project management at the NCI, and data analyses. ES carried out the biological tests and laboratory work. JAD assisted in PK analyses. RS undertook the statistical analyses. JAC assisted in protocol development and data analyses. All of the authors approved the final manuscript and agreed upon its submission to *BMC Pharmacology and Toxicology*.

Acknowledgements
Universidad Nacional de Colombia DIB, School of Science project 202010015111–2010 and Instituto Nacional de Cancerología project 41030310169 by means of the inter-agency teaching assistance agreement with the Universidad Nacional de Colombia in Bogota. VITALIS SACI from the "Research Development Endowment" agreement signed by VITALIS SACI and the Facultad de Ciencias of the Universidad Nacional de Colombia. The group of researchers wants to give special thanks to Dr. Maria Judith Arias for their invaluable support in the administration of the project from her work group in the company VITALIS SACI.

Author details
[1]Universidad Nacional de Colombia, Facultad de Medicina, Bogotá, Colombia. [2](GREICAH): Grupo de Investigación en Enfermedades Infecciosas en Cáncer y alteraciones hematológicas, Bogotá, Colombia. [3]Instituto Nacional de Cancerología, Bogotá, Colombia. [4]Departamento de Farmacia, Facultad de Ciencias, Universidad Nacional de Colombia, Bogotá, Colombia. [5]Departamento de Medicina, Facultad de Medicina, Ciudad Universitaria, Carrera 30 No. 45-03, edificio 471, oficina 510, Bogotá A. A. 14490, Colombia.

References
1. Garzón JR, Cuervo MS, Gómez J, Cortés JA, Farmacocinética y farmacodinamia de antimicrobianos: a propósito de pacientes con

neutropenia y fiebre: Pharmacokinetics and pharmacodynamics of antimicrobials: a report of patients with neutropenia and fever. *Rev Chilena Infectol* 2011, **28**:537–545.

2. Theuretzbacher U: Pharmacokinetic and pharmacodynamic issues for antimicrobial therapy in patients with cancer. *Clin Infect Dis* 2012, **54**:1785–1792.

3. Freifeld AG, Bow EJ, Sepkowitz KA, Boeckh MJ, Ito JI, Mullen CA: Clinical practice guideline for the use of antimicrobial agents in neutropenic patients with cancer: 2010 update by the infectious diseases society of America. *Clin Infect Dis* 2011, **52**:e56–e93.

4. Drusano GL, DeJongh C, Newman K, Joshi J, Wharton R, Moody MR: Moxalactam and Piperacillin: a study of in vitro characteristics and pharmacokinetics in cancer patients. *Infection* 1985, **13**:20–26.

5. Drusano GL, Forrest A, Plaisance KI, Wade JC: A prospective evaluation of optimal sampling theory in the determination of the steady-state pharmacokinetics of piperacillin in febrile neutropenic cancer patients. *Clin Pharmacol Ther* 1989, **45**:635–641.

6. Levey AS, Coresh J, Bolton K, Culleton B, Schiro K, Alp T: Guidelines for chronic kidney disease: evaluation, classification and stratification. *Am J Kidney Dis* 2002, **39**(Suppl 1):S1–S266.

7. Infante-Rivard C, Esnaola S, Villeneuve JP: Clinical and statistical validity of conventional prognostic factors in predicting short-term survival among cirrhotics. *Hepatology* 1987, **7**:660–664.

8. Ritschel WA, Kearns JL: *Handbook of Basic Pharmacokinetics*. 4th edition. American Pharmacists Association: Washington; 1992.

9. Mattoes HM, Capitano B, Kim MK, Xuan D, Quintiliani R, Nightingale CH: Comparative pharmacokinetic and pharmacodynamic profile of piperacillin/tazobactam 3.375G Q4H and 4.5G Q6h. *Chemother* 2002, **48**:59–63.

10. Strayer AH, Gilbert DH, Pivarnik P, Medeiros AA, Zinner SH, Dudley MN: Pharmacodynamics of piperacillin alone and in combination with tazobactam against piperacillin-resistant and -susceptible organisms in an in vitro model of infection. *Antimicrob Agents Chemother* 1994, **38**:2351–2356.

11. Shea KM, Cheatham C, Matthew F, Wack M, Smith DW, Sowinski KM, Kays MB: Steady-state pharmacokinetics and pharmacodynamics of piperacillin/tazobactam administered via prolonged infusion in hospitalised patients. *Internat J Antimicrob Agents* 2009, **34**:429–433.

12. Auclair B, Ducharme MP: Piperacillin and tazobactam exhibit linear pharmacokinetics after multiple standard clinical doses. *Antimicrob Agents Chemother* 1999, **43**:1465–1468.

13. Benet LZ, Kroetz DL, Sheiner LB: *Pharmacokinetics*, Goodman & Gilman's the pharmacological basis of therapeutics, Volume 1.1. 2nd edition. Philadelphia: McGraw Hill; 2011:3–29.

14. Langgartner J, Lehn J, Glück T, Herzig H, Kees F: Comparison of the pharmacokinetics of piperacillin and sulbactam during intermittent and continuous intravenous infusion. *Chemother* 2007, **53**:370–377.

18

Pharmacoepidemiology of common colds and upper respiratory tract infections in children and adolescents in Germany

Nathalie Eckel[1], Giselle Sarganas[2], Ingrid-Katharina Wolf[2] and Hildtraud Knopf[2]*

Abstract

Background: Medicines to treat common colds (CC) and upper respiratory tract infections (URTI) are widely used among children, but there are only few data about treatments actually applied for these diseases. In the present study we analyze the prevalence and correlations of self-medicated and prescribed drug use for the treatment of CCs and URTIs among children and adolescents in Germany.

Methods: Medicine use during the week preceding the interview was recorded among 17,450 children (0–17 years) who participated in the drug interview of the 2003–2006 German Health Interview and Examination Survey for Children and Adolescents (KiGGS). The definition of CCs and URTIs in the present study included the WHO-ICD-10 codes J00, J01.0, J01.9, J02.0, J02.9, J03.0, J03.9, J04.0, J06.8, J06.9, J11.1, J11.8, R05 and R07.0. Using the complex sample method, the prevalence and associated socio-demographic factors of self-medication, prescribed medicines and antibiotics were defined.

Results: 13.8% of the participating girls and boys use drugs to treat a CC or an URTI. About 50% of this group use prescribed medications. Among the users of prescribed medication, 11.5% use antibiotics for the treatment of these diseases. Looking at all prescribed medicines we find associations with younger age, immigration background, and lower social status. Antibiotic use in particular is associated with female sex, higher age, residency in the former East Germany and immigration background.

Conclusions: The use of medicines to treat CCs or URTIs is widespread among children and adolescents in Germany. Thus, longitudinal studies should investigate the risks associated with this drug use. Differences in socio-demographic variables regarding exposure to antibiotic use indicate that there could be an implausible prescribing behavior among physicians in Germany.

Keywords: Common cold, Upper respiratory tract infection, Cough & cold medicines, Pharmacotherapy, Antibiotics, Children, KiGGS

Background

Common colds (CCs) and other upper respiratory tract infections (URTIs) are usually self-limiting conditions with a high prevalence worldwide. Earlier analyses of the German Health Interview and Examination Survey for Children and Adolescents (KiGGS) indicate that the 1-year-average-prevalence of CCs among children and adolescents amounts to 88.5%, with the highest prevalence among children aged 3 to 6 years - almost 94% [1]. According to the literature, an average child undergoes a minimum of 4 to 8 URTIs per year [2-4]. Due to missing or low immunity in the first years of life, children are particularly vulnerable to viral infections [5].

Medicines against CCs and its symptoms are widely marketed, e.g. cough medicines, nasal decongestants, throat medicines, but also vitamins and herbal or homeopathic medicines. Data of the statutory health insurance document that 9 of the 20 most often prescribed drugs for children and adolescents belong to cough&cold medicines (CCMs) [6]. Additionally, many of these

* Correspondence: knopfh@rki.de
[2]Robert Koch-Institute, Department of Epidemiology and Health Monitoring, General-Pape-Str. 62-66 12101, Berlin, Germany
Full list of author information is available at the end of the article

drugs are acquired over-the-counter (OTC) [7]. Analyzing children's and adolescents' use of medications to treat CCs and URTIs throws light on the prevalence and related factors of drug use and is an essential step for understanding issues concerning their safety. Data from health insurances and sales figures are not able to completely provide this transparency as they do not necessarily correspond to the actual medication usage. In the USA, serious adverse events and even some deaths are associated with the use of OTC CCMs [8,9]. About 7% of all pediatric prescriptions for the respiratory tract system are not officially licensed for use in children, which means that they have never been tested rigorously for pediatric safety and efficacy [10]. Earlier analyses of KiGGS suggest that about 30% of the medicines are used off-label in terms of under-dosing, over-dosing, untested indication, or age [11].

Antibiotics are usually not indicated for viral infections such as uncomplicated URTIs or CCs. Antibiotics do not lead to an improvement of CC and URTI symptoms, but they yield potential side effects [12,13]. Nevertheless, their use is common: Data from the statutory health insurance show that an URTI is the main reason for an antibiotic prescription. The data also indicate that antibiotic use is highest among children aged 0 to 4 years [14]. High and unnecessary antibiotic consumption is not only a problem for the individual but for the whole population, as this is one of the main reasons for antibiotic resistances [15].

However, national representative data regarding the pharmacoepidemiology of CCs and URTIs in the child population of Germany are lacking. By analyzing data of the KiGGS survey we attempt to fill this knowledge gap. We describe prevalence rates, investigate socio-demographic characteristics and analyze factors associated with the use of CC and URTI medicines. The analyses are differentiated into the use of overall CCMs, prescribed CCMs, self-medicated CCMs, and antibiotic use.

Methods

KiGGS, a nationwide representative Health Interview and Examination Survey for children and adolescents, was conducted by the Robert Koch Institute between May 2003 and May 2006. The target population comprised all non-institutionalized residents of Germany between 0 and 17 years of age. Therefore, children and adolescents with a foreign nationality were also included. A detailed description of the methods of KiGGS have been published elsewhere [16]. Briefly, two-stage sampling procedures were applied. In the first stage 167 municipalities were drawn. This sample was representative for municipality sizes and structures in Germany. In the second stage, samples of children and adolescents aged

between 0 and 17 years were drawn randomly from the corresponding local population registries. In total, 17,641 participants were included in the survey which equated to a response rate of 66.6%. Nonresponse analysis showed only little differences in socio-demographic and health-related variables between responders and non-responders. The survey was approved by the Ethics Committee of the Virchow Hospital, Humboldt University Berlin and federal data-protection officials. The children's parents/guardians and/or children aged 14 years or older were informed about all aspects of the survey and they submitted a written consent [17].

Standardized, age-specified self-administered questionnaires filled out by parents/guardians and children aged 11 years or older were used to collect socio-demographic data, family background and health-related issues. The children's age was categorized in 5 age groups: 0–2, 3–6, 7–10, 11–13, and 14–17 years. Children with immigration background were defined as those who had no German nationality themselves or whose parents had no German nationality. In order to calculate the socio-economic status according to Winkler, the parents' education, professional classification and household net income were inquired [16]. Medicine use was investigated in a standardized computer-assisted face-to-face-interview by a physician. Information on medicine use was collected by asking the parents and the children themselves. The participants were asked to bring all of the original packages of medicines used in the last 7 days to the interview. Drug use was assessed by the following question: *"Has your child taken any medicines in the last 7 days? Please also mention any ointments, lineaments, contraceptive pills, vitamin and mineral supplements, medicinal teas, herbal medicines and homeopathic medicines."* For all of the used drugs further information was collected, such as the form of administration, frequency of intake, origin ('prescribed by a doctor', 'prescribed by a non-medical practitioner', 'bought over the counter', 'obtained from other sources'), duration of use, improvement of the condition(s) treated, and degree of tolerability. In addition, up to two conditions for which the medication was taken were registered. The reported medicines were classified according to the Anatomical Therapeutic Chemical (ATC) codes and the conditions treated according to the WHO International Classification of Diseases-10 codes (WHO ICD-10 codes) [18]. To evaluate the medication used for CCs or URTIs we included the following conditions (WHO-ICD-10 codes in brackets): CC (J00), acute sinusitis (J01.0, J01.9), acute pharyngitis (J02.0, J02.9), acute tonsillitis (J03.0, J03.9), acute laryngitis (J04.0), acute respiratory tract infections (J06.8, J06.9), influenza (J11.1, J11.8), cough (R05) and sore throat (R07.0).

All statistical analyses were performed using SPSS statistical software 18.0. The analyses were performed with a weighting factor to adjust for deviations in demographic characteristics (age, sex, residence in West or former East Germany, level of urbanity) in comparison to the national child population. Descriptive statistics were used to estimate the prevalence of medication use to treat CCs or URTIs according to sex, age, region of residence, immigration background, and social status. Prevalence of self-medication, prescribed medicines and antibiotic use were estimated among those children who used drugs to treat CCs or URTIs. Odds Ratios (ORs) were obtained from multivariate logistic regression models to depict associations between socio-demographic factors and self-medication, use of prescribed medicines and antibiotic use. Results with a probability level of $p < 0.05$ and 95% confidence intervals (CIs) not including the value 1 were considered as statistically significant.

Results

Characteristics of the study population stratified by gender are listed in Table 1. 16.5% of all participants are living in the former East Germany and about 17% have an immigration background. The largest part of the boys and girls come from families with an intermediate social status. No significant differences are observed between girls and boys regarding the listed socio-demographic characteristics.

2,595 children and adolescents used 3,648 medicines to treat a CC or URTI during the last 7 days. The vast majority of these medicines are drugs acting on the respiratory system (ATC code R00, 84.0%), followed by homeopathic medicines (Z00, 5.0%) and anti-infectives for systemic use (J00, 4.7%). 21% of the used medicines are not recorded on the last 5th level of the ATC-codes (level of the chemical substance), because participants forgot the brand names. Therefore, only 2,887 medicines could get analyzed on the basis of their active ingredients. The 10 most frequently used active ingredients are shown in Figure 1.

Table 2 illustrates the prevalence rates of drug use to treat CCs or URTIs during the last 7 days. 14.3% (95% CI 13.2%, 15.5%) of the study participants use medicines to treat a CC or an URTI. The use of those medicines decreases with rising age. All other socio-demographic variables (region, immigration background and social status) show no statistically significant differences. About half of the children using

Table 1 Socio-demographic characteristics of survey participants by gender

	Boys		Girls	
	n	% (95% CI)	n	% (95% CI)
Age (years)				
0-2	1397	13.6 (13.2, 13.9)	1373	13.6 (13.2, 14.0)
3–6	1925	21.0 (20.7, 21.3)	1907	21.1 (20.8, 21.4)
7-10	2103	21.7 (21.4, 22.1)	2004	21.8 (21.4, 22.1)
11-13	1572	17.3 (17.0, 17.6)	1468	17.3 (17.0, 17.7)
14-17	1883	26.4 (25.8, 27.0)	1818	26.3 (25.7, 26.9)
Region				
East	2889	16.5 (12.3, 21.9)	2847	16.5 (12.3, 21.9)
West	5991	83.5 (78.1, 87.7)	5723	83.5 (78.1, 87.7)
Urbanity				
Rural town	1958	17.9 (12.6, 27.8)	1939	17.9 (12.6, 24.8)
Small town	2337	27.6 (20.9, 35.6)	2229	27.2 (20.5, 35.1)
Medium-sized town	2498	29.0 (22.2, 37.0)	2475	29.3 (22.4, 37.2)
Large city	2087	25.5 (25.5, 19.0)	1927	25.6 (19.1, 33.5)
Immigration background				
Yes	1350	17.4 (15.4, 19.6)	1230	16.9 (14.9, 19.1)
No	7498	82.6 (80.4, 84.6)	7592	83.1 (80.9, 85.1)
Social class				
Low	2454	27.7 (26.1, 29.4)	2306	27.3 (25.9, 28.8)
Intermediate	4011	45.2 (43.7, 46.8)	3890	45.7 (44.1, 47.2)
High	2185	27.0 (25.2, 29.0)	2181	27.1 (25.2, 29.0)
Total	8880	100	8570	100

n unweighted; % weighted.
German Health Interview and Examination Survey for Children and Adolescents (KiGGS), 2003–2006.

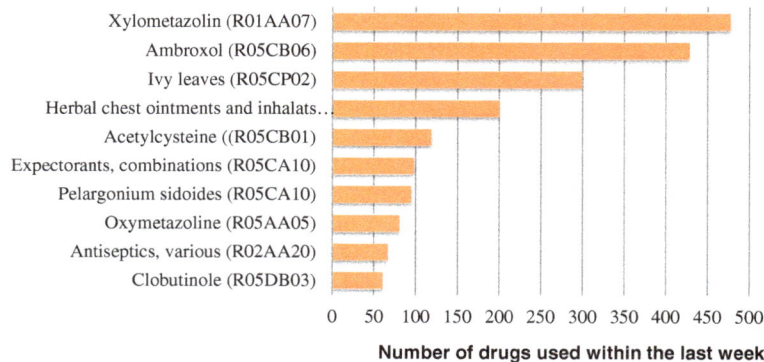

Figure 1 The 10 most frequently used active ingredients to treat common colds (CCs) or upper respiratory tract infections (URTIs).
German Health Interview and Examination Survey for Children and Adolescents (KiGGS), 2003-2006.

drugs to treat CCs or URTIs, utilize drugs prescribed by a physician (Table 2). The proportion decreases with rising age. Furthermore, we observed a statistically significant association between the use of prescribed medicine and immigration background as well as lower socio-economic status. The proportion of using self-medication to treat CCs and URTIs amounts to 57.6%. This proportion increases with higher age and is also higher for children without migration background and for children from families with a high social status (Table 2). Among those children and adolescents who use prescribed drugs, the antibiotic use is 11.6% (95% CI 9.8%, 13.7%). The antibiotic use in the descriptive analysis is significantly associated with immigration background and older age.

Multivariate logistic regression models show that the use of self-medication is significantly associated with

Table 2 Prevalence rates, proportions of overall prescribed medicines, proportion of self-medication and proportion of prescribed antibiotics to treat common colds (CCs) or upper respiratory tract infections (URTIs) (n = 17,450)

	Prevalence rates		Proportions of prescribed medicine		Proportions of self-medication use		Proportions of prescribed antibiotic	
	n	% (95% CI)	n	% (95% CI)	n	% (95% CI)	n	% (95% CI)
Gender								
Boys	1255	14.0 (12.7, 15.3)	655	50.3 (47.1, 53.6)	688	56.4 (53.1, 59.6)	69	9.5 (7.5, 12.0)
Girls	1340	14.7 (13.5, 16.1)	685	49.8 (46.1, 53.5)	772	58.8 (55.4, 62.1)	97	13.6 (10.8, 17.0)
Age (years)								
0 - 2	610	22.0 (19.9, 24.2)	416	66.1 (61.1, 70.7)	249	42.0 (37.1, 47.0)	32	6.1 (3.9, 9.5)
3 - 6	855	23.0 (20.9, 25.2)	473	55.4 (51.6, 59.1)	451	52.9 (48.8, 56.9)	53	11.0 (8.1, 14.7)
7 - 10	520	12.3 (10.8, 14.1)	223	42.4 (37.1, 47.8)	328	63.1 (58.6, 67.4)	29	9.8 (6.2, 15.0)
11 - 13	303	9.7 (8.3, 11.2)	118	38.9 (33.4, 44.7)	209	69.7 (63.5, 75.3)	24	18.9 (11.6, 29.1)
14 - 17	307	8.2 (7.1, 9.5)	110	34.2 (27.8, 41.1)	223	73.4 (67.3, 78.7)	28	24.8 (16.8, 35.0)
Region								
East	834	13.3 (11.6, 15.2)	439	52.6 (46.8, 58.4)	468	57.1 (52.3, 61.8)	70	15.0 (11.9, 18.6)
West	1761	14.5 (13.3, 15.9)	901	49.6 (46.7, 52.5)	992	57.6 (54.8, 60.5)	96	10.9 (8.9, 13.3)
Immigration background								
Yes	352	12.0 (11.2, 14.4)	225	63.0 (57.2, 68.4)	150	43.3 (38.3, 48.4)	39	18.2 (13.2, 24.5)
No	2229	14.6 (13.2, 15.5)	1108	47.7 (44.9, 50.5)	1305	60.2 (57.6, 62.9)	127	10.1 (8.3, 12.2)
Social status								
Low	683	13.8 (12.8, 15.6)	408	57.6 (53.4, 61.7)	319	48.0 (44.0, 52.1)	53	12.3 (9.4, 15.9)
Intermediate	1151	13.9 (12.7, 15.2)	582	48.8 (45.1, 52.5)	669	59.7 (56.2, 63.0)	76	13.0 (10.0, 16.7)
High	712	16.0 (14.4, 17.6)	315	43.6 (39.6, 47.7)	456	64.4 (60.3, 68.4)	31	8.0 (5.3, 11.9)
Total	2595	14.3 (13.2, 15.5)	1340	50.1 (47.5, 52.7)	1460	57.6 (55.0, 60.1)	166	11.6 (9.8, 13.7)

German Health Interview and Examination Survey for Children and Adolescents (KiGGS), 2003–2006.

higher age (OR 2.40; 95% CI 1.87, 3.07), no immigration background (OR 1.64; 95% CI 1.28, 2.11) and high (OR 1.77; 95% CI 1.42, 2.20) or intermediate (OR 1.44; 95% CI 1.16, 1.82) social status. In contrast, use of prescribed medicines is significantly associated with immigration background (OR 1.60; 95% CI 1.21, 2.11), younger age (OR 2.27; 95% CI 1.81, 2.85) and lower socio-economic status (OR 1.58; 95% CI 1.25, 1.99). Antibiotic use is significantly associated with immigration background (OR 2.37; 95% CI 1.51, 3.73), female gender (OR 1.52, 95% CI 1.05, 2.18), older age (OR 1.45; 95% CI 1.01, 2.08) and residency in former East Germany (OR 1.67; 95% CI 1.19, 2.34) (Table 3).

Discussion

The present study documents a high prevalence of medicine use to treat CCs or URTIs among children and adolescents in Germany. About 14% of the boys and girls use at least one of these medicines within a given week. The most frequently used medicines are drugs acting on the respiratory system followed by homeopathic medicines and anti-infectives for systemic use. About half of

Table 3 Socio-economic characteristics associated with the use of self-medication, prescribed medicine and antibiotics to treat common colds (CCs) and upper respiratory tract infections (URTIs) (n = 17,450)

	Self-medication[1]	Prescribed medicine[1]	Antibiotic use[1]
	OR	OR	OR
Sex			
Boys	Reference	Reference	Reference
Girls	1.04 (0.87, 1.25)	1.04 (0.86, 1.26)	1.52 (1.05, 2.18)
Age (years)			
0-10	Reference	2.27 (1.81, 2.85)	Reference
11-17	2.40 (1.87, 3.07)	Reference	1.45 (1.01, 2.08)
Region			
East	Reference	1.23 (0.94, 1.60)	1.67 (1.19, 2.34)
West	1.14 (0.90, 1.45)	Reference	Reference
Immigration background			
Yes	Reference	1.60 (1.21, 2.11)	2.37 (1.51, 3.73)
No	1.64 (1.28, 2.11)	Reference	Reference
Social status			
Low	Reference	1.58 (1.25, 1.99)	1.57 (0.93, 2.64)
Intermediate	1.44 (1.16, 1.80)	1.55 (0.98, 2.53)	1.55 (0.87, 2.75)
High	1.77 (1.42, 2.20)	Reference	Reference

Odds ratios and 95% confidence intervals were obtained from multivariate regression models [1]includes WHO-ICD-10 codes J00, J01.0, J01.9, J02.0, J02.9, J03.0, J03.9, J04.0, J06.8, J06.9, J11.1, J11.8, R05 and R07.0.
German Health Interview and Examination Survey for Children and Adolescents (KiGGS), 2003–2006.

the children with medicine use to treat CCs and URTIs use prescribed medicine. Almost 60% of children with CCMs use self-medication. Self-medication is associated with higher age, no immigration background, and high or intermediate social-status. In contrast, children of younger age, with an immigration background, and from families with low social-status use significantly more often prescribed drugs. Furthermore, antibiotic use is significantly associated with higher age, female sex, immigration background, and residency in former East Germany.

Data of medicine use based on treated conditions are sparse worldwide. The Slone Survey (1999–2006), a representative random-digit-dialing survey collecting data on medication use among the USA population during the last 7 days, observes a prevalence of children's exposure to CCMs of 10.1%. The definition CCMs includes all oral medications containing ≥ 1 antitussive, decongestant, expectorant or first-generation-antihistamine [19]. In KiGGS, expectorants are more frequently used than antitussives (6.7 vs. 1%), whereas in the Slone Survey, antitussives are more often used than expectorants (4.1 vs. 1.5%). Furthermore, there are differences regarding the active ingredients for certain medications, such as in antitussives and expectorants. The Slone Survey shows a high usage of dextromethorphan in antitussives and guafenisin in expectorants, whereas in our study, the most frequent active ingredients in expectorants are ambroxol, ivy leafs and acetylcystein and the most often used active ingredient in antitussives is clobutinol. The use of clobutinol has ceased since the year 2007 when all medicines containing clobutinol were withdrawn from the market. Data from a cohort study in South-West England, which were collected by self-administered questionnaires, yield exposure prevalences of 43.1% to CCMs, 5.0% to rhinologicals and 4.3% to throat medicines in the last 12 months among children aged up to 7.5 years [20]. However, comparability of these results with our prevalence rates (8.9% for CCMs, 5.9% for rhinologicals, 1.0% for throat medicines) is limited, mainly because of the difference in the reference periods. Longer observation periods lead to higher prevalence rates but also increase susceptibility for recall-bias. Despite of a much shorter observation period in our survey, the prevalence rate of rhinological use is higher in our study. This implies the probability of a higher 12 month prevalence in Germany compared to South-West England.

In our study self-medication for treating URTI is more common among children with higher age and among those without immigration background. These findings correspond to earlier analyses of KiGGS data looking at overall self-medication [7]. Moreover, our results suggest that self-medication is associated with a higher social-status. The same results are reported by a study looking at overall self-medication in Dutch adolescents [21]. In contrast to self-medication, the prevalence of using prescribed medicine is decreasing with higher age in our study, which is in accordance with results of the SLONE survey and a cohort study in three European countries [19,22]. Furthermore, in the present study the use of prescribed medication to treat CCs and URTIs is strongly associated with having an immigration background and a lower social-status. This finding is partly in line with earlier studies. A study in Poland observes positive associations between physician consultations and low school-leaving qualifications, as well as between use of OTC medicines and a high household income when treating respiratory tract infections in adults [23]. An Israeli cross-sectional study analyzes reasons why patients with flu-like symptoms consult a doctor. The reason "to get a prescription" is associated with low school-leaving qualifications, low income and unemployment [24]. However, Dutch secondary data analysis observes no association between use of prescription medicines and social-status by adolescents for all conditions [21].

Earlier findings looking at prevalence rates for antibiotic use among children in Europe and in the USA range from 31% to 38% [25-27]. However, these data refer to patients who were visiting a physician, thus comparability to our findings is limited. Our results suggest an increasing antibiotic use with higher age and with female sex. A previous study based on KiGGS data shows that children of younger age are more often exposed to antibiotic use compared to older children [28]. However, this study analyses the overall antibiotic use while the present study only looks at antibiotic use for treatment of CCs and URTIs. Our findings are probably influenced by not having included otitis media in the definition of URTIs, as the prevalence of otitis media is strongly decreasing with higher age [1]. Health insurance data on antibiotic use in Germany does not differentiate according to age or indication [14]. Gender differences concerning antibiotic use are already known: Data from the National Ambulatory Medical Care Survey from 1992 in the USA indicate a significant positive association between antibiotic consumption and female sex [29]. Moreover, findings from Abbas et al. suggest higher antibiotic use for girls compared to boys in all age groups except for 2-4-years old children [30]. Our results regarding regional differences are in line with the results of the EVA survey (Einflüsse auf die ärztliche Verschreibung von Antibiotika in Deutschland) which investigates influences on prescribing patterns by physicians in Germany. This survey demonstrates that physicians in the eastern part of Germany prescribe antibiotics more frequently than in the western part [31]. Moreover, our results suggest an association between antibiotic use for CCs and URTIs and children with immigration background. The findings of earlier studies investigating this association are inconsistent. Neither a Swedish prospective cohort study nor a Norwegian survey

observes an association between antibiotic consumption and immigration background [32,33]. A Cyprian cross-sectional-study finds a higher inappropriate antibiotic use by children with immigration background [34]. Furthermore, data of an Italian cohort-study suggests a significant higher antibiotic prescribing rate for URTIs for children with immigration background [27]. Altiner et al. report as a result of a qualitative study that physicians often tend to misinterpret the patients' demands and often feel urged by the patients to give them an antibiotic prescription. This pressure is especially felt in consultations with Turkish immigrants [35,36].

A major strength of our study is the large number of population-representative data with a high response-rate including non-responder-analyses and quality assurances measures. The parents or the adolescents themselves were asked to bring the packages of the medicines used in the previous week to the interview. In contrast to health-insurance data, we analyze the medication actually used by children and adolescents, not only prescribed and potentially never used medicines. However, our study has some limitations. Although the personal interview was conducted by a physician, indications were only reported by the parents or adolescents and were not validated. Because of language difficulties and possible cultural differences in symptom reporting, this might result in more imprecisely measured data particularly among children with immigration background. Recall bias has to be considered which would result in underreporting. By limiting the observation period to 7 days prior to the interview we tried to minimize recall bias. Because of the cross-sectional design of the survey it is not possible to draw conclusions on the risks children and adolescents are to exposed to the used medicines. A longitudinal study is required to examine this. Furthermore, although all reported conditions were documented and confirmed by medical professionals, a standardized severity assessment was not carried out. Thus, we are not able to asses if the antibiotic prescribing was unnecessary.

Conclusions

In summary, our study shows that the medicine use to treat CCs or URTIs is highly prevalent among children in Germany. Thus, longitudinal studies should investigate potential risks concerning this drug use. Furthermore, differences in socio-demographic variables, particularly sex, age, immigration background, and the difference between West and former East Germany, regarding antibiotic use indicate that there could be an implausible prescribing behavior among physicians in Germany. Thus, physicians should get trained to follow established guidelines when prescribing antibiotics for CCs and URTIs.

Competing interests
The authors declare that they have no competing interests.

Authors' contributions

NE and HK coordinated the conceptualization and conduction of the project. NE performed the statistical analysis, wrote and finalized the manuscript. HK provided specific knowledge, assisted in analyzing the data and interpreting the results and contributed writing to the manuscript. GS assisted in analyzing the data and interpreting the results. IKW provided specific knowledge, assisted in interpreting the results and finalizing the manuscript. All authors read and approved the final manuscript.

Acknowledgments

The German Health Interview and Examination Survey for Children and Adolescents (KiGGS) was funded by the German Federal Ministry of Health and the Ministry of Education and Research. There was no funding for the present study.

Author details

[1]German Institute of Human Nutrition Potsdam-Rehbrücke, Department of Molecular Epidemiology, Arthur-Scheunert-Allee 114-116, 14558 Nuthetal, Potsdam, Germany. [2]Robert Koch-Institute, Department of Epidemiology and Health Monitoring, General-Pape-Str. 62-66 12101, Berlin, Germany.

References

1. Kamtsiuris P, Atzpodien K, Ellert U, Schlack R, Schlaud M: [Prevalence of somatic diseases in German children and adolescents. Results of the German health interview and examination survey for children and adolescents (KiGGS)]. *Bundesgesundheitsblatt Gesundheitsforschung Gesundheitsschutz* 2007, **50:**686–700.
2. Padberg J, Bauer T: [Common cold]. *Dtsch Med Wochenschr* 2006, **131:**2341–2349.
3. Stickler GB, Smith TF, Broughton DD: **Review: the common cold.** *Eur J Pediatr* 1985, **144:**4–8.
4. Lorber B: **Perspectives: the common cold.** *J Gen Intern Med* 1996, **11:**229–236.
5. Gebel J, Teichert-Barthel U, Hornbach-Beckers S, Vogt A, Kehr B, Littmann M, Kupfernagel F, Ilschner C, Simon A, Exner M: [Hygiene tips for kids. Concept and examples of realisation]. *Bundesgesundheitsblatt Gesundheitsforschung Gesundheitsschutz* 2008, **51:**1304–1313.
6. Jahnsen K: **Arzneimitteltherapie im Kindes- und Jugendalter [in German].** *GEK-Arzneimittelreport* 2008, **61:**98–111.
7. Du Y, Knopf H: **Self-medication among children and adolescents in Germany: results of the National Health Survey for Children and Adolescents (KiGGS).** *Br J Clin Pharmacol* 2009, **68:**599–608.
8. Rimsza ME, Newberry S: **Unexpected infant deaths associated with use of cough and cold medications.** *Pediatrics* 2008, **122:**318–322.
9. Schaefer MK, Shehab N, Cohen AL, Budnitz DS: **Adverse events from cough and cold medications in children.** *Pediatrics* 2008, **121:**783–787.
10. Bücheler R, Meisner C, Kalchthaler B, Mohr H, Schröder H, Mörike K, Schwoerer P, Schwab M, Gleiter CH: **"Off-label"Verschreibung von Arzneimitteln in der ambulanten Versorgung von Kindern und Jugendlichen [in German].** *Dtsch Med Wochenschr* 2002, **127:**2551–2557.
11. Knopf H, Wolf IK, Sarganas G, Zhuang W, Rascher W, Neubert A: **Off-label medicine use in children and adolescents: results of a population-based study in Germany.** *BMC Public Health* 2013, **13:**631.
12. Arroll B, Kenealy T, Falloon K: **Are antibiotics indicated as an initial treatment for patients with acute upper respiratory infections? A review.** *NZJM* 2008, **121:**63–70.
13. Fahey T, Stocks N, Thomas T: **Systematic review of the treatment of upper respiratory tract infection.** *Arch Dis Child* 1998, **79:**225–230.
14. Kern WV: **Antibiotika und Chemotherapeutika [in German].** In *Arzneiverordnungs-Report 2007: Aktuelle Daten, Kosten, Trends und Kommentare.* Edited by Schwabe U, Paffrath D. Berlin Heidelberg NewYork Tokyo: Springer Verlag; 2008:287–311.
15. Schröder H, Nink K, Günther J, Kern WV: **Antibiotika: Solange sie noch wirken...** [in German]. *GGW* 2003, **3:**7–16.
16. Kurth BM, Bergmann KE, Hölling H: **The National child and adolescent health survey. The complete concept.** *Gesundheitswesen* 2002, **64**(Suppl 1):3–11.
17. Kamtsiuris P, Lange M, Schaffrath Rosario A: [The German health interview and examination survey for children and adolescents (KiGGS): sample design, response and nonresponse analysis]. *Bundesgesundheitsblatt Gesundheitsforschung Gesundheitsschutz* 2007, **50:**547–556.
18. Knopf H: [Medicine use in children and adolescents. Data collection and first results of the German health interview and examination survey for children and adolescents (KiGGS)]. *Bundesgesundheitsblatt Gesundheitsforschung Gesundheitsschutz* 2007, **50:**863–870.
19. Vernacchio L, Kelly JP, Kaufman DW, Mitchell AA: **Medication use among children <12 years of age in the United States: results from the Slone Survey.** *Pediatrics* 2009, **124:**446–454.
20. Headley J, Northstone K: **Medication administered to children from 0 to 7.5 years in the Avon longitudinal study of parents and children (ALSPAC).** *Eur J Clin Pharmacol* 2007, **63:**189–195.
21. Tobi H, Meijer WM, Tuinstra T, de Jong-van den Berg LT: **Socio-economic differences in prescription and OTC drug use in Dutch adolescents.** *Pharm World Sci* 2003, **25:**203–206.
22. Sturkenboom MCJM, Verhamme KMC, Nicolosi A, Murray ML, Neubert A, Caudri D, Picelli G, Sen EF, Giaquinto C, Cantarutti L, Baiardi P, Felisi MG, Ceci A, Wong ICK: **Drug use in children: cohort study in three European countries.** *BMJ* 2008, **337:**2245–2245.
23. Baran S, Teul I, Ignys-O'Byrne A: **Use of over-the-counter medications in prevention and treatment of upper respiratory tract infections.** *J Physiol Pharmacol* 2008, **59:**135–143.
24. Kahan E, Giveon SM, Zalevsky S, Imber-Shachar Z, Kitai E: **Behavior of patients with flu-like symptoms: consultation with physician versus self-treatment.** *IMAJ* 2008, **2:**421–425.
25. Nash DR, Harman J, Wald ER, Kelleher KJ: **Antibiotic prescribing by primary care physicians for children with upper respiratory tract infections.** *Arch Pediatr Adolesc Med* 2002, **156:**1114–1119.
26. Meropol SB, Chen Z, Metlay JP: **Reduced antibiotic prescribing for acute respiratory infections in adults and children.** *Br J Gen Pract* 2009, **59:**e321–e328.
27. Moro ML, Marchi M, Gagliotti C, Di Mario S, Resi D, Progetto Bambini a Antibiotici [ProBA]" Regional Group: **Why do paediatricians prescribe antibiotics? Results of an Italian regional project.** *BMC PEdiatr* 2009, **9:**69.
28. Robert Koch-Institut, Bundeszentrale für gesundheitliche Aufklärung: *Erkennen – Bewerten – Handeln: Zur Gesundheit von Kindern und Jugendlichen in Deutschland [in German].* Berlin: Robert Koch-Institut; 2008.
29. Gonzales R, Steiner JF, Sande MA: **Antibiotic prescribing for adults with colds, upper respiratory tract infections, and bronchitis by ambulatory care physicians.** *JAMA* 1997, **278:**901–904.
30. Abbas S, Ihle P, Heymans L, Kupper-Nybelen J, Schubert I: [Differences in antibiotic prescribing between general practitioners and pediatricians in Hessen, Germany]. *Dtsch Med Wochenschr* 2010, **135:**1792–1797.
31. Velasco E, Eckmanns T, Espelage W, Barger A, Krause G: *Einflüsse auf die ärztliche Verschreibung von Antibiotika in Deutschland (EVA-Studie): Abschlussbericht an das Bundesministerium für Gesundheit [in German],* Report from the Department for Infectious Disease Epidemiology. Berlin: Robert Koch-Institut; 2009.
32. Hedin K, Andre M, Hakansson A, Mölstad S: **A population based study of different antibiotic prescribing in different areas.** *Br J Gen Pract* 2006, **56:**680–685.
33. Soma M, Slapgård H, Lerberg M, Lindbaek M: [Patients' expectations of antibiotics for acute respiratory tract infections]. *Tidsskr Nor Laegeforen* 2005, **125:**1994–1997.
34. Rousounidis A, Papaevangelou V, Hadjipanayis A, Panagakou S, Theodoridou M, Syrogiannopoulos G, Hadjichristodoulou C: **Descriptive study on parents' knowledge, attitudes and practices on antibiotic use and misuse in children with upper respiratory tract infections in Cyprus.** *Int J Environ Res Public Health* 2011, **8:**3246–3262.
35. Altiner A, Knauf A, Moebes J, Sielk M, Wilm S: **Acute cough: a qualitative analysis of how GPs manage the consultation when patients explicitly or implicitly expect antibiotic prescriptions.** *Fam Pract* 2004, **21:**500–506.
36. Sahlan S, Wollny A, Brockmann S, Fuchs A, Altiner A: **Reducing unnecessary prescriptions of antibiotics for acute cough: adaptation of a leaflet aimed at Turkish immigrants in Germany.** *BMC Fam Pract* 2008, **9:**57.

19

Randomized pharmacokinetic evaluation of different rifabutin doses in African HIV- infected tuberculosis patients on lopinavir/ritonavir-based antiretroviral therapy

Suhashni Naiker[1], Cathy Connolly[2], Lubbe Wiesner[3], Tracey Kellerman[3], Tarylee Reddy[2], Anthony Harries[4], Helen McIlleron[3], Christian Lienhardt[5] and Alexander Pym[1,6]*

Abstract

Background: Pharmacokinetic interactions between rifampicin and protease inhibitors (PIs) complicate the management of HIV-associated tuberculosis. Rifabutin is an alternative rifamycin, for patients requiring PIs. Recently some international guidelines have recommended a higher dose of rifabutin (150 mg daily) in combination with boosted lopinavir (LPV/r), than the previous dose of rifabutin (150 mg three times weekly {tiw}). But there are limited pharmacokinetic data evaluating the higher dose of rifabutin in combination with LPV/r. Sub-optimal dosing can lead to acquired rifamycin resistance (ARR). The plasma concentration of 25-O-desacetylrifabutin (d-RBT), the metabolite of rifabutin, increases in the presence of PIs and may lead to toxicity.

Methods and results: Sixteen patients with TB-HIV co-infection received rifabutin 300 mg QD in combination with tuberculosis chemotherapy (initially pyrazinamide, isoniazid and ethambutol then only isoniazid), and were then randomized to receive isoniazid and LPV/r based ART with rifabutin 150 mg tiw or rifabutin 150 mg daily. The rifabutin dose with ART was switched after 1 month. Serial rifabutin and d-RBT concentrations were measured after 4 weeks of each treatment. The median AUC_{0-48} and Cmax of rifabutin in patients taking 150 mg rifabutin tiw was significantly reduced compared to the other treatment arms. Geometric mean ratio (90% CI) for AUC_{0-48} and Cmax was 0.6 (0.5-0.7) and 0.5 (0.4-0.6) for RBT 150 mg tiw compared with RBT 300 mg and 0.4 (0.4-0.4) and 0.5 (0.5-0.6) for RBT 150 mg tiw compared with 150 mg daily. 86% of patients on the tiw rifabutin arm had an AUC0-24 < 4.5 μg.h/mL, which has previously been associated with acquired rifamycin resistance (ARR). Plasma d-RBT concentrations increased 5-fold with tiw rifabutin dosing and 15-fold with daily doses of rifabutin. Rifabutin was well tolerated at all doses and there were no grade 4 laboratory toxicities. One case of uveitis (grade 4), occurred in a patient taking rifabutin 300 mg daily prior to starting ART, and grade 3 neutropenia (asymptomatic) was reported in 4 patients. These events were not associated with increases in rifabutin or metabolite concentrations.

Conclusions: A daily 150 mg dose of rifabutin in combination with LPV/r safely maintained rifabutin plasma concentrations in line with those shown to prevent ARR.

Trial registration: ClinicalTrials.gov Identifier: NCT00640887

Keywords: Rifabutin, Pharmacokinetics, Lopinavir, Tuberculosis, HIV, DDI, Randomized, Clinical trial, Neutropenia, Uveitis

* Correspondence: alex.pym@k-rith.org
[1]TB Research Unit, Medical Research Council, Durban, South Africa
[6]KwaZulu-Natal Research Institute for Tuberculosis and HIV (K-RITH), University of KwaZulu-Natal, Durban, South Africa
Full list of author information is available at the end of the article

Background

Treating HIV associated tuberculosis remains a formidable challenge. In 2014, 13% of the 9 million incident cases of tuberculosis, and 25% of deaths from tuberculosis were in HIV-infected patients [1]. Combining efavirenz-based first-line antiretroviral therapy (ART) with rifampicin based tuberculosis chemotherapy significantly reduces mortality in these patients [2-4] and is safe and efficacious. However, as public sector ART expands in developing countries, an increasing number of patients are developing virological failure and require second-line ART with protease inhibitors [5,6]. Combining rifampicin and protease inhibitor-based second-line ART is problematic as rifampicin significantly reduces the bioavailability and increases the clearance of protease inhibitors by accelerating their metabolism via induction of cytochrome 3A4 (CYP3A4) enzymes. Increasing the dose of the protease inhibitor or co-administering higher doses of a CYP3A4 inhibitor to ameliorate this adverse drug-drug interaction have been thwarted by hepatotoxicity and other problems with tolerability [7,8].

Rifabutin, a less potent inducer of CYP3A4 [9,10], is recommended at 300 mg daily as prophylaxis and treatment of *Mycobacterium avium* complex (MAC) and for the treatment of drug susceptible tuberculosis. Plasma concentrations of rifabutin are increased in the presence of protease inhibitors [11] therefore dose adjustments are recommended when rifabutin is combined with a protease inhibitor. Some recent guidelines recommend dosing rifabutin 150 mg daily (QD) in combination with a ritonavir-boosted protease inhibitor [12], but others still recommend 150 mg three time weekly (tiw) [13]. These differences in guidelines are due to the limited pharmacokinetic studies comparing the 2 dosing regimens of rifabutin and persisting concerns about the tolerability and toxicity of using higher doses of rifabutin [14]. Previous reports suggested that less frequent dosing at 150 mg in HIV-positive tuberculosis patients can result in inadequate rifamycin concentrations [15,16], relapse [17] and acquired rifamycin resistance (ARR) [18]. Patients with rifabutin $AUC_{0-24} < 4.5$ µg.h/mL were identified as at the highest risk of ARR. The optimum pharmacokinetic parameter associated with treatment efficacy is unknown.

Elimination of rifabutin is primarily by metabolism via various routes, with deacetylation to d-RBT considered the most important. The d-RBT metabolite is known to have antibacterial activity [19] but may also contribute to toxicity, and is thought to be metabolized further in the liver by CYP 3A4. The present study was therefore undertaken to compare the bioavailability of rifabutin and d-RBT after two different dosing regimens of rifabutin (150 mg tiw and 150 mg daily) in combination with ritonavir boosted lopinavir (LPV/r), the protease inhibitor most commonly used to treat HIV infection in South Africa.

Methods

Study design

An open-label, randomized, three-period, crossover drug interaction study was undertaken to investigate the pharmacokinetics of rifabutin with and without PI-based ART (Figure 1). The secondary objective was to assess the tolerability and safety of rifabutin and LPV/r. The Biomedical Research Ethics Committees of the Universities of Kwa-Zulu Natal and Cape Town, and the Ethics Committee of the International Union against Tuberculosis and Lung Disease (Paris) and the South African Medicines Control Council approved the study. The trial registration number was NCT00640887 (https://clinical-trials.gov/).

Recruitment

Patients were recruited from local tuberculosis clinics in Kwa-Zulu Natal, South Africa. The study ran from February 2009 until October 2010. All patients provided written informed consent. Eligibility requirements were a diagnosis of pulmonary tuberculosis confirmed by microscopy or culture, HIV infection with CD4 lymphocyte count ≥ 50 and ≤ 200 cells/mm^3, weight ≥ 50 kg or a BMI ≥ 18, a Karnofsky score Q $\geq 80\%$ and no grade 3 or 4 clinical or laboratory findings according to DAIDS tables [20]. The CD4 restrictions for this study were a reflection of the South African guidelines for the initiation of ART in TB patients at the time the study was conducted [21]. Patients with CD4 counts below 50 were recommended to initiate therapy immediately whereas those with CD4 count between 50 and 200 were initiated at 2 months of TB therapy.

Only patients who completed and adhered to 6 weeks of standard intensive phase chemotherapy and had not received ART therapy in the preceding three months were enrolled. Patients with a previous tuberculosis episode within three years prior to the current episode, a history of prior treatment for MDR tuberculosis, concomitant opportunistic infection requiring additional antimicrobial treatment, a formal contraindication to any trial medication, diabetes mellitus requiring treatment, recreational drug or alcohol abuse, mental illness, total neutrophil count <1200 cells/L, hemoglobin <6.8 g/dL, or liver function tests > grade 2, pregnancy or lactating women were excluded.

Treatments under study

At enrollment, six weeks after starting standard tuberculosis chemotherapy, rifampicin was switched to rifabutin 300 mg daily (Figure 1). After two weeks of rifabutin, pyrazinamide and ethambutol were stopped and patients continued with daily doses of rifabutin 300 mg in combination with isoniazid 300 mg. After two more weeks, the first pharmacokinetic evaluation (PK1) was carried

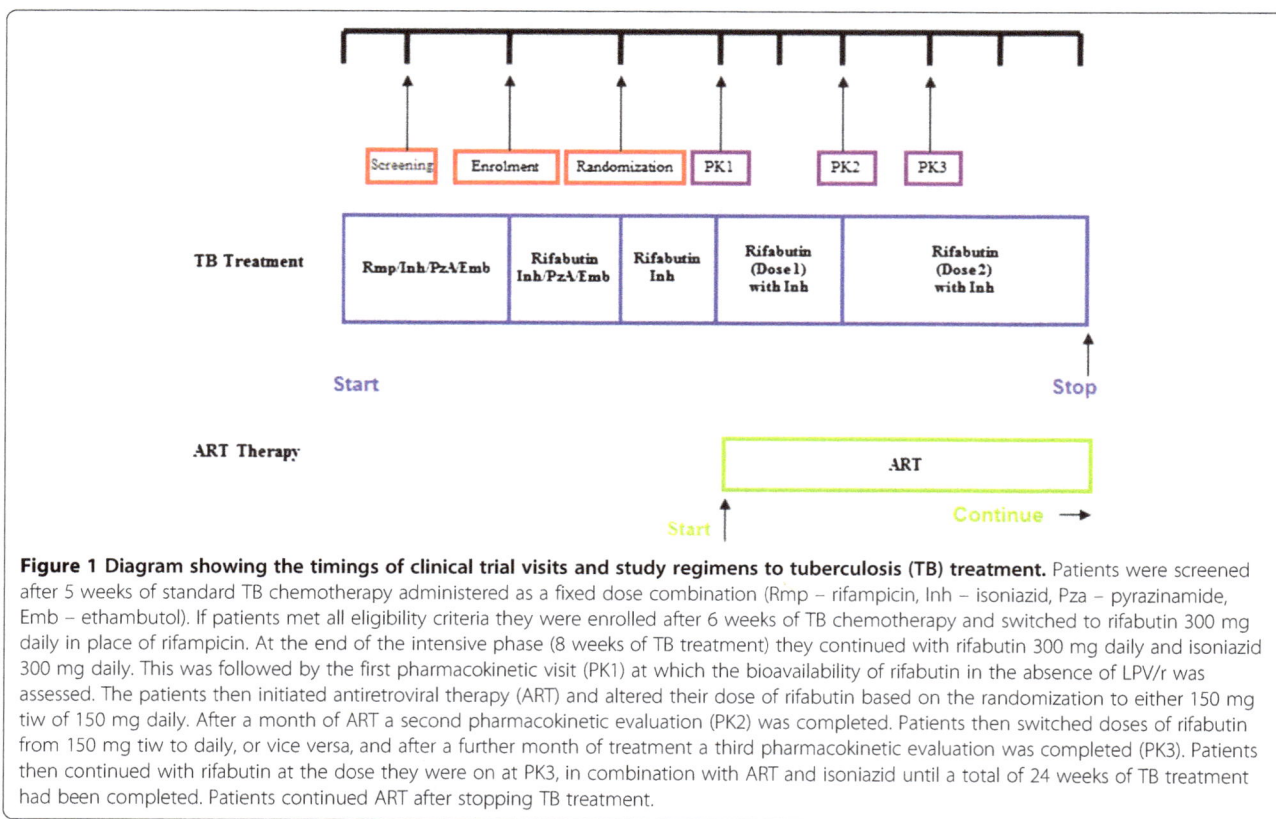

Figure 1 Diagram showing the timings of clinical trial visits and study regimens to tuberculosis (TB) treatment. Patients were screened after 5 weeks of standard TB chemotherapy administered as a fixed dose combination (Rmp – rifampicin, Inh – isoniazid, Pza – pyrazinamide, Emb – ethambutol). If patients met all eligibility criteria they were enrolled after 6 weeks of TB chemotherapy and switched to rifabutin 300 mg daily in place of rifampicin. At the end of the intensive phase (8 weeks of TB treatment) they continued with rifabutin 300 mg daily and isoniazid 300 mg daily. This was followed by the first pharmacokinetic visit (PK1) at which the bioavailability of rifabutin in the absence of LPV/r was assessed. The patients then initiated antiretroviral therapy (ART) and altered their dose of rifabutin based on the randomization to either 150 mg tiw of 150 mg daily. After a month of ART a second pharmacokinetic evaluation (PK2) was completed. Patients then switched doses of rifabutin from 150 mg tiw to daily, or vice versa, and after a further month of treatment a third pharmacokinetic evaluation was completed (PK3). Patients then continued with rifabutin at the dose they were on at PK3, in combination with ART and isoniazid until a total of 24 weeks of TB treatment had been completed. Patients continued ART after stopping TB treatment.

out and patients were randomized to one of two different rifabutin dose sequences together with daily doses of isoniazid and ART comprising LPV/r (400/100 mg) plus lamivudine (150 mg bd) and stavudine (30 mg bd). Half the patients received rifabutin 150 mg tiw for 4 weeks before being switched to rifabutin 150 mg daily after a second pharmacokinetic evaluation (PK2). A third pharmacokinetic evaluation (PK3) took place after 4 weeks and they remained on this dose of rifabutin until completion of tuberculosis treatment. Half the patients received the two rifabutin doses in a reverse sequence.

Physical examinations and laboratory investigations were done at screening, after 1 month of rifabutin (trial day 28 – PK1), after 1 month of ART and rifabutin (trial day 56 – PK2), after 2 months of ART and rifabutin (trial day 84 – PK2) and 2 weeks before the end of TB treatment (trial day 112) as shown in Figure 1. Upon completion of the trial, patients were referred to local antiretroviral clinics for further management. Pfizer (South Africa) supplied the rifabutin (Mycobutin®) 150 mg capsules and the new film-coated tablet formulation of LPV/r, Aluvia® was purchased from Abbott Laboratories (USA).

Sample size
Based on the AUC_{0-24} for rifabutin determined in previous studies, it was estimated that a sample size of 12

participants had a power of 80% to detect a 20% difference between the mean AUC_{0-24} for rifabutin with and without ART. The sample size was calculated on the assumption that 16 enrolled participants would result in a minimum of 12 evaluable subjects. The additional 4 patients in each arm were recruited as it was thought that there may be drop out of patients before completing 3 full pharmacokinetic visits.

Pharmacokinetic sampling
All patients were admitted before each pharmacokinetic occasion and were fasted from midnight. A standard hospital breakfast (oats with 2 slices of toast and tea) was served 2 h after drug ingestion. Blood draws were done at 0, 2, 3, 4, 5, 6, 8, 12, 24 and 48 h after drug ingestion. The samples were placed on ice immediately and centrifuged at 3000 rpm at 4°C for 10 minutes. Separated plasma was stored immediately at −70°C until batch analysis.

Drug analyses
Rifabutin and d-RBT were analyzed with a validated LC/MS/MS assay [14]. Rifaximin was used as internal standard at a concentration of 100 ng/ml. Gradient chromatography was performed on a Phenomenex, Luna 5 μm PFP (2), 100 A, 50 mm × 2 mm analytical column, using

acetonitrile and 0.1% formic acid as mobile phase, and a flow rate of 500 μl/min. An AB Sciex API 3200 mass spectrometer monitored protonated ions at m/z 847.4 to the product ions at m/z 95.1 for rifabutin, at m/z 805.4 to the product ions at m/z 95.1 for d-RBT, and at m/z 786.3 to the product ions m/z 151.1 for rifaximin. Rifabutin and d-RBT accuracies were between 99.1% and 109.0% during inter-batch validation. The co-efficient of variation during inter-batch validation was less than 9.2%. The calibration range for rifabutin was between 3.91 ng/ml and 1000 ng/ml, and for d-RBT between 0.780 ng/ml and 200 ng/ml. The intra- and inter-batch accuracy statistics of the rifabutin and d-RBT assay validation were between 93.3% and 111.5%, and between 99.1% and 109%. The co-efficient of variation was less than 13.8%.

Plasma lopinavir concentrations were quantified by a validated LCMS/MS method previously described by Chi et al. [22]. The calibration curve was linear over the range from 0.05 to 20 mg/L. Samples with a concentration of >20 mg/L, were diluted and re-analyzed. Any sample below the LLQ was reported as 0.5 X LLQ for analysis. The intra- and inter-batch accuracy statistics of the lopinavir assay validation were between 95.0% and 96.4%, and between 96.2% and 99.1%. The coefficient of variation (%CV) was less than 3.9%.

Pharmacokinetic analysis

The main pharmacokinetic measures for rifabutin, d-RBT and lopinavir were derived by non-compartmental analysis using Stata (StataCorp. 2009. *Stata Statistical Software: Release 11.* College Station, TX: StataCorp LP). The peak concentration (C_{max}), and time to C_{max} (T_{max}) were obtained directly from concentration-time profiles. Drug concentrations at the end of a dosing interval are reported as C_{min} and pre-dose concentrations as C_0. The steady-state AUC from time 0 h to the last quantifiable sample at 24 h (AUC_{0-24}) or 48 h (AUC_{0-48}) for rifabutin and 12 h (AUC_{0-12}) for LPV/r were calculated by the linear trapezoidal method. The apparent total oral clearance of rifabutin from plasma at steady state (CL/F) was calculated by dose/AUC.

Statistics

For statistical analysis, the AUC_{0-24} was log-transformed. A linear mixed model with two doses (high and low), day (2 and 3), the sequence of the doses, log AUC_{0-24} and id nested within sequence was used. As there was no significant effect of sequencing of the doses (whether the patients received the tiw dose before the daily dose of rifabutin or vice versa), the two corresponding doses from each arm were pooled for further analysis. A paired t-test was used to compare the AUC_{0-24} for the 150 mg daily dose with that for 150 mg tiw and 300 mg daily doses. An AUC_{0-48}

was derived for the 150 mg daily and 300 mg daily doses by doubling the AUC_{0-24}. This was compared with the AUC_{0-48} for the 150 mg tiw dose using a paired t-test. The dosing interval is 48 hours for the tiw dose for 2 of 3 doses.

To calculate geometric mean ratios (GMR) for AUC, log means and 90% confidence limits were back transformed and presented in their original units as geometric means. Geometric mean ratios for the AUC of rifabutin: 150 mg daily with LPV/r / 300 mg daily, and 150 mg tiw with LPV/300 mg daily, respectively, were computed. A P-value < 0.05 was considered significant. Inter-patient variability was measured by co-efficient of variation (%CV) that was calculated as {100 X (e (var est) -1)$^{1/2}$}. Baseline and final log viral loads and $CD4^+$ counts were compared using paired t-tests.

Results

Patient demographics

Sixteen patients received LPV/r therapy with rifabutin. Two patients were prematurely withdrawn from the study and were therefore not evaluable for pharmacokinetic analysis, one due to uveitis and another due to non-compliance with trial medication. All patients were Black South Africans and (64%) were male. All patients had not previously received any antiretroviral therapy. The evaluable subjects' mean (SD) age was 31.5 (5.8) years, weight was 59.9 (9.7) kg, height was 160 (7.7) cm, BMI was 23.3 (2.6), Karnofsky score Q was 100% (100) and $CD4^+$ lymphocyte count was 150.9 (12.1) cells/mm^3.

Rifabutin and 25-O-desacetylrifabutin pharmacokinetic analysis

The main pharmacokinetic parameters for rifabutin and d-RBT are summarized in Table 1 and shown graphically in Figures 2 and 3. The AUC_{0-24} of rifabutin 150 mg daily with LPV/r was significantly higher when compared to the AUC_{0-24} of rifabutin 300 mg daily in the absence of LPV/r (p = 0.004). In contrast, the AUC_{0-48} of rifabutin 150 mg tiw with LPV/r was significantly lower than the AUC_{0-48} of rifabutin 300 mg daily (p = 0.0001). These differences were large as demonstrated by the GMR (Table 2). The GMR (90% CI) for AUC_{0-48} was 0.6 (0.5-0.7) and 0.5 (0.4-0.6) for rifabutin 150 mg tiw compared with rifabutin 300 mg. For the comparison of the 150 mg daily dose of rifabutin with the 300 mg dose the GMR of the AUC_{0-24} was 1.6 (1.4-1.9). Wide inter-patient variability was observed in rifabutin AUC for all three doses (Table 2). The %CV was 24% for the 300 mg dose, 46% for rifabutin 150 mg daily plus LPV/r and 52% for rifabutin 150 mg tiw plus LPV/r.

The C_{max} of rifabutin 150 mg tiw with LPV/r was also significantly lower when compared to the 150 mg daily dose with LPV/r (P = 0.01) and the 300 mg daily dose

Table 1 Pharmacokinetic parameters for rifabutin and 25-O-desacetylrifabutin for each study treatment

Treatment period	Rifabutin 300 mg	Rifabutin 150 mg tiw plus LPV/r	Rifabutin 150 mg daily plus LPV/r
Rifabutin (n = 14)			
AUC_{0-24} (ng.h/mL)	3052.9 (2650.2-3431.5)	2307.5 (1767.5-3884.0)	4766.0 (3950.5-6099.5)
AUC_{0-48} (ng.h/mL)	6105.8 (5300.4-6863.0)*	3402.1 (2809.2-6092.0)	9532.0 (2238.2-22425.4)*
C_{max} (ng/mL)	291.5 (250.0-377.0)	167.5 (87.8-294.0)	311.0 (258.0-376.0)
T_{max} (h)	3.0 (3.0-4.0)	3.5 (3.0-5.0)	3.0 (3.0-4.0)
C_0 (ng/mL)	59.0 (36.4-78.6)	49.1 (27.7-58.9)	176.5 (149.0-195.0)
C_{min} 24 h (ng/mL)	60.7 (40.6-68.8)	70.7 (45.7-96.6)	133.0 (105.0-191.0)
C_{min} 48 h (ng/mL)	-	37.0 (26.6-70.0)	-
CL/F (L/h)	98.3 (87.4-113.2)	65.2 (38.6-85.0)	31.5 (25.0-38.0)
AUC_{0-24} (ng.h/mL) (Rifabutin + Metabolite)	3402.3 (2900.3-3717.2)	3937.2 (2424.6-6772.7)	8753.0 (7771.7-11 505.0)
d-RBT (n = 14)			
AUC_{0-24} (ng.h/mL)	273.3 (235.7-344.1)	1565.5 (1105.5-2567.3)	4118.0 (2678.2-5405.5)
AUC_{0-48} (ng.h/mL)	546.6 (471.4-688.2)*	2318.2 (1722.9-4685.9)	8236.0 (5356.4-10811.0)*
C_{max} (ng/mL)	32.5 (25.2-37.7)	77.2 (58.6-128)	236.5 (159.0-274.0)
T_{max} (h)	3.0 (3.0-4.0)	5.0 (4.0-6.0)	4.0 (3.0-3.0)
C_0 (ng/mL)	5.1 (2.7-6.6)	44.6 (31.7-68.9)	186.0 (115.0-232.0)
C_{min} 24 h (ng/mL)	5.0 (3.4 -5.8	63.9 (42.7-101.0)	155.0 (53.6-206.0)
C_{min} 48 h (ng/mL)	-	35.4 (27.7-81.0)	-

Parameters are median values (interquartile range).
*calculated by 2X AUC_{0-24}.
RBT = rifabutin.
d-RBT =25-O-desacetylrifabutin.
LPV/r = lopinavir/ritonavir based ART.
tiw = three times per week.
AUC = area under the curve.
C_{max} = maximum concentration in plasma.
T_{max} = time at which maximum plasma attained.
CL/F = clearance.
C_0 = pre-dose concentration.
C_{min} = trough concentration.

without LPV/r (P = 0.01). The GMR (90% CI) for Cmax was 0.5 (0.4-0.6) for RBT 150 mg tiw compared with RBT 300 mg and 0.5 (0.5-0.6) for RBT 150 mg tiw compared with 150 mg daily. The median C_{min} for rifabutin 300 mg was 60.7 ng/mL (IQR, 40.6-68.8 ng/mL). The C_{min} values increased in the presence of LPV/r with daily dosing of rifabutin but dropped significantly with the tiw dose. Rifabutin clearance was significantly reduced in the presence of LPV/r (p = 0.001 for daily and p = 0.002 tiw rifabutin dosing) compared to 300 mg rifabutin given alone.

Without lopinavir, d-RBT concentrations were 11% of the parent drug. Plasma d-RBT concentrations increased 5-fold with tiw rifabutin dosing and 15-fold with daily doses of rifabutin (Figure 3). The total antimicrobial moiety (combined AUC_{0-24} of rifabutin and metabolite) for rifabutin at 150 mg tiw with ART was 1.2 times greater than for 300 mg rifabutin and 2.6 times less than for 150 mg daily with ART.

Lopinavir pharmacokinetic analysis

Lopinavir pharmacokinetic measures are shown in Table 3 and Figure 4. Median lopinavir trough (C_0) concentrations were above the recommended lower limit for ART-naïve patients of 1 μg/ [23]. Although there was a trend to higher lopinavir concentrations with the once daily dosing of rifabutin, the differences in AUC_{0-12} and C_{max} between the two doses were not significant. Double peaks were observed in the individual lopinavir concentration-time profiles with both doses of rifabutin.

Response to TB/HIV treatment

Three patients were culture positive after two months of tuberculosis therapy and none culture positive at the end of therapy. The mean final $CD4^+$ count at the end of tuberculosis therapy was 253.8 (42.4) cells/mm^3, and significantly higher (p = 0.03) than baseline. The mean (SD) viral load dropped significantly (p < 0.001) by 2.7 log10 copies and 8 patients had viral loads < 500 copies/ml.

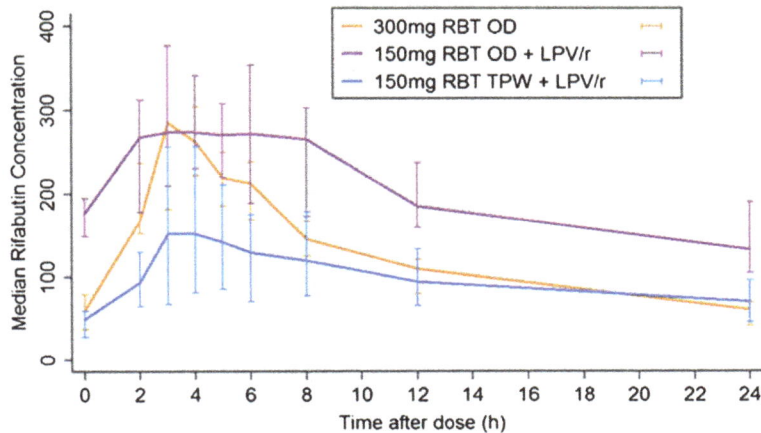

Figure 2 Rifabutin median concentration-time profiles. Median rifabutin (RBT) concentrations for the three pharmacokinetic evaluations in 14 patients. The orange line corresponds to the dosing of RBT at 300 mg without ART; the blue line to RBT dosing at 150 mg tiw with ART and the purple line to dosing with 150 mg of RBT daily with ART. The bars represent interquartile range (IQR).

Adverse events

Adverse events (AE) were analyzed for all sixteen patients. Rifabutin was well tolerated at all doses and there was only one withdrawal because of an adverse event (uveitis). There were two serious adverse events (bacterial meningitis and pyelonephritis), both considered unrelated to rifabutin by the study team. Grade 2 uveitis occurred in one patient after 1 month of rifabutin, coinciding with the start of ART, and resolved with no sequelae after withdrawal of medication. Her AUC_{0-24} and C_{max} values for rifabutin were within the interquartile range. The commonest laboratory AE was neutropenia. Grade 3 neutropenia occurred on 7 occasions in 5 patients (Table 4). There were 2 grade 3 elevations in transaminases and amylase. There were no grade 4 laboratory events.

Discussion

The results of this study show that there are substantial differences in the AUC_{0-24} of rifabutin obtained with the two different dosing regimens in combination with LPV/r. The daily dose of 150 mg resulted in a more than two fold increase in the AUC_{0-24} when compared to the three times a week dose. The difference between the two doses was even greater when comparing the AUC_{0-48}. There is a lack of conventional efficacy data in support of a particular dose or target pharmacokinetic parameter for rifabutin [24], but there is convincing evidence that intermittent rifamycin therapy is associated with tuberculosis relapse and rifamycin resistance, especially in subjects with low CD4 counts [17,18,25-27]. In TBTC study [18], TB-HIV co-infected patients who had $AUC_{0-24} < 4.5$ µg.h/mL were

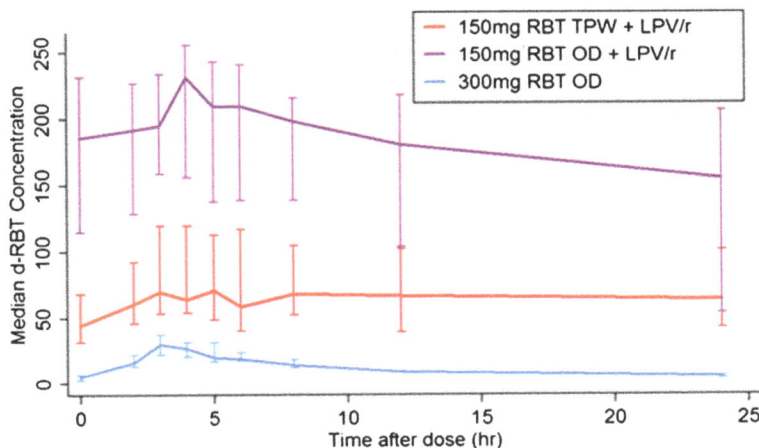

Figure 3 25-O-desacetylrifabutin median concentration-time profiles. Median 25-O-desacetylrifabutin (d-RBT) concentrations for the three pharmacokinetic evaluations in 14 patients. The bars represent interquartile range (IQR). The blue line corresponds to the dosing of RBT at 300 mg without ART; the red line to RBT dosing at 150 mg tiw with LPV/r based ART and the purple line to dosing with 150 mg of RBT daily.

Table 2 Geometric mean ratios of rifabutin and 25-O-desacetylrifabutin parameters with and without antiretroviral therapy

	GMR (90% CI)		
	RBT 150 mg tiw with RBT 300 mg daily	RBT 150 mg tiw with RBT 150 mg daily	RBT 150 mg daily with RBT 300 mg daily
AUC_{0-24}	0.8 (0.7 – 0.9)	0.4 (0.5 – 0.5)	1.6 (1.4 – 1.9)
AUC_{0-48}*	0.6 (0.5 – 0.7)	0.4 (0.4 – 0.4)	n/a
C_{max}(ng/mL)	0.5 (0.4 – 0.6)	0.5 (0.5 – 0.6)	1.0 (0.9 – 1.0)
C_0(ng/mL)	0.7 (0.5 – 0.9)	0.2 (0.1 – 0.3)	3.4 (3.7 – 3.1)
C_{min}24h(ng/mL)	1.2 (1.0 – 1.4)	0.5 (0.4 – 0.5)	2.7 (2.2 – 3.2)

*calculated by 2 times the AUC_{0-24} for the RBT 300 mg daily and RBT 150 mg daily arms.
n/a – Not applicable.
GMR – Geometric mean ratio.
90% CI – 90% confidence interval.
RBT 150 mg tiw – rifabutin dose of 150 mg three times per week (tiw) in combination with lopinavir/ritonavir based ART and isoniazid.
RBT 150 mg daily – rifabutin dose of 150 mg daily in combination with lopinavir/ritonavir based ART and isoniazid.
RBT 300 mg daily – rifabutin dose of 300 mg daily in combination with isoniazid.

at higher risk of ARR. Of the patients who relapsed or failed therapy 83% developed ARR as opposed to 33% who had AUC's above this threshold value. In this study, 71% patients on rifabutin 150 mg daily had AUC_{0-24} values >4.5 μg.h/mL compared to 14% on rifabutin tiw dosing. Similarly the C_{min} values of rifabutin 48 hours after dosing tiw are significantly lower than the C_{min} values for 300 mg daily and 150 mg daily. On the basis of prevention of resistance our data support the guidelines that recommend a dose of rifabutin 150 mg daily in combination with protease inhibitors [28].

The AUC_{0-24} and C_{max} of d-RBT were significantly increased in the presence of LPV/r in keeping with previous treatment [29,30] and healthy volunteer studies [11,31,32]. There were respective increases in exposure

Table 3 Pharmacokinetic parameters for lopinavir for each study treatment

	Median (Interquartile range)	
Parameter	RBT 150 mg tiw plus LVP/r	RBT 150 mg daily plus LPV/r
AUC_{0-12} (μg.h/mL)	139.5 (103.8-163.9)	160.1 (129.1-181.9)
C_{max} (ng/mL)	15.8 (12.9-17.1)	18.1 (14.5-19.6)
T_{max} (h)	2.0 (2.0-3.0)	2.0 (2.0-3.0)
C_0(μg/mL)	9.8 (3.5-14.0)	11.4 (9.9-15.2)
C_{min} (μg/mL)	7.4 (4.5-10.0)	9.4 (7.2-11.6)

RBT = rifabutin.
LPV/r = lopinavir/ritonavir.
tiw = three times per week.
AUC = area under the curve.
C_{max} = maximum concentration in plasma.
T_{max} = time at which maximum plasma attained.
C_0 = pre-dose concentration.
C_{min} = trough concentration.

to the metabolite of approximately 5- and 15-fold when rifabutin 150 mg was given tiw or daily with LPV/r and are probably due to the presence of ritonavir. Ritonavir is a potent inhibitor of CYP3A4, which metabolizes d-RBT. d-RBT is known to have significant anti-mycobacterial activity and could contribute to the regimen efficacy [19]. These elevations of the d-RBT metabolite could led to an increase in adverse drug reactions. We were unable to show a significant association between plasma rifabutin and d-RBT concentration and adverse events such as neutropenia or elevated transaminases however the numbers of patients are few and larger studies are required to establish the safety of the rifabutin 150 mg daily dose. It will also be important to investigate the interaction of RBT in combination with other antiretrovirals [33].

Although the currently recommended dose of rifabutin for the treatment of pulmonary tuberculosis is 300 mg daily there are few pharmacokinetic data from HIV infected African tuberculosis patients treated with this dose. The median rifabutin AUC_{0-24} and C_{max} values from this study are comparable to previous studies of rifabutin 300mg daily in HIV-infected patients [15,34-36]. The pharmacodynamic-pharmacokinetic (PKPD) relationship for rifabutin has not been comprehensively studied so it is not clear how the reduced AUC of the 150 mg tiw dose relative to the 300 mg dose without ART reported here would impact on tuberculosis treatment outcomes. It is still uncertain if C_{max} or AUC is the critical pharmacodynamic measure for rifamycins. Mitchison [37] and others reported the C_{max}/MIC to be the best PKPD measure whereas subsequent murine and hollow fibre models [38,39], and early bactericidal activity studies in humans [40] found that the AUC_{0-24}/MIC ratio was a superior parameter.

Previous studies of the pharmacokinetic interaction of rifabutin with LPV/r in HIV infected individuals have mostly been small case series or involved an adaptive design in which only selected patients were exposed to the higher dose of rifabutin [15,16,41]. One previous study has reported on the rifabutin pharmacokinetics in combination with LPV/r (Aluvia) but in patients initiating rifabutin at the start of therapy [42]. This study was conducted in Vietnam in a different population group but also reported that the 150 mg tiw dose was potentially sub therapeutic when compared to the 150 mg daily dose or the 300 mg dose without ART. Similar to that study we adopted a cross-over design in which all patients received 3 full pharmacokinetic assessments with rifabutin alone and at two different rifabutin doses in combination with ART allowing us to formally compare the different dosing strategies and reduce intra-patient variability. However there are limitations to our study. Although patients received rifabutin for a total of 18 weeks our numbers are small so it is necessary to be cautious in

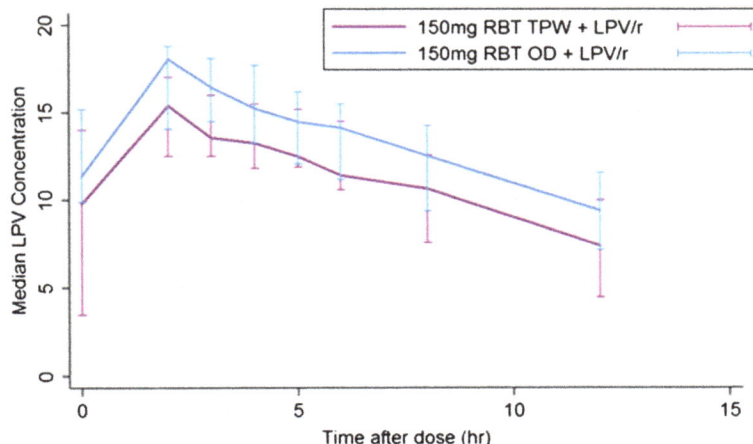

Figure 4 Median concentration-time profile of boosted lopinavir administered with two different doses of rifabutin. The median lopinavir (LPV) concentrations for 14 patients administered 2 different concentrations of rifabutin (RBT). Blue line corresponds to a RBT dose of 150 mg daily and the purple line to 150 mg tiw. LPV/r corresponds to boosted lopinavir. The bars represent interquartile range (IQR).

drawing definitive conclusions about the safety of rifabutin at the higher dose. We included immune-suppressed HIV positive patient but not those with CD4 count less than 50, and it is conceivable that the pharmacokinetics and tolerability of rifabutin may be different in the most highly immune-suppressed group of patients.

Although the higher dose (150 mg daily) used in this study resulted in rifabutin levels that reduce the risk of resistance it is important to emphasis that the approximately 15 fold increase in the d-RBT metabolite might result in an increase in adverse events. Neutropenia and uveitis have previously been identified as severe adverse events associated with the co-administration of rifabutin with a CYP3A4 inhibitor [43-47]. A recent paediatric clinical trial of rifabutin in combination with LPV/r was stopped due to a high frequency of grade 4 neutropenia [14]. An advantage of this study is that patients remained on study doses for sixteen weeks allowing a safety evaluation to be made over a longer duration. In this study the combinations of rifabutin and LPV/r were generally well tolerated with no grade 4 toxicities apart from 2 clinical serious adverse events reported by the study investigators as unrelated to rifabutin. Neutropenia was a common adverse event and has been reported predominantly in previous studies on healthy volunteers, but there were no grade 4 cases. Although there was a significant fall in the neutrophil count during the course of the trial most of this decline occurred in the first few weeks of rifabutin therapy prior to the initiation of ART and we did not find a significant association between neutropenia and plasma

Table 4 Timing of selected grade 3 laboratory adverse events

Subject	AE Grade	AE	RBT dose at time of AE	Arm	Days on RBT
148	3	AST increased	150 mg daily	Low-High	106
148	3	Amylase increased	150 mg daily	Low-High	113
171	3	Neutropenia	300 mg daily	Low-High	29
182	3	Neutropenia	300 mg daily	Low-High	27
204	3	Neutropenia	150 mg daily	High-Low	57
204	3	Neutropenia	150 mg tiw	High-Low	112
242	3	Neutropenia	300 mg daily	High-Low	28
242	3	Neutropenia	150 mg daily	High-Low	53
242	3	AST increased	150 mg tiw	High-Low	96
242	3	Amylase increased	150 mg tiw	High-Low	119
250	3	Neutropenia	150 mg daily	Low-High	77

AE – adverse event.
RBT – rifabutin.
ARM – refers to the sequencing order of the rifabutin dosing in combination with ART.
tiw- three times per week.

rifabutin concentrations. Neutropenia is also the most common side effect of cotrimoxazole therapy in HIV- infected patients [48] and all patients in the present study were prescribed cotrimoxazole 960 mg daily as prophylaxis. The majority of the patients started cotrimoxazole at enrollment and this would have contributed to the declining neutrophil count seen in this study. Uveitis occurred only once in a participant who had been taking 300 mg rifabutin and was not associated with high serum concentrations of drug suggesting it could have been HIV related rather than drug related. However the number of patients are small in this study so the safety of the 150 mg daily rifabutin dose needs to be established in a larger cohort.

The activity of protease inhibitors is influenced by their concentrations in plasma [49] therefore the pharmacokinetics of LPV/r were evaluated in the presence of rifabutin. The median LPV/r AUC_{0-12}, C_{max}, C_0 and C_{12} obtained in this study when LPV/r was administered with two different doses of rifabutin are consistent with historical control data [50]. Secondary peaks were observed in the time-concentration profiles of LPV/r, usually within 4 hours of drug ingestion, similar to patterns observed in other studies. In both dosing arms, median LPV/r trough (C_0) concentrations at steady state were above the recommended lower limit for ART-naïve patients of 1 μg/mL [23] and therapeutic LPV/r trough (C_0) and C_{min} (C_{12}) concentrations were achieved in all participants with both doses of rifabutin.

Conclusions

In conclusion this study supports the recent change to some guidelines for the dosing of rifabutin in combination with LPV/r [28]. The high proportion of participants on the 150 mg tiw arm who failed to achieve rifabutin concentrations that prevented the emergence of drug resistance when the drug is dosed twice weekly is concerning. Although escalating the rifabutin dose after therapeutic drug monitoring is a viable option in resource rich settings, it is impractical in many regions of the world where HIV and TB are endemic. Our study was too small to address all concerns about the toxicity of the higher dose rifabutin with LPV/r, most notably the decrease in neutrophil count, which requires further evaluation.

Competing interests
The authors declare that they have no competing interests.

Authors' contributions
SN, CC, HM, TR, AP carried out data analysis, SN, CC, HM, AH, CL, AP wrote the manuscript, SN, CL, AH, AP managed and provided oversight of the clinical aspects of the study. AP, CL, HM conceived and designed the study. LW, TK, HM carried out the pharmacological analysis. All authors read and approved the final manuscript.

Acknowledgements
We wish to thank the following: Roxana Rustomjee for support in carrying out the study and to the patients and their families who participated in the study. We also like to thank the following for donation of study medications: Pfizer South Africa (Rifabutin), Aspen South Africa (Lamivudine, Stavudine), MSD South Africa (Efavirenz). We also acknowledge Devola Phillips who was the physician who cared for the patients during the study. The study was funded by ANRS (Agence Nationale de Recherche Sur le Sida et les Hépatites Virales). Open access publication of this article has been made possible through support from the Victor Daitz Information Gateway, an initiative of the Victor Daitz Foundation and the University of KwaZulu-Natal.

Author details
[1]TB Research Unit, Medical Research Council, Durban, South Africa. [2]Biostatistics Unit, Medical Research Council, Durban, South Africa. [3]Division of Clinical Pharmacology, Department of Medicine, University of Cape Town, Cape Town, South Africa. [4]International Union Against Tuberculosis and Lung Disease, Paris, France. [5]WHO STOP Tuberculosis Programme, Geneva, Switzerland. [6]KwaZulu-Natal Research Institute for Tuberculosis and HIV (K-RITH), University of KwaZulu-Natal, Durban, South Africa.

References
1. World Health Organization, Global Tuberculosis report: *WHO/HTM/TB/ 2014.08*. 20 Avenue Appia, 1211 Geneva 27, Switzerland: WHO Press, World Health Organization; 2014.
2. Abdool Karim SS, Naidoo K, Grobler A, Padayatchi N, Baxter C, Gray A, Gengiah T, Nair G, Bamber S, Singh A, Khan M, Pienaar J, El-Sadr W, Friedland G, Abdool Karim Q: Timing of initiation of antiretroviral drugs during tuberculosis therapy. *N Engl J Med* 2010, 362:697–706.
3. Blanc FX, Sok T, Laureillard D, Borand L, Rekacewicz C, Nerrienet E, Madec Y, Marcy O, Chan S, Prak N, Kim C, Lak KK, Hak C, Dim B, Sin CI, Sun S, Guillard B, Sar B, Vong S, Fernandez M, Fox L, Delfraissy JF, Goldfeld AE: Earlier versus later start of antiretroviral therapy in HIV-infected adults with tuberculosis. *N Engl J Med* 2011, 365:1471–1481.
4. Havlir DV, Kendall MA, Ive P, Kumwenda J, Swindells S, Qasba SS, Luetkemeyer AF, Hogg E, Rooney JF, Wu X, Hosseinipour MC, Lalloo U, Veloso VG, Some FF, Kumarasamy N, Padayatchi N, Santos BR, Reid S, Hakim J, Mohapi L, Mugyenyi P, Sanchez J, Lama JR, Pape JW, Sanchez A, Asmelash A, Moko E, Sawe F, Andersen J, Sanne I: Timing of antiretroviral therapy for HIV-1 infection and tuberculosis. *N Engl J Med* 2011, 365:1482–1491.
5. World Health Organization: *Global HIV/AIDS response: epidemic update and health sector progress towards universal access. Progress report.* 20 Avenue Appia, 1211 Geneva 27, Switzerland: WHO Press, World Health Organization; 2011.
6. Gupta RK, Jordan MR, Sultan BJ, Hill A, Davis DH, Gregson J, Sawyer AW, Hamers RL, Ndembi N, Pillay D, Bertagnolio S: Global trends in antiretroviral resistance in treatment-naive individuals with HIV after rollout of antiretroviral treatment in resource-limited settings: a global collaborative study and meta-regression analysis. *Lancet* 2012, 380:1250–1258.
7. Burman WJ, Gallicano K, Peloquin C: Comparative pharmacokinetics and pharmacodynamics of the rifamycin antibacterials. *Clin Pharmacokinet* 2001, 40:327–341.
8. Murphy RA, Marconi VC, Gandhi RT, Kuritzkes DR, Sunpath H: Coadministration of lopinavir/ritonavir and rifampicin in HIV and tuberculosis co-infected adults in South Africa. *PLoS One* 2012, 7:e44793.
9. Della Bruna C, Schioppacassi G, Ungheri D, Jabès D, Morvillo E, Sanfilippo A: LM 427, a new spiropiperidylrifamycin: in vitro and in vivo studies. *J Antibiot* 1983, 36:1502–1506.
10. Sanfilippo A, Della Bruna C, Marsili L, Morvillo E, Pasqualucci C, Schioppacassi G, Ungheri D: Biological activity of a new class of rifamycins. Spiro-piperidyl-rifamycins. *J Antibiot* 1980, 33:1193–1198.
11. Polk RE, Brophy DF, Israel DS, Patron R, Sadler BM, Chittick GE, Symonds WT, Lou Y, Kristoff D, Stein D: Pharmacokinetic Interaction between amprenavir and rifabutin or rifampin in healthy males. *Antimicrob Agents Chemother* 2001, 45:502–508.
12. CDC: *Managing Drug Interactions in the Treatment of HIV-Related Tuberculosis.* 1600 Clifton Rd., NE MS E10 Atlanta, GA 30333: Centers for Disease Control and Prevention, Division of Tuberculosis Elimination (DTBE); 2013. Available from URL: http://www.cdc.gov/tb/?404;http://www.cdc.gov:80/tb/TB_HIV_Drugs/default.htm.

13. European AIDS Clinical Society: *Guidelines version 7.02*. Pierre - PL 709 Rue Haute 322 1000 Brussels, Belgium: European AIDS Clinical Society (EACS) CHU; 2014. http://eacsociety.org/Portals/0/140601_EACS%20EN7.02.pdf.

14. Moultrie H, McIlleron H, Sawry S, Kellermann T, Wiesner L, Kindra G, Gous H, Van Rie A: Pharmacokinetics and safety of rifabutin in young HIV-infected children receiving rifabutin and lopinavir/ritonavir. *J Antimicrobial Chemother* 2014,

15. Boulanger C, Hollender E, Farrell K, Stambaugh JJ, Maasen D, Ashkin D, Symes S, Espinoza LA, Rivero RO, Graham JJ, Peloquin CA: Pharmacokinetic evaluation of rifabutin in combination with lopinavir-ritonavir in patients with HIV infection and active tuberculosis. *Clin Infect Dis: Off Publ Infect Dis Soc Am* 2009, 49:1305–1311.

16. Khachi H, O'Connell R, Ladenheim D, Orkin C: Pharmacokinetic interactions between rifabutin and lopinavir/ritonavir in HIV-infected patients with mycobacterial co-infection. *J Antimicrobial Chemother* 2009, 64:871–873.

17. Jenny-Avital ER, Joseph K: Rifamycin-resistant Mycobacterium tuberculosis in the highly active antiretroviral therapy era: a report of 3 relapses with acquired rifampin resistance following alternate-day rifabutin and boosted protease inhibitor therapy. *Clin Infect Dis* 2009, 48:1471–1474.

18. Weiner M, Benator D, Burman W, Peloquin CA, Khan A, Vernon A, Jones B, Silva-Trigo C, Zhao Z, Hodge T: Association between acquired rifamycin resistance and the pharmacokinetics of rifabutin and isoniazid among patients with HIV and tuberculosis. *Clin Infect Dis* 2005, 40:1481–1491.

19. Ungheri D, Franceschi G, Dellaa Bruna C: Main Urinary metabolites of the spiropiperidyl rifamycin LM 427: isolation and biological properties. In *Recent Advances in Chemotherapy*. Edited by Ishigami J. Tokyo: Tokyo Press; 1986:1917–1918.

20. ACTG: *AIDS Clinical Trials Group, Division of AIDS table for grading the severity of adult and pediatric adverse events*. Rockville, MD: National Institutes of Health, National Institute of Allergy and Infectious Diseases, Division of AIDS; 2004.

21. Republic of South Africa Department of Health: *South African National Tuberculosis Management Guidelines*. Private Bag X828 Pretoria 0001 South Africa: Directorate of TB Control and Management; 2009.

22. Chi J, Jayewardene AL, Stone JA, Motoya T, Aweeka FT: Simultaneous determination of five HIV protease inhibitors nelfinavir, indinavir, ritonavir, saquinavir and amprenavir in human plasma by LC/MS/MS. *J Pharm Biomed Anal* 2002, 30:675–684.

23. La Porte C, Back D, Blaschke T, Boucher C, Fletcher C, Flexner C, Gerber J, Kashuba A, Schapiro J, Burger D: Updated guideline to perform therapeutic drug monitoring for antiretroviral agents. *Rev Antivir Ther* 2006, 3:4–14.

24. Davies G, Cerri S, Richeldi L: Rifabutin for treating pulmonary tuberculosis. *Cochrane Database Syst Rev* 2007, 4:1–21.

25. Li J, Munsiff SS, Driver CR, Sackoff J: Relapse and acquired rifampin resistance in HIV-infected patients with tuberculosis treated with rifampin-or rifabutin-based regimens in New York City, 1997–2000. *Clin Infect Dis* 2005, 41:83–91.

26. Nettles RE, Mazo D, Alwood K, Gachuhi R, Maltas G, Wendel K, Cronin W, Hooper N, Bishai W, Sterling TR: Risk factors for relapse and acquired rifamycin resistance after directly observed tuberculosis treatment: a comparison by HIV serostatus and rifamycin use. *Clin Infect Dis* 2004, 38:731–736.

27. Spradling P, Drociuk D, McLaughlin S, Lee L, Peloquin C, Gallicano K, Pozsik C, Onorato I, Castro K, Ridzon R: Drug-drug interactions in inmates treated for human immunodeficiency virus and Mycobacterium tuberculosis infection or disease: an institutional tuberculosis outbreak. *Clin Infect Dis* 2002, 35:1106–1112.

28. Panel on Antiretroviral Guidelines for Adults and Adolescents: *Guidelines for the use of antiretroviral agents in HIV-1-infected adults and adolescents*. Section accessed Nov 2014, AIDSinfo P.O. Box 4780 Rockville, MD, USA: Department of Health and Human Services; Available at http://aidsinfo.nih. gov/contentfiles/lvguidelines/adultandadolescentgl.pdf.

29. Benator DA, Weiner MH, Burman WJ, Vernon AA, Zhao ZA, Khan AE, Jones BE, Sandman L, Engle M, Silva-Trigo C: Clinical Evaluation of the Nelfinavir-Rifabutin Interaction in Patients with Tuberculosis and Human Immunodeficiency Virus Infection. *Pharmacother: J Human Pharmacol Drug Ther* 2007, 27:793–800.

30. Hamzeh FM, Benson C, Gerber J, Currier J, McCrea J, Deutsch P, Ruan P, Wu H, Lee J, Flexner C: Steady-state pharmacokinetic interaction of modified-dose indinavir and rifabutin*. *Clin Pharmacol Ther* 2003, 73:159–169.

31. Ford SL, Chen Y-C, Lou Y, Borland J, Min SS, Yuen GJ, Shelton MJ: Pharmacokinetic interaction between fosamprenavir-ritonavir and rifabutin in healthy subjects. *Antimicrob Agents Chemother* 2008, 52:534–538.

32. Sekar V, Lavreys L, Van de Casteele T, Berckmans C, Spinosa-Guzman S, Vangeneugden T, De Pauw M, Hoetelmans R: Pharmacokinetics of darunavir/ritonavir and rifabutin coadministered in HIV-negative healthy volunteers. *Antimicrob Agents Chemother* 2010, 54:4440–4445.

33. Dooley KE, Sayre P, Borland J, Purdy E, Chen S, Song I, Peppercorn A, Everts S, Piscitelli S, Flexner C: Safety, tolerability, and pharmacokinetics of the HIV integrase inhibitor dolutegravir given twice daily with rifampin or once daily with rifabutin: results of a phase 1 study among healthy subjects. *JAIDS J Acquir Immune Defic Syndr* 2013, 62:21–27.

34. Colborn D, Lampiris H, Lee B, Lewis R, Sullam P, Narang PK: Concomitant cotrimoxazole (CTX) does not affect rifabutin (RBT) kinetics in HIV+ patients. *Clin Pharmacol Therapuet* 1996, 59:PI49–PI49.

35. Li RC, Nightingale S, Lewis RC, Colborn DC, Narang PK: Lack of effect of concomitant zidovudine on rifabutin kinetics in patients with AIDS-related complex. *Antimicrob Agents Chemother* 1996, 40:1397–1402.

36. Moyle G, Buss N, Goggin T, Snell P, Higgs C, Hawkins D: Interaction between saquinavir soft-gel and rifabutin in patients infected with HIV. *Br J Clin Pharmacol* 2002, 54:178–182.

37. Mitchison D, Dickinson JM: Laboratory aspects of intermittent drug therapy. *Postgrad Med J* 1971, 47:737.

38. Gumbo T, Louie A, Deziel MR, Liu W, Parsons LM, Salfinger M, Drusano GL: Concentration-dependent Mycobacterium tuberculosis killing and prevention of resistance by rifampin. *Antimicrob Agents Chemother* 2007, 51:3781–3788.

39. Jayaram R, Gaonkar S, Kaur P, Suresh B, Mahesh B, Jayashree R, Nandi V, Bharat S, Shandil R, Kantharaj E: Pharmacokinetics-pharmacodynamics of rifampin in an aerosol infection model of tuberculosis. *Antimicrob Agents Chemother* 2003, 47:2118–2124.

40. Diacon A, Patientia R, Venter A, Van Helden P, Smith P, McIlleron H, Maritz J, Donald P: Early bactericidal activity of high-dose rifampin in patients with pulmonary tuberculosis evidenced by positive sputum smears. *Antimicrob Agents Chemother* 2007, 51:2994–2996.

41. Tanuma J, Sano K, Teruya K, Watanabe K, Aoki T, Honda H, Yazaki H, Tsukada K, Gatanaga H, Kikuchi Y, Oka S: Pharmacokinetics of rifabutin in Japanese HIV-infected patients with or without antiretroviral therapy. *PLoS One* 2013, 8:e70611.

42. Lan NT, Thu NT, Barrail-Tran A, Duc NH, Lan NN, Laureillard D, Lien TT, Borand L, Quillet C, Connolly C, Lagarde D, Pym A, Lienhardt C, Dung NH, Taburet AM, Harries AD: Randomised pharmacokinetic trial of rifabutin with lopinavir/ritonavir-antiretroviral therapy in patients with HIV-associated tuberculosis in Vietnam. *PLoS One* 2014, 9:e84866.

43. Apseloff G, Foulds G, LaBoy-Goral L, Kraut E, Vincent J: Severe neutropenia caused by recommended prophylactic doses of rifabutin. *Lancet* 1996, 348:685.

44. Flexner C, Barditch-Crovo PA: Severe neutropenia among healthy volunteers given rifabutin in clinical trials*. *Clin Pharmacol Ther* 2003, 74:592–593.

45. Griffith DE, Brown BA, Girard WM, Wallace RJ: Adverse events associated with high-dose rifabutin in macrolide-containing regimens for the treatment of Mycobacterium avium complex lung disease. *Clin Infect Dis* 1995, 21:594–598.

46. Griffith DE, Brown BA, Wallace RJ: Varying dosages of rifabutin affect white blood cell and platelet counts in human immunodeficiency virus-negative patients who are receiving multidrug regimens for pulmonary Mycobacterium avium complex disease. *Clin Infect Dis* 1996, 23:1321–1322.

47. Shafran SD, Singer J, Zarowny DP, Deschênes J, Phillips P, Turgeon F, Aoki FY, Toma E, Miller M, Duperval R: Determinants of rifabutin-associated uveitis in patients treated with rifabutin, clarithromycin, and ethambutol for Mycobacterium avium complex bacteremia: a multivariate analysis. *J Infect Dis* 1998, 177:252–255.

48. Moh R, Danel C, Sorho S, Sauvageot D, Anzian A, Minga A, Gomis OB, Konga C, Inwoley A, Gabillard D: Haematological changes in adults receiving a zidovudine-containing HAART regimen in combination with co-trimoxazole in Côte d'Ivoire. *Antivir Ther* 2005, 10:615–624.

49. Kempf DJ, Marsh KC, Kumar G, Rodrigues AD, Denissen JF, McDonald E, Kukulka MJ, Hsu A, Granneman GR, Baroldi PA: Pharmacokinetic

enhancement of inhibitors of the human immunodeficiency virus protease by coadministration with ritonavir. *Antimicrob Agents Chemother* 1997, **41**:654–660.

50. Crommentuyn KM, Mulder JW, Mairuhu A, Van Gorp E, Meenhorst PL, Huitema A, Beijnen JH: **The plasma and intracellular steady-state pharmacokinetics of lopinavir/ritonavir in HIV-1-infected patients.** *Antivir Ther* 2004, **9**:779–786.

20

Overuse of antibiotics for the common cold – attitudes and behaviors among doctors in rural areas of Shandong Province, China

Qiang Sun[1*], Oliver J Dyar[2], Lingbo Zhao[1], Göran Tomson[3], Lennart E Nilsson[4], Malin Grape[5], Yanyan Song[6], Ling Yan[7] and Cecilia Stålsby Lundborg[8]

Abstract

Background: Irrational antibiotic use is common in rural areas of China, despite the growing recognition of the importance of appropriate prescribing to contain antibiotic resistance. The aim of this study was to analyze doctors' attitudes and prescribing practices related to antibiotics in rural areas of Shandong province, focusing on patients with the common cold.

Methods: A survey was conducted with doctors working at thirty health facilities (village clinics, township health centers and county general hospitals) in three counties within Shandong province. Questions were included on knowledge and attitudes towards antibiotic prescribing. Separately, a random selection of prescriptions for patients with the common cold was collected from the healthcare institutions at which the doctors worked, to investigate actual prescribing behaviors.

Results: A total of 188 doctors completed the survey. Most doctors (83%, 149/180) had attended training on antibiotic use since the beginning of their medical practice as a doctor, irrespective of the academic level of their undergraduate training. Of those that had training, most had attended it within the past three years (97%, 112/116). Very few doctors (2%, 3/187) said they would give antibiotics to a patient with symptoms of a common cold, and the majority (87%, 156/179) would refuse to prescribe an antibiotic even if patients were insistent on getting them. Doctors who had attended training were less likely to give antibiotics in this circumstance (29% vs. 14%, $p < 0.001$). A diagnosis of common cold was the only diagnosis reported on 1590 out of 8400 prescriptions. Over half (55%, 869/1590) of them included an antibiotic. Prescriptions from village clinics were more likely to contain an antibiotic than those from other healthcare institutions (71% vs. 44% [township] vs. 47% [county], $p < 0.001$).

Conclusions: Most doctors have recently attended training on antibiotic use and report they would not prescribe antibiotics for patients with a common cold, even when placed under pressure by patients. However, more than half of the prescriptions from these healthcare institutions for patients with the common cold included an antibiotic. Exploring and addressing gaps between knowledge and practice is critical to improving antibiotic use in rural China.

Keywords: Antibiotics, Attitudes and behavior, Prescription, Rural area, China

* Correspondence: qiangs@sdu.edu.cn
[1]Center for Health Management and Policy, Key Lab of Health Economics and Policy Research of Ministry of Health, Shandong University, 250012 Jinan, Shandong, China
Full list of author information is available at the end of the article

Background

Inappropriate antibiotic use is a global problem [1,2]. Several studies in China, the most populated country in the world, have found significant overuse of antibiotics for upper respiratory tract infections [3-5]. Many policies on improving antibiotic use have been issued in China, from the first policy on rational use of antibiotics issued by the Ministry of Health in 1989, to the most strict policy on antibiotic use, launched in 2012. Implementation is lagging behind, however, and irrational use of antibiotic remains common [6].

A detailed context-specific examination of factors which cause high levels of inappropriate antibiotic prescribing is warranted. Few studies to date have been conducted in rural areas of China, although this is where the majority of China's 1.35 billion inhabitants live [6]. The knowledge, attitudes, and actions of a wide variety of stakeholders including patients, clinicians, and pharmaceutical companies are critical factors that can be modified to improve antibiotic use [7,8]. The present study is part of the ongoing "Sino-Swedish Bilateral Cooperation on Management of Antibiotic Resistance" with the aim of understanding the problems of antibiotic resistance in China and Sweden and developing interventions to address different aspects of the problems. The purpose of this paper is to analyze attitudes and behaviors of doctors at different levels of the rural health care system in relation to antibiotic use, with a focus on patients with the common cold, at health facilities in three counties in Shandong province.

Methods

Study sites

The study was conducted in 2012 in Shandong Province, located in the eastern part of China. A total of 3 county general hospitals, 9 township health centers and 18 village clinics were selected as study sites using a multistage sampling based on the vertical administrative structure in rural China (see Figure 1). First, three counties (JN, NY and YG) were purposely selected out of a total of 91 counties in Shandong Province, based on geographic location and feasibility of the study. These three counties had around 2.47 million inhabitants in 2012. Secondly, three administrative units were randomly selected in each county. Each administrative unit consists of a town and its surrounding villages. Thirdly, two villages were randomly selected from within each administrative unit. The only county general hospital in each county was included in the study, alongside the only township health centers in each participating administrative unit, and the village clinic within each village.

Data collection

The data in this paper are from two sources: (i) a survey of doctors and (ii) collection of prescriptions.

Survey of doctors

A questionnaire concerning knowledge and attitudes of antibiotic prescribing, particularly in the context of patients with the common cold, was developed jointly between the collaborators in Sweden and China, based on a review of the relevant literature [4,6,8]. It was developed in Chinese and translated into English for the collaborators to discuss. The survey consisted of closed-ended questions with preset alternatives. It was tested for language understanding and face validity, and piloted with doctors from the county hospitals and township health centers. The questionnaire was self-completed and paper-based.

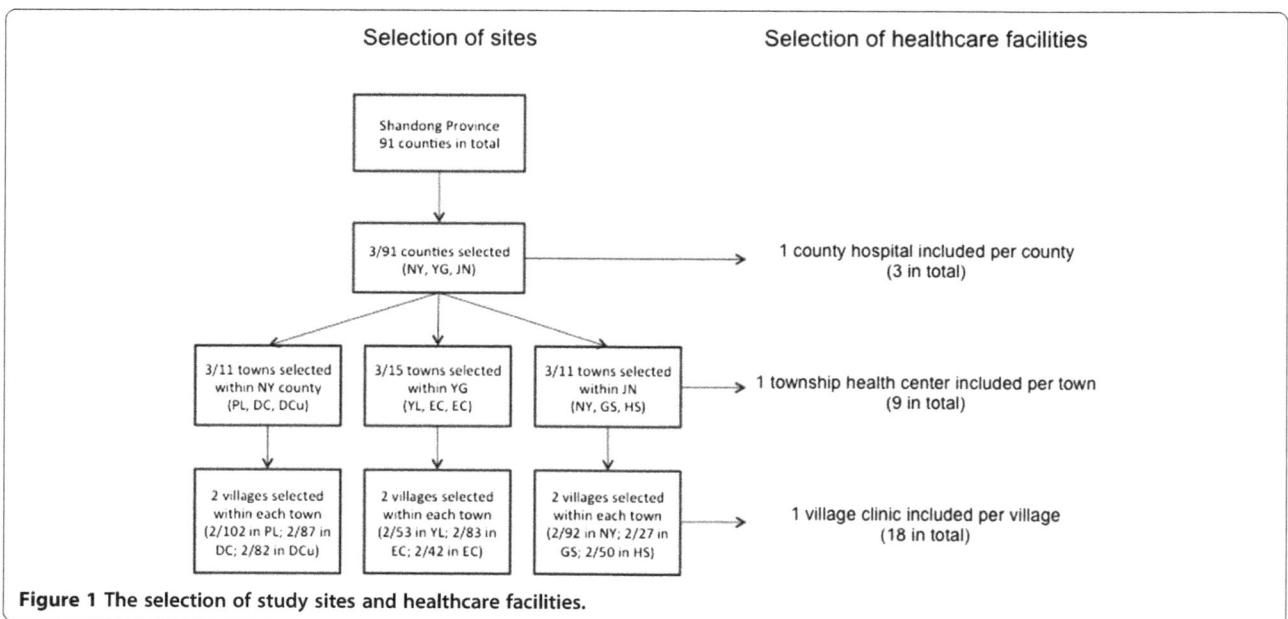

Figure 1 The selection of study sites and healthcare facilities.

The study was limited to clinical doctors who were working with patients, and who had a right to prescribe antibiotics. All doctors working at the selected township health centers and village clinics, and at the county hospitals in the departments of internal medicine, surgery, pediatrics and obstetrics & gynecology, were invited to participate.

Collection of prescriptions

Outpatient prescriptions were collected from the selected healthcare institutions in the month prior to the survey (September 2012), in order to analyze actual prescribing behaviors. All available prescriptions were collected from the selected township health centers and village clinics. At the county hospitals, where there was a much higher number of prescriptions than at other institutions, a systematic random sampling methodology was used to generate a maximum of 200 sample prescriptions from each department. The information on the prescriptions included patient name, age, gender, diagnosis, the drug prescribed and medical cost. The name of the prescriber was not collected for individual prescriptions.

For this paper, all prescriptions that included only the single diagnosis of common cold ("Gan Mao") were analyzed; prescriptions with more than one diagnosis were excluded. No attempt at external validation of diagnosis was made, although it is likely that if the doctor found a more severe disease then they would have written this on the prescription instead.

Data management and analysis

Data collection was carried out by ten master's students and researchers from the Center for Health Management and Policy at Shandong University. They were trained by the first author in questionnaire use and the methodology for sampling prescriptions; they also participated in the pilot survey. The first author checked all of the questionnaires on the survey days for quality control of the data collection. Each prescribed antibiotic was coded according to the World Health Organization (WHO) Collaborating Centre for Drug Statistics Methodology, Anatomical Therapeutic Chemical (ATC) classification [9]. All data were entered and validated by two separate data collectors using the EpiData software, and analyzed using STATA 12 software and Microsoft Excel 2010. Categorical data were compared using the Chi-square test, with comparisons made against village clinics unless otherwise stated. The cut-off point for statistical significance was set at $p < 0.05$.

Ethics Statement

Ethical approval was granted by the ethical committee of the School of Public Health, Shandong University. All of the doctors signed an informed consent form before the start of the questionnaire, and were aware they could withdraw at any point. There was no compensation for participation.

Results

Characteristics of the doctors

All eligible doctors working on the day in which the questionnaire was distributed at each facility completed the survey, resulting in a total of 188 completed questionnaires from the different health institutions in the three counties. A summary of the characteristics of the doctors is shown in Table 1. The gender distribution, average age and work experience were broadly similar across all counties. Almost all doctors (99%, 186/187) had a major in Western medicine alone.

Attitudes of doctors towards patients with a common cold

The doctors were asked what action they would take when they see a patient with a common cold, with symptoms such as a mild headache, myalgia and malaise. Most doctors (80%, 150/187) suggested that they would encourage the patient to drink water and rest. Many doctors said they would use antipyretics, analgesics or antivirals (67%, 126/187), and only a very small number said they would consider giving an antibiotic (2%, 3/187). Furthermore, the majority of doctors (87%, 156/179)

Table 1 Characteristics of the doctors completing the questionnaire

	Healthcare institution			TOTAL
	County hospital	Township health center	Village clinic	
Total number of doctors	60	98	30	188
YG county	20	22	9	51
NY county	20	40	11	71
JN county	20	36	10	66
Male (%)	26 (43)	49 (50)	22 (73)	97 (52)
Average age in years	35	36	48	38
Average working experience in years	11	14	26	15
Doctors with degree of bachelor or above (%)	46 (77)	32 (33)	0 (0)	78 (41)

stated they would still refuse to give antibiotics when facing a patient who was insisting on having antibiotics. Doctors were more likely to give antibiotics in this circumstance if they had not attended training (29% vs. 14%, p < 0.001), or worked in a county hospital (23% vs. 12% [township] vs. 13% [village clinic], p < 0.05).

Table 2 shows the results from the questionnaire according to county and healthcare facility type.

General attitudes and knowledge of doctors towards antibiotics

Most doctors (83%, 149/180) stated that they had participated in some training on antibiotic use since becoming a doctor; doctors in township health centers were less likely to have attended training that doctors at the other institution types (74% vs. 93% [village clinics] vs. 92% [county hospitals], p < 0.001). There was also some variation between the three counties, with training attendance rates highest amongst doctors from JN (93% vs. 80% [YG] and 74% [NY]). Doctors with a bachelor's degree were as likely to have attended training as those without a degree. Of the doctors who provided dates for the training, 97% (112/116) had had training within the three years prior to the survey.

Almost all doctors (98%, 182/186) did not think that newer antibiotics are more effective, and most doctors (87%, 156/179) did not think that antibiotics having a broader antimicrobial spectrum imply a better effect. There was no difference in these responses if the doctors had received training, nor if they had a bachelor's degree. Doctors in the county hospitals were less likely to think

that broader spectrum antibiotics had better effects (6% vs. 15% [township center] and 21% [village clinic], p < 0.01).

The vast majority of doctors (99%, 182/184) were aware that antibiotic guidelines exist either at a county or hospital level. Most doctors (86%, 160/185) were aware that different levels of doctor have different rights to prescribe antibiotics (for instance, prescription of some antibiotics is restricted to certain specialists). Village clinic doctors were more likely to be unaware of the different prescribing rights compared with doctors in the other healthcare institutions (17% vs. 2% [township center doctors] and 0% [county hospital doctors], p < 0.001); there was no variation based on training received.

A quarter of doctors (27%, 51/188) said that they had not had clinical experiences with antibiotic-resistant bacteria. Doctors were more likely to say they had encountered resistant bacteria if they had a bachelor's degree (81% vs. 65%, p < 0.001), had attended training on antibiotic use (79% vs. 47%, p < 0.001), or worked at a county hospital (83% vs. 66% [township] vs. 69% [village], p < 0.001).

Analysis of prescriptions

A total of 8400 prescriptions were analyzed from the healthcare institutions. Of these, 1590 (19%) cited a single diagnosis of the common cold, with over half (55%, 869/1590) of these prescriptions including an antibiotic (Table 3). Common cold prescriptions from village clinics were more likely to contain a prescription for an antibiotic than prescriptions from other institutions (71% vs. 44% [township] vs. 47% [county], p < 0.001).

Table 2 Attitudes and knowledge of doctors towards antibiotic use and patients with the common cold

	YG			NY			JN			Total		
	CH	THC	VC	CH	THC	VC	CH	THC	VC	CH	THC	VC
No. of doctors	20	22	9	20	40	11	20	36	10	60	98	30
Self-reported behaviour of doctors for patients with symptoms of the common cold:												
Would recommend to drink water and rest (%)	75	73	100	100	74	73	85	89	40	87	79	70
Would give an analgesic, antipyretic or antiviral (%)	55	68	67	30	74	73	80	75	80	55	73	73
Would use antibiotics (%)	0	0	0	5	3	9	0	0	0	2	1	3
Would still refuse to give antibiotics if a patient insisted on receiving antibiotics (%)	80	95	100	100	78	82	50	94	80	77	88	87
General attitudes and knowledege of doctors towards antibiotics:												
Believe that newer antibiotics are more effective (%)	0	0	0	5	0	10	0	6	0	2	2	3
Believe that broader specturm antibiotics are more effective (%)	16	18	22	0	15	40	0	11	0	6	15	21
Are aware that antibiotic treatment guidelines exist at a county or hospital level (%)	100	100	100	100	95	100	100	100	100	100	98	100
Are aware that different levels of doctor have different prescribing rights for antibiotics (%)	100	100	67	100	79	55	95	86	67	98	86	62
Have clinical experience of resistant bacteria (%)	90	59	89	85	44	40	74	92	80	83	66	69
Have participated in training on the use of antibiotics since starting work as a doctor (%)	20	5	0	0	23	18	50	6	20	23	12	13

Abbreviations: CH County Hospital, THC Township Health Centre, VC Village Clinic.

Table 3 Common cold prescriptions: amounts and classes of antibiotics

	Healthcare institution			
	County hospital	Township health center	Village clinic	TOTAL
Number of healthcare institutions	3	6	18	27
Total number of prescriptions	1303	4799	2298	8400
Total number of common cold prescriptions	122	839	629	1590
Number of cold prescriptions with antibiotic (%)	57 (47)	366 (44)	446 (71)	869 (55)
Mean number of antibiotics prescribed	1.01	1.17	1.11	1.12
Amount of types of antibiotics prescribed for the diagnosis of common cold				
Other beta-lactam antibacterials (J01D)	22	156	210	388
Macrolides, lincosamides and streptogramins (J01F)	31	158	145	334
Beta-lactam antibacterials, penicillins (J01C)	3	76	77	156
Quinolone antibacterials (J01M)	1	14	30	45
Other antibacterials (J01X)	1	18	18	37
Sulfonamides and trimethoprim (J01E)	0	3	6	9
Aminoglycoside antibacterials (J01G)	0	1	7	8
Tetracyclines (J01A)	0	1	0	1

A total of 979 antibiotics were prescribed, with a mean of 1.12 antibiotics per prescription. At county hospitals, five classes of antibiotics were prescribed, compared with eight in the township health centers, and seven in the village clinics. The most frequently used classes of antibiotics across all healthcare institutions were 'other beta-lactam antibacterials' (J01D), including cephalosporins and carbapenems; 'macrolides, lincosamides and streptogramins' (J01F); and 'beta-lactam antibacterials, and penicillins' (J01C) (Table 3).

Discussion

To date, few studies have investigated the attitudes and practices of doctors concerning antibiotic use in rural China [6,10]. In our study we have combined analysis of prescription data and doctors' attitudes and knowledge on antibiotics from three different levels of rural health-care institutions, within three counties in Shandong province. Although almost all doctors stated they would not use antibiotics for a patient with a common cold in our questionnaire, we found that at least one antibiotic was present on over half of all prescriptions for patients with a common cold taken from the institutions these doctors work at. Gaps between reported knowledge and actual practice within antibiotic prescribing are commonly encountered. This high prescription rate of antibiotics in the context of viral upper respiratory tract infections is in line with the results of a recent systematic review suggesting that almost half of all outpatient appointments in China result in a prescription for an antibiotic [6]. At the time of the current study, doctors were able to make a profit from individual drug prescriptions, including antibiotics, and this may have

stimulated over-prescribing of antibiotics [11-13]. This is particularly important at the current stage of comprehensive health system reform occurring now in China.

Reynolds *et al.* carried out semi-structured interviews with doctors from a variety of healthcare institutions in Guizhou province in southern China [14]. Their findings suggest that although doctors are aware that antibiotics are not needed to treat the common cold, antibiotics are often given under the belief that they might speed recovery, and also in response to patient expectations. A recent study of caregivers in rural China [15] found that 80% of parents thoughts that antibiotics help with viral infections. Undergraduate education and postgraduate training of doctors can help address such misconceptions, and provide strategies to respond to patient expectations [16,17]. A high proportion of doctors in our study have attended training on antibiotics since qualifying, and for the vast majority this training has occurred recently. It is unclear why doctors from township health centers were less likely to have attended such training than village doctors or doctors from county hospitals. It may be that doctors from township health centers have received less encouragement or have fewer opportunities to attend training than doctors from other health facility levels.

Our study has assessed attitudes and practice across three rural counties and three levels of the healthcare system, with a high response rate. It has, however, several important limitations. Firstly, the questionnaire was self-completed and consequently some individuals may have modified their answers to meet social expectations. Secondly, it was not possible to validate the diagnosis of common cold on the prescriptions, nor was data available on clinical outcomes. Thirdly, it is possible that some patients attended the healthcare institutions and received a diagnosis of common cold, but did not receive a prescription; however, all patients will generally get a prescription at these healthcare facilities. Fourthly, although the prescriptions analyzed are all from healthcare institutions where the survey respondents worked, we are unable to guarantee that the doctors who responded to the survey are responsible for all of the prescriptions analyzed. In future studies researchers should consider collecting the name of the prescriber from each prescription, enabling further investigation of the relationship between self-reported knowledge and attitudes and actual practice at the level of the individual.

Conclusions

This study showed a substantial gap between rural doctors' attitudes and practice regarding antibiotic prescribing. Attitudes were in line with recommendations, whereas practice showed a high level of inappropriate prescribing of antibiotics for the common cold. Exploring and addressing gaps between knowledge and practice is critical to improving antibiotic use in rural China.

Competing interests
The authors declare that they have no competing interests.

Authors' contributions
QS, GT, LZ, LEN, MG, and YYS were involved in conception and design of this project, QS, LBZ, YS, MG and LEG were involved in the implementation of the project, QS, OJD, LZ, YS, MG, LEG, GT YL and CSL were involved in the analysis and interpretation of data. QS, OJD, LBZ, and CSL have drafted the manuscripts, while GT and LEN have provided critical comments. All authors approved the final version of the manuscript.

Acknowledgments
This work was supported by National Nature Science Foundation of China, "The Study on rational use of antibiotic and resistance evaluation in rural China (71073098)" and the Swedish International Development Cooperation Agency (Sida), in accordance with the agreement between Sida and the former Swedish Institute for Communicable Disease Control (SMI) (now Public Health Agency of Sweden; Sida contribution number 2010–001861). We are grateful to the managers of the county Centres for Disease Prevention and Control in the study sites for their contributions to data collection. We would also like to acknowledge the faculty members and graduate students from Shandong University, Jinan, China, for their work in data collection, management and analysis. Finally, we would like to thank Anna Dyar for language revision of the manuscript.

Author details
[1]Center for Health Management and Policy, Key Lab of Health Economics and Policy Research of Ministry of Health, Shandong University, 250012 Jinan, Shandong, China. [2]Medical Education Centre, North Devon District Hospital, Raleigh Park, Barnstaple, Devon EX31 4JB, UK. [3]Department of Public Health Sciences, Department of Learning, Informatics, Management, Tomtebodavägen 18 A; Medical Management Centre (MMC), Ethics Karolinska Institutet, 171 77 Stockholm, Sweden. [4]Department of Clinical and Experimental Medicine, Clinical Microbiology, Faculty of Health Sciences, Linköping University, 581 85 Linköping, Sweden. [5]Antibiotics and Infection Control Unit, Public Health Agency of Sweden, 17182 Solna, Sweden. [6]School of Public Health, Shandong University, Jinan, Shandong 250012, China. [7]Jinan Central Hospital, Jinan, Shandong 250013, China. [8]Department of Public Health Sciences, Global Health (IHCAR), Tomtebodavägen 18 A, Karolinska Institutet, 1771 77 Stockholm, Sweden.

Reference
1. Cars O, Högberg LD, Murray M, Nordberg O, Sivaraman S, Lundborg CS, et al. Meeting the challenge of antibiotic resistance. BMJ. 2008;337:1438–41.
2. WHO. The evolving threat of antimicrobial resistance: options for action. Geneva: World Health Organisation; 2012.
3. Zheng Y, Zhou Z. The root causes of the abuse of antibiotics, harm and the rational use of the strategy. Hospital Manage Forum. 2007;123(1):23–7.
4. Sun Q, Yan Y, Wang W, Bogg L, Tang S. Analyzing the status of drug use in medical institutions at county, township and village level in Shandong and Ningxia. Chinese J Health Manage. 2010;8:535–8.
5. Yin J. Study on drug use in rural area, Shandong province and Ningxia Autonomous Region. Jinan, China: Shandong University; 2009.
6. Yin X, Song F, Gong Y, Tu X, Wang Y, Cao S, et al. A systematic review of antibiotic utilization in China. J Antimicrob Chemother. 2013;68(11):2445–52.
7. Tomson G, Vlad I. Strengthening the rational use of drugs: International perspective and its implications for China. Chinese J Health Policy. 2012;5(10):6–9.
8. Ebert SC. Factors contributing to excessive antimicrobial prescribing. Pharmacotherapy. 2007;27(10 Pt 2):126S–30.
9. WHO. Anatomical Therapeutic Chemical (ATC) classification system: guidelines for ATC classification and DDD assignment 2009. Geneva: World Health Organisation; 2009.
10. Dong L, Yan H, Wang D. Antibiotic prescribing patterns in village health clinics across10 provinces of Western China. J Antimicrob Chemother. 2008;62(2):410–5.
11. Sun Q, Santoro MA, Meng Q, Liu C, Eggleston K. Pharmaceutical policy in China. Health Aff. 2008;27(4):1042–50.
12. Li C, Sun Q, Li K, Yang H, Zuo G, Meng Q. Analysis of the prescription quality before and after the essential medicine system implementation in township health centers of Anhui Province. Chinese Health Econ. 2012;31 (4):68–9.
13. Yip WC, Hsiao WC, Chen W, Hu S, Ma J, Maynard A. Early appraisal of China's huge and complex health-care reforms. Lancet. 2012;379(9818):833–42.
14. Reynolds L, McKee M. Factors influencing antibiotic prescribing in China: an exploratory analysis. Health Policy. 2009;90(1):32–6.
15. Yu M, Zhao G, Stålsby Lundborg C, Zhu Y, Zhao Q, Xu B. Knowledge, attitudes, and practices of parents in rural China on the use of antibiotics in children: a cross-sectional study. BMC Infect Dis. 2014;14(1):112.
16. Pulcini C, Gyssens IC. How to educate prescribers in antimicrobial stewardship practices. Virulence. 2013;4(2):192–202.
17. Wang H, Li N, Zhu H, Xu S, Lu H, Feng Z. Prescription pattern and its influencing factors in Chinese county hospitals: a retrospective cross-sectional study. PLoS One. 2013;8(5):e63225.

21

Indoxyl sulfate promotes apoptosis in cultured osteoblast cells

Young-Hee Kim[1], Kyung-Ah Kwak[1], Hyo-Wook Gil[2*], Ho-Yeon Song[1] and Sae-Yong Hong[2]

Abstract

Background: Indoxyl sulfate (IS), an organic anion uremic toxin, promotes the progression of renal dysfunction. Some studies have suggested that IS inhibits osteoclast differentiation and suppresses parathyroid hormone (PTH)-stimulated intracellular cAMP production, decreases PTH receptor expression, and induces oxidative stress in primary mouse calvaria osteoblast cell culture. However, the direct effects of IS on osteoblast apoptosis have not been fully evaluated. Hence, we investigated whether IS acts as a bone toxin by studying whether IS induces apoptosis and inhibits differentiation in the cultured osteoblast cell line MC3T3-E1.

Methods: We assessed the direct effect of IS on osteoblast differentiation and apoptosis in the MC3T3-E1 cell line. We examined caspase-3/7 activity, apoptosis-related proteins, free radical production, alkaline phosphatase activity, and mRNA expression of type 1 collagen and osteonectin. Furthermore, we investigated the uptake of IS via organic anion transport (OAT).

Results: We found that IS increased caspase activity and induced apoptosis. Production of free radicals increased depending on the concentration of IS. Furthermore, IS inhibited the expression of mRNA type 1 collagen and osteonectin and alkaline phosphatase activity. The expression of OAT, which is known to mediate the cellular uptake of IS, was detected in in the MC3T3-E1 cell line. The inhibition of OAT improved cell viability and suppressed the production of reactive oxygen species. These results suggest that IS is transported in MC3T3-E1 cells via OAT, which causes oxidative stress to inhibit osteoblast differentiation.

Conclusions: IS acts as a bone toxin by inhibiting osteoblast differentiation and inducing apoptosis.

Keywords: Uremia, Renal osteodystrophy, Apoptosis, Cell differentiation, Organic anion transporters

Background

Indoxyl sulfate (IS) is an organic anion uremic toxin belonging to the family of protein-bound retention solutes [1]. IS is synthesized in the liver from indole, which is produced from the metabolism of dietary tryptophan in the body. The studies performed to date have shown that IS accumulates in blood and promotes the progression of renal dysfunction [2-5]. IS may also act as a vascular toxin [2-4,6]. It directly stimulates rat vascular smooth muscle cell proliferation in a concentration-dependent manner. Furthermore, Dahl salt-sensitive hypertensive rats administered IS in combination with a high-salt diet have been found to show an increase in aortic wall thickness and severe aortic calcification, with colocalization of osteoblast-specific proteins such as Cbfa-1, osteonectin, and alkaline phosphatase [7]. In a recent study, Iwasaki et al. reported that when rats with renal dysfunction and low bone turnover were administered an oral adsorbent, their blood IS level decreased and osteoblastic cell function improved [8]. Iwasaki et al. have also shown that in primary mouse calvaria osteoblast cell culture, addition of IS suppresses parathyroid hormone (PTH)-stimulated intracellular cAMP production, decreases PTH receptor expression, and induces oxidative stress [9]. IS inhibits osteoclast differentiation and bone-resorbing activity, which could affect bone remodeling in chronic kidney disease patients [10]. Limited data suggest that IS could act as a bone toxin by affecting both osteoblast and osteoclast activities. To

* Correspondence: hwgil@schmc.ac.kr
[2]Department of Internal Medicine, Soonchunhyang University Cheonan Hospital, 31 Soonchunhyang 6gil, Dongnam-gu, Cheonan, Chungnam 330-721, Korea
Full list of author information is available at the end of the article

date, the direct effects of IS on osteoblast apoptosis have not been fully evaluated.

Hence, we investigated whether IS acts as a bone toxin by studying whether IS induces apoptosis and inhibits differentiation in a cultured osteoblast cell line.

Methods

Chemicals

L-Ascorbic acid, β-glycerophosphate, probenecid, probucol, N-acetylcysteine (NAC), and IS were all obtained from Sigma (St. Louis, MO, USA). All cell culture media and supplements were from Hyclone (Logan, UT, USA). Reagents for reverse transcription and those for real-time PCR reactions were from Toyobo (Osaka, Japan). Anti-Bax, Anti-Bcl-2, and anti-p53 mouse monoclonal antibodies were purchased from Santa Cruz (Santa Cruz, CA, USA). Secondary goat anti-rabbit IgG was obtained from Thermo Fisher Scientific (Rockford, USA). The assay kit for caspase-3/7 activity was purchased from Promega (Mannheim, Germany).

Cells and osteogenic induction

Newborn mouse calvaria-derived MC3T3-E1 subclone 14 pre-osteoblastic cells (ATCC, USA) were cultured in α-MEM medium (Hyclone) supplemented with 10% fetal bovine serum (Hyclone), 100 U/mL penicillin, and 100 mg/mL streptomycin (Hyclone) at 37°C in an atmosphere with 100% humidity and 5% CO_2. Osteoblast differentiation was induced by the addition of 10 mM β-glycerophosphate, as described previously [11].

Cell viability

Cell viability was assessed using the 3-(4,5-dimethyl-thiazol-2-yl)-2,5-diphenyltetrazolium bromide (MTT) assay, as described previously [12]. MC3T3-E1 cells were incubated in osteogenic induction medium with or without IS at 37°C for 72 h. After the cells were lysed with DMSO solution, the optical density was measured at 590 nm using the optical density at 630 nm as reference (VICTOR™X3; PerkinElmer, USA).

Bone differentiation

Alkaline phosphatase (ALP) activity was measured in cells treated with 0–1.5 mM IS and in control cells incubated for 3, 5, 7, and 10 d. Cells were washed with PBS and were lysed with a solution containing 0.1% Triton X-100 at the same time as the cellular alkaline phosphatase activity and cell protein content were determined. The enzymatic reaction was started by the addition of 50 µL of substrate/buffer mixture (equal volumes of p-nitrophenol phosphate substrate [N 1891; Sigma Chemicals, St. Louis, MO] and alkaline buffer solution [A9226; Sigma Chemicals]). After 30 min of incubation at 37°C, the reaction was stopped by adding an equal volume of

0.05 M NaOH. The lysate from the wells was collected into individual Eppendorf tubes and vortexed. The ALP activity was determined colorimetrically at 405 nm using p-nitrophenol (PNP) standards (0–50 nmol, N7660; Sigma Chemicals). The protein concentration in the lysate was determined using the Bradford assay. ALP activity is expressed as nanomoles of PNP released per milligram of protein.

Assessment of cellular oxidative stress

Production of intracellular reactive oxygen species was detected using the nonfluorescent cell-permeating compound, 2′-7′-dichlorofluorescein diacetate (DCF-DA). DCF-DA is hydrolyzed by intracellular esterases, and is then oxidized by reactive oxygen species (ROS) to a fluorescent compound, 2′-7′-dichlorofluorescein (DCF). After treatment with 0–1.5 mM IS, MC3T3-E1 cells were treated with DCF-DA (10 µM) for 30 min at 37°C. Following DCF-DA exposure, the cells were rinsed and then scraped into PBS with 0.2% Triton X-100. Fluorescence was measured with a plate reader (VICTOR™X3) with excitation at 485 nm and emission at 535 nm.

Flow cytometry analysis of apoptosis

Quantification of cells undergoing programmed cell death was conducted using an annexin V-propidium iodide apoptosis kit (Invitrogen). Analyzed cells were washed once in phosphate-buffered saline and resuspended in the binding buffer provided. Annexin V (Alexa 488-conjugated) and propidium iodide were added and incubated for 15 min at room temperature in the dark. The cells were analyzed using a FACS Calibur flow cytometer and CellQuest software.

Apoptosis measurement: caspase-3/7 activity, and immunoblot assay for apoptosis-related factors p53, Bcl-2, and Bax

Caspase-3/7 activity was detected using a Caspase-Glo 3/7 Assay system (Promega) after preincubating the MC3T3-E1 cells (2×10^5/96-well plate), followed by treatment with various IS concentrations (control, 0.5 mM, 1 mM) for 3, 6, 9, 12, and 24 h. The background luminescence associated with the cell culture and assay reagent (blank reaction) was subtracted from the experimental values. The activity of caspase-3/7 is presented as the mean value of triplets for the given cells. The intensity of the emitted fluorescence was determined at a wavelength of 521 nm with the use of luminometry (VICTOR™X3).

The immunoblot assay was conducted as follows. After stimulation, cells were washed once with phosphate-buffered saline and lysed with radioimmunoprecipitation assay (RIPA) lysis buffer (ROCKLAND, USA) and placed on ice for 30 min. Total cell extracts were centrifuged at

14 000 g (for 20 min at 4°C), and protein-containing supernatants were collected. Equal amounts of proteins (40 μg) were resolved by sodium dodecyl sulfate–polyacrylamide gel electrophoresis, transferred to a nitrocellulose membrane, and immunoblotted with specific antibodies against Bax, Bcl-2, and p53. Secondary antibodies were obtained from Thermo Fisher Scientific. Equal loading was confirmed using a β-actin antibody. Protein expression levels were quantified using a densitometer (ChemiDoc™ XPS + with Image Lab™ Software, Bio-Rad). The data are represented as the ratio of expression of the target protein to that of β-actin.

RNA isolation, cDNA synthesis, and PCR analysis

Total RNA was isolated using an RNeasy Mini Kit (QIA-GEN, Tokyo, Japan) according to the manufacturer's instructions. Total RNA (1 μg) was used as the template for cDNA synthesis in a 50-μL reaction mixture using a reverse transcriptase-PCR kit (TOYOBO) according to the manufacturer's instructions. Real-time PCR was performed on a CFX96™ (BIO-RAD). The PCR reactions consisted of Power SYBR Green PCR Master Mix (Applied Biosystems, UK), 0.1 mM (10 pM) specific primers, and 50 ng of cDNA. The primer sequences, designed with Beacon Designer 7.6 software (Bio-Rad), were as follows: mouse osteonectin, 5′-TCTCAACAAACAAATCAGGGAT-3′ and 5′-TGGCAG-CACATTCATCTATG-3′; collagen 1, 5′-ATCACCAAACT CAGAAGATGTAG-3′ and 5′-CAGGAAGTCCAGGCTG TC-3′; organic anion transport 1 (OAT1), 5-ATG CCT ATC CAC ACC CGT GC-3 and 5-GGC AAA GCT AGT GGC AAA CC-3); OAT3, 5-CAG TCT TCA TGG CAG GTA TAC TGG-3 and 5-CTG TAG CCA GCG CCA CTG AG-3; and GAPDH, 5′-CAAGAAGGTGGTGAAGCA-3′ and 5′-TGTTGAAGTCGCAGGAGA-3′.

Statistical analysis

All results are expressed as the mean ± standard error of the mean (SEM) values. The mean values of the groups were compared by analysis of variance, and a P-value <0.05 was considered significant.

Results

Effect of indoxyl sulfate on cell viability in the MC3T3-E1 cell line

To determine cytotoxicity, the effect of IS on the cell proliferation of MC3E3-T1 was studied using an MTT assay. As shown in Figure 1, IS, at the concentration range of 0.1–1.5 mM, inhibited cell proliferation at 72 h.

Gene expression of OATs in the MC3T3-E1 cell line

Because other studies have shown that IS is transported into osteoblasts and renal tubule cells via OAT, gene expression of OAT-1 and OAT-3 was investigated by real time PCR using RNA extracts. The expression of OAT-3 was relatively higher than that of OAT-1 in the MC3T3-E1 cell line (Figure 2A). After confirming the expression of the OAT gene in the MC3T3-E1 cell line, we investigated whether blocking OAT could prevent IS toxicity. To confirm the role of OAT in MC3T3-E1 cells, probenecid, a transporter inhibitor, was added to the cells during pretreatment with 1 mmol/L of IS. Blocking OAT in MC3T3-E1 cells improved cell survival (Figure 2B). ROS production was inhibited by probenecid. The effect obtained was similar to that obtained on pretreatment with the antioxidants NAC (500 μM) and probucol (62.5 μM) (Figure 2C). Probenecid works by interfering with the OAT in the kidneys, which blocks the efflux of IS in cells. Probucol is a phenolic lipid-lowering agent with antioxidant and anti-inflammatory properties. N-acetylcysteine (NAC) is the

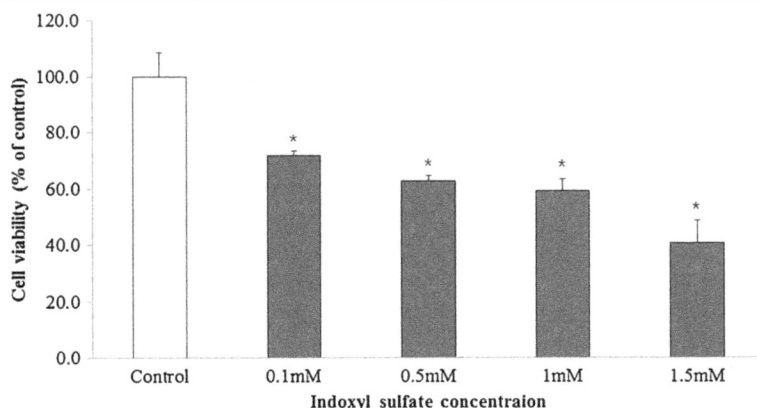

Figure 1 Effect of IS on the viability of MC3T3-E1 cells. Cell number was measured 24 h after the addition of IS at concentrations ranging from 0.1 to 1.5 mM and was expressed as the percentage of control cells not pretreated with IS (open bar). The cell toxicity of IS was found to be dose dependent. The data represent the mean ± SEM from 8 replicates in each group. *P < 0.05 vs. control cells.

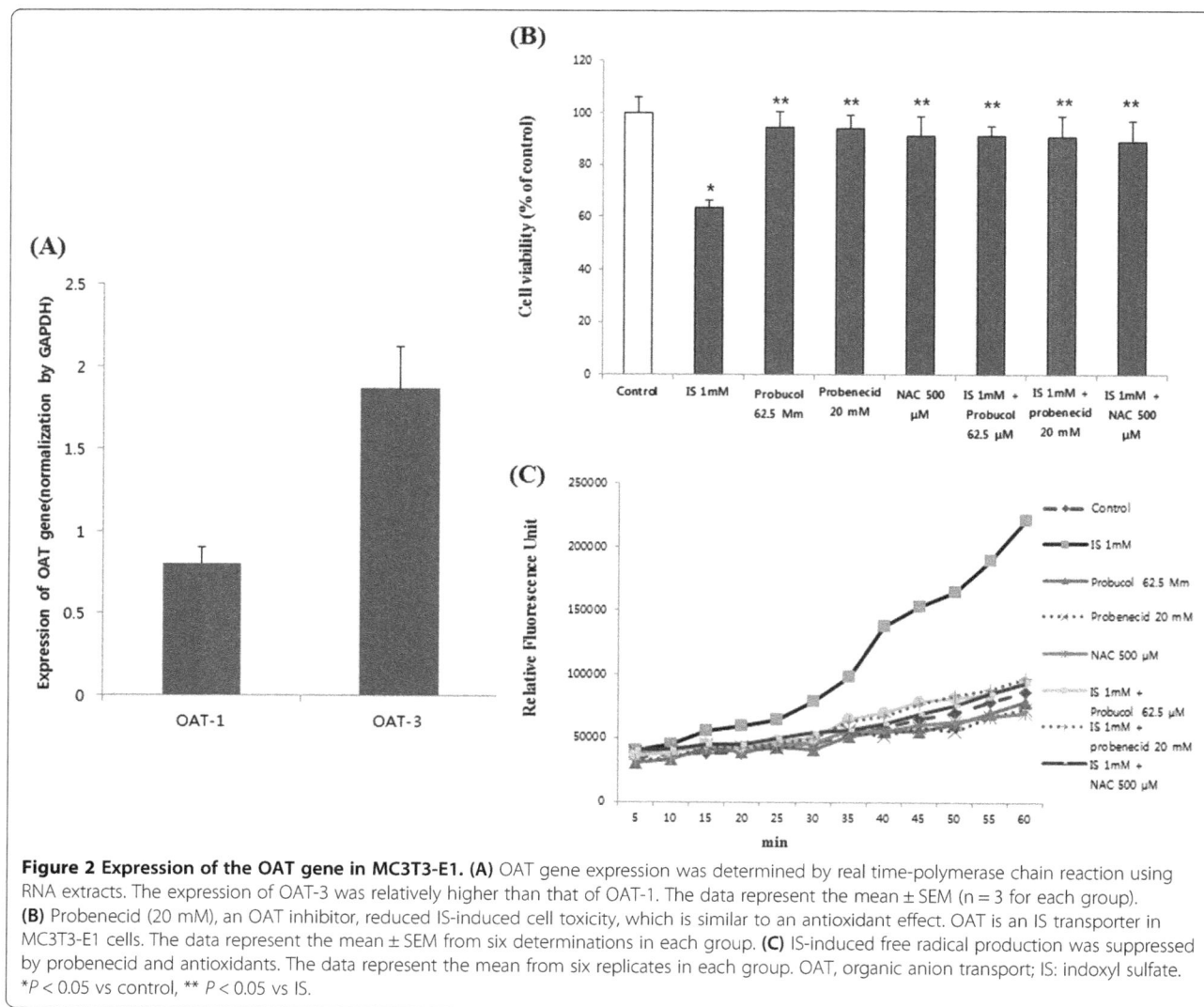

Figure 2 Expression of the OAT gene in MC3T3-E1. (A) OAT gene expression was determined by real time-polymerase chain reaction using RNA extracts. The expression of OAT-3 was relatively higher than that of OAT-1. The data represent the mean ± SEM (n = 3 for each group). **(B)** Probenecid (20 mM), an OAT inhibitor, reduced IS-induced cell toxicity, which is similar to an antioxidant effect. OAT is an IS transporter in MC3T3-E1 cells. The data represent the mean ± SEM from six determinations in each group. **(C)** IS-induced free radical production was suppressed by probenecid and antioxidants. The data represent the mean from six replicates in each group. OAT, organic anion transport; IS: indoxyl sulfate. *$P < 0.05$ vs control, ** $P < 0.05$ vs IS.

precursor of L-cysteine and therefore of reduced glutathione and has been widely used as an antioxidant.

Intracellular oxidative stress

As shown in Figure 3, IS increased cellular oxidative stress in a concentration-dependent manner. Addition of antioxidants or the OAT inhibitor suppressed free radical production (Figure 2C, Figure 3).

Inhibition of osteoblast differentiation by IS

To determine the differentiation of the pre-osteoblast cell line, ALP activity was measured in osteogenic induction medium with or without IS. As shown in Figure 4, ALP activity was suppressed above 1 mM IS. Collagen 1 and osteonectin were produced only in differentiated osteoblasts. To determine whether the osteoblasts had differentiated, the expression of collagen 1 and

osteonectin mRNA was analyzed using real-time PCR. At 5 d, the production of collagen 1 and osteonectin mRNA was significantly inhibited by the addition of IS, as shown in Figure 5.

Apoptosis induction by IS

To determine whether IS induces apoptosis, the cells were incubated with different concentrations of IS for 12 h, stained, and subjected to Fluorescence-activated cell sorting (FACS) analysis to measure apoptosis and necrosis. IS increased the proportion of apoptotic cells, particularly in osteoblasts (Figure 6). To elucidate the role of caspases in osteoblasts, we first examined the activity of the executioner caspase-3/7 in response to IS in osteoblasts. The activity of caspases was determined using fluorometric peptide substrates specific to caspase. As shown in Figure 7, the activity of caspase-3/7 peaked

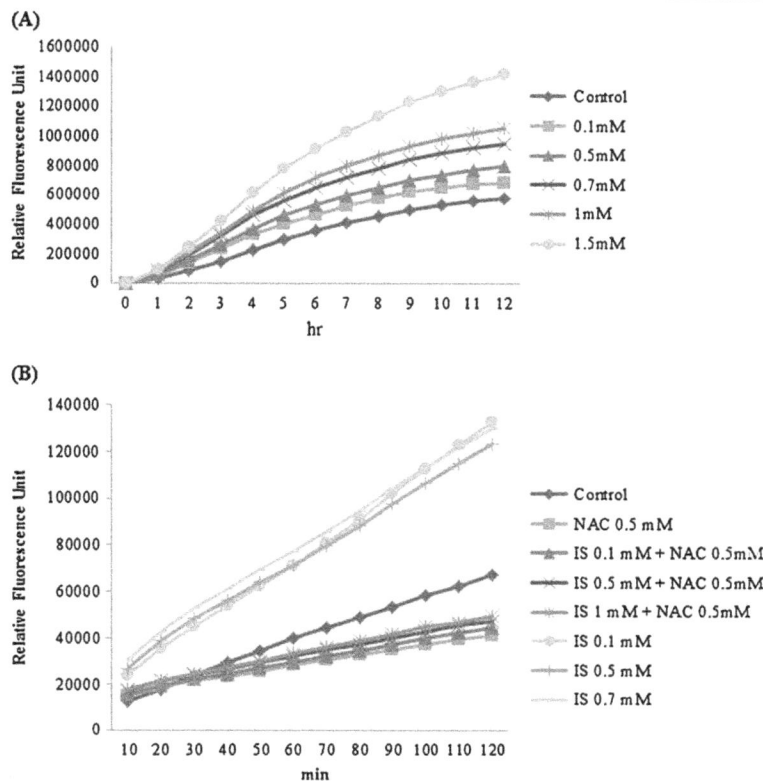

Figure 3 Free radical production induced by the addition of IS. MC3T3-E1 cells were seeded in 96-well plates, IS was added, and free radical production was measured after the indicated time. **(A)** Free radical production increased with time in a dose-dependent manner. **(B)** IS-induced free radical production was suppressed by 0.5 mM N-acetylcysteine (NAC). The data represent the mean from six replicates ns in each group.

at 6 h of incubation with IS (1.0 mM). Caspase-dependent apoptosis thus appears to be involved in IS-induced osteoblast toxicity. To determine which apoptosis-related factors may be acting upstream of caspase activation, the expression of p53, Bcl2, and Bax was measured after the addition of IS (1.0 mM). IS increased the expression of Bax and p53, which play a role in

apoptosis. However, Bcl-2 was not influenced by IS (1.0 mM) at 1, 3, and 6 h (Figure 8).

Discussion

In the present study, we studied whether the uremic toxin IS directly suppressed osteoblast differentiation and induced osteoblast apoptosis via caspase activity.

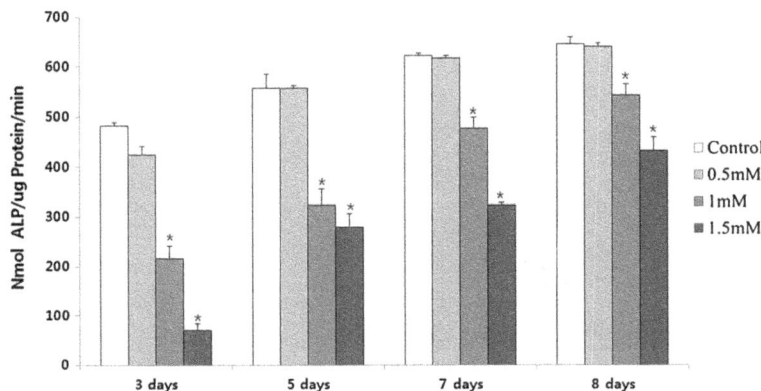

Figure 4 Effect of IS addition on ALP activity in MC3T3-E1 cells. ALP activity was suppressed by IS at concentrations greater than 1 mM. ALP activity is expressed as nanomoles of p-nitrophenol released per milligram of protein. ALP, alkaline phosphatase *$P < 0.05$ vs. control cells at each time point. The data represent the mean ± SEM (n = 6 for each group).

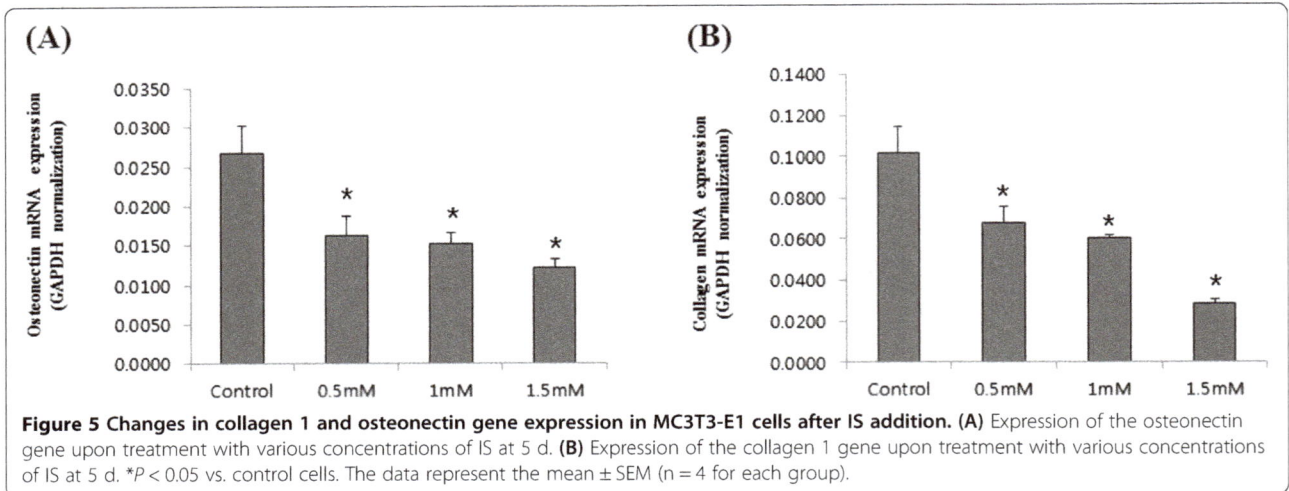

Figure 5 Changes in collagen 1 and osteonectin gene expression in MC3T3-E1 cells after IS addition. (A) Expression of the osteonectin gene upon treatment with various concentrations of IS at 5 d. **(B)** Expression of the collagen 1 gene upon treatment with various concentrations of IS at 5 d. *$P < 0.05$ vs. control cells. The data represent the mean ± SEM ($n = 4$ for each group).

Bone toxicity is mediated by IS-induced free radical production, which evokes apoptosis. Our data emphasize the fact that several uremic toxins could affect osteoblast differentiation and function. Recently, several reports have shown that IS may be a bone toxin [8-10]. Iwasaki et al. [8] showed that oral administration of the indole-absorbing Kremezin prevents the progression of renal failure and improves bone formation in a rat model of chronic kidney disease (CKD) with low bone turnover.

This group also demonstrated that the IS taken up by osteoblasts via the OAT-3 present in these cells augments oxidative stress to impair osteoblast function and downregulate PTH receptor expression [9]. These findings suggested that IS may be a bone toxin that is taken up via OAT-3 in osteoblasts and inhibits bone turnover by free radicals produced because of IS. Our data support the previous studies and suggest that IS itself could induce apoptosis via the production of free radicals.

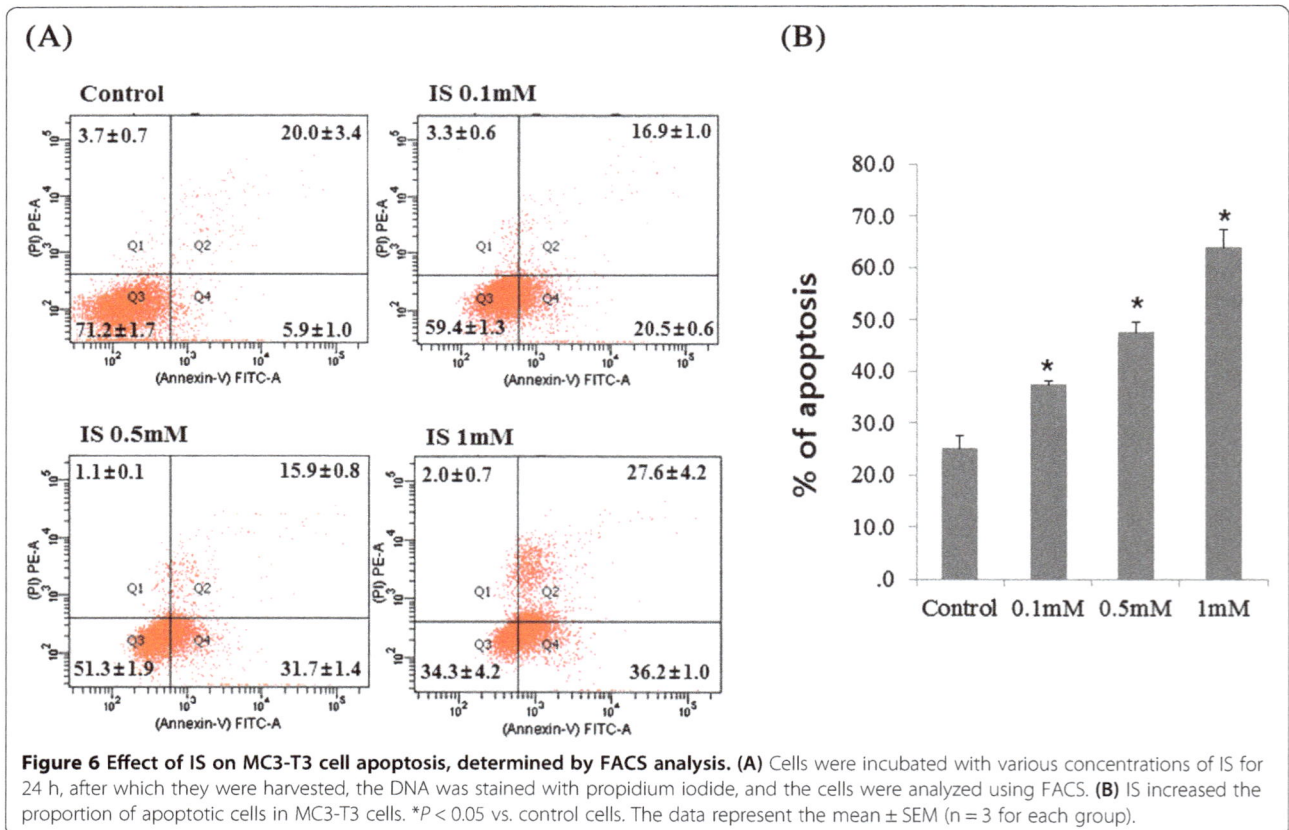

Figure 6 Effect of IS on MC3-T3 cell apoptosis, determined by FACS analysis. (A) Cells were incubated with various concentrations of IS for 24 h, after which they were harvested, the DNA was stained with propidium iodide, and the cells were analyzed using FACS. **(B)** IS increased the proportion of apoptotic cells in MC3-T3 cells. *$P < 0.05$ vs. control cells. The data represent the mean ± SEM ($n = 3$ for each group).

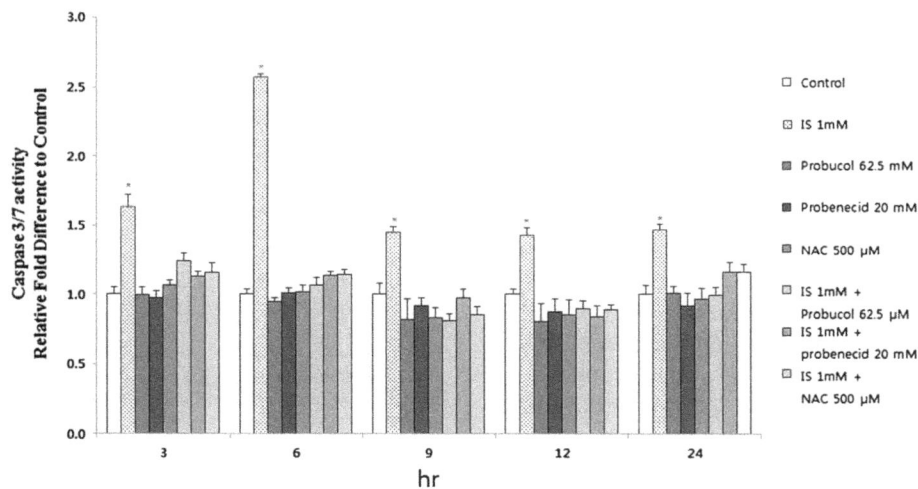

Figure 7 Effect of IS on caspase-3/7 activity. Caspase-3/7 activity was analyzed using a Promega Caspase Glo 3/7 kit (described in the Materials and Methods) Caspase-3/7 activity peaked at 6 h at 1 mM IS. IS increased caspase-3/7 activity, but probenecid (20 mM), an OAT inhibitor, attenuated IS-induced caspase-3/7 activity, which is similar to an antioxidant effect. The data represent the mean ± SEM (n = 6 for each group). $*P < 0.05$ vs. control cells at each time point.

Our data showed that IS-induced apoptosis is mediated by caspases. It is well established that p53 positively regulates Bax, but negatively regulates Bcl-2 expression [13]. IS-elicited changes in the Bax protein level are likely to be the result of an increase in p53 [14]. The Bcl-2 family plays a prominent antiapoptotic role by acting upstream of caspase activation. Our data showed that the expression of Bcl-2 is not influenced at 1, 3, or 6 h. The proapoptotic factors Bax and p53 may play a predominant role in IS-induced osteoblast apoptosis, which is activated via the caspase pathway.

Mozar et al. showed that IS inhibits osteoclast differentiation and bone-resorbing activity [10]. Goto et al. [15] reported that IS levels correlated negatively with 2

serum markers of bone formation (alkaline phosphatase and bone-specific alkaline phosphatase) independently of intact PTH, but not with a serum marker of bone resorption (TRAP 5b). Although serum markers may not be ideal for testing bone turnover, on the basis of their results, they suggested that IS may promote low-turnover bone disease outcomes (such as adynamic bone disease) observed in CKD patients.

With CKD progression, the ability of the kidneys to maintain systemic mineral homeostasis gradually decreases, resulting in the various abnormalities of bone and vascular physiology observed in CKD-MBD (CKD associated with mineral and bone disorders) [16]. In high-turnover bone disease, e.g., secondary

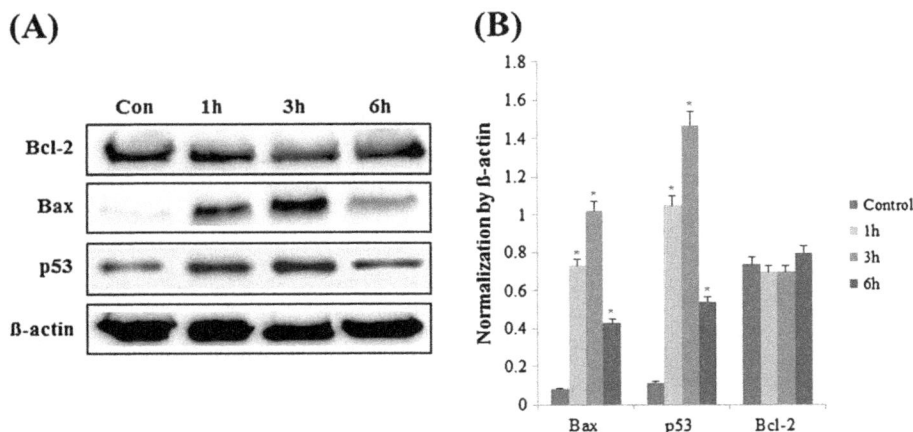

Figure 8 Effect of IS on the protein expression of Bcl-2, Bax, and p53 in MC3-T3 cells. (A) Representative immunoblots with anti-Bcl-2, anti-Bax, anti-p53, and anti-β-actin at 1 mM IS. **(B)** Densitometric analysis of Bcl-2, Bax, and p53, normalized by the data for β-actin. The data represent the mean ± SEM (n = 3 for each group).

hyperparathyroidism in CKD patients, PTH can be controlled by many drugs, including phosphate binders, vitamin D, and cinacalcet. However, no treatment specific to low-turnover bone disease is available. Elimination of uremic toxins could be an option for controlling low-turnover bone disease in CKD patients.

Our study suggested that IS-induced apoptosis might be mediated by free radical production. These findings are supported by many previous reports [15,16]. Several studies have shown that IS induces NADPH oxidase mRNA expression and increases its activity in various types of cells [17-19]. Namikoshi et al. reported that decreasing the serum concentration of IS by administrating the oral adsorbent AST-120 reduces the expression of the NADPH oxidase component and alleviates oxidative stress in the aorta [20]. In our study, we did not determine NADPH mRNA expression or its activity, but it appears that increasing free radical production by adding IS may occur through an activation pathway of NADPH oxidase.

A list of uremic toxins has been provided by EUTox. The normal concentration of IS is 0.53 mg/L (2 μM). The mean concentration of IS in uremic patients is 23.1 mg/L (~100 μM), and the maximum concentration found in uremic patients was 44.5 mg/L [21].

Conclusions

Our data confirm that IS acts as a bone toxin by inhibiting osteoblast differentiation and inducing apoptosis via the caspase pathway. Further studies are required to elucidate whether elimination of IS could improve osteoblast differentiation in chronic renal failure.

Abbreviations
ALP: Alkaline phosphatase; DCF-DA: 2'-7'-dichlorofluorescein diacetate; CKD: Chronic kidney disease; CKD-MBD: CKD associated with mineral and bone disorders; IS: Indoxyl sulfate; MTT: 3-[4,5-dimethylthiazol-2-yl]-2,5-diphenyltetrazolium bromide; OAT: Organic anion transport; PNP: p-nitrophenol; PTH: Parathyroid hormone; RIPA: Radio-immunoprecipitation assay; ROS: Reactive oxygen species.

Competing interests
All the authors declare that they have no competing interests.

Authors' contributions
KYH carried out the molecular studies and PCR array. KKA carried out the molecular studies, FACS scan. GHW conceived of the study, and participated in its design and coordination. SHY participated in the design of the study and performed the statistical analysis. SHY participated in the design of the study and performed the statistical analysis. All authors read and approved the final manuscript.

Acknowledgement
This work was supported by the Soonchunhyang University Research Fund.

Author details
[1]Department of Microbiology, Soonchunhyang University Medical college, Cheonan, Korea. [2]Department of Internal Medicine, Soonchunhyang University Cheonan Hospital, 31 Soonchunhyang 6gil, Dongnam-gu, Cheonan, Chungnam 330-721, Korea.

References
1. Raff AC, Meyer TW, Hostetter TH: New insights into uremic toxicity. Curr Opin Nephrol Hypertens 2008, 17:560–565.
2. Barreto FC, Barreto DV, Liabeuf S, Meert N, Glorieux G, Temmar M, Choukroun G, Vanholder R, Massy ZA, European Uremic Toxin Work Group (EUTox): Serum indoxyl sulfate is associated with vascular disease and mortality in chronic kidney disease patients. Clin J Am Soc Nephrol 2009, 4:1551–1558.
3. Jourde-Chiche N, Dou L, Cerini C, Dignat-George F, Brunet P: Vascular incompetence in dialysis patients–protein-bound uremic toxins and endothelial dysfunction. Semin Dial 2011, 24:327–337.
4. Yu M, Kim YJ, Kang DH: Indoxyl sulfate-induced endothelial dysfunction in patients with chronic kidney disease via an induction of oxidative stress. Clin J Am Soc Nephrol 2011, 6:30–39.
5. Shoji T, Wada A, Inoue K, Hayashi D, Tomida K, Furumatsu Y, Kaneko T, Okada N, Fukuhara Y, Imai E, Tsubakihara Y: Prospective randomized study evaluating the efficacy of the spherical adsorptive carbon AST-120 in chronic kidney disease patients with moderate decrease in renal function. Nephron Clin Pract 2007, 105:c99–c107.
6. Peng YS, Lin YT, Chen Y, Hung KY, Wang SM: Effects of indoxyl sulfate on adherens junctions of endothelial cells and the underlying signaling mechanism. J Cell Biochem 2012, 113:1034–1043.
7. Adijiang A, Goto S, Uramoto S, Nishijima F, Niwa T: Indoxyl sulphate promotes aortic calcification with expression of osteoblast-specific proteins in hypertensive rats. Nephrol Dial Transplant 2008, 23:1892–1901.
8. Iwasaki Y, Yamato H, Nii-Kono T, Fujieda A, Uchida M, Hosokawa A, Motojima M, Fukagawa M: Administration of oral charcoal adsorbent (AST-120) suppresses low-turnover bone progression in uraemic rats. Nephrol Dial Transplant 2006, 21:2768–2774.
9. Nii-Kono T, Iwasaki Y, Uchida M, Fujieda A, Hosokawa A, Motojima M, Yamato H, Kurokawa K, Fukagawa M: Indoxyl sulfate induces skeletal resistance to parathyroid hormone in cultured osteoblastic cells. Kidney Int 2007, 71:738–743.
10. Mozar A, Louvet L, Godin C, Mentaverri R, Brazier M, Kamel S, Massy ZA: Indoxyl sulphate inhibits osteoclast differentiation and function. Nephrol Dial Transplant 2012, 27:2176–2181.
11. Wang A, Ding X, Sheng S, Yao Z: Bone morphogenetic protein receptor in the osteogenic differentiation of rat bone marrow stromal cells. Yonsei Med J 2010, 51:740–745.
12. Jung KY, Takeda M, Shimoda M, Narikawa S, Tojo A, Kim DK, Chairoungdua A, Choi BK, Kusuhara H, Sugiyama Y, Sekine T, Endou H: Involvement of rat organic anion transporter 3 (rOAT3) in cephaloridine-induced nephrotoxicity: in comparison with rOAT1. Life Sci 2002, 70:1861–1874.
13. Miyashita T, Krajewski S, Krajewska M, Wang HG, Lin HK, Liebermann DA, Hoffman B, Reed JC: Tumor suppressor p53 is a regulator of bcl-2 and bax gene expression in vitro and in vivo. Oncogene 1994, 9:1799–1805.
14. Muteliefu G, Shimizu H, Enomoto A, Nishijima F, Takahashi M, Niwa T: Indoxyl sulfate promotes vascular smooth muscle cell senescence with upregulation of p53, p21, and prelamin A through oxidative stress. Am J Physiol Cell Physiol 2012, 303:C126–C134.
15. Goto S, Fujii H, Hamada Y, Yoshiya K, Fukagawa M: Association between indoxyl sulfate and skeletal resistance in hemodialysis patients. Ther Apher Dial 2010, 14:417–423.
16. Brancaccio D, Cozzolino M: CKD-MBD: an endless story. J Nephrol 2011, 24(Suppl 18):S42–S48.
17. Dou L, Jourde-Chiche N, Faure V, Cerini C, Berland Y, Dignat-George F, Brunet P: The uremic solute indoxyl sulfate induces oxidative stress in endothelial cells. J Thromb Haemost 2007, 5:1302–1308.
18. Gelasco AK, Raymond JR: Indoxyl sulfate induces complex redox alterations in mesangial cells. Am J Physiol Renal Physiol 2006, 290:F1551–F1558.
19. Muteliefu G, Enomoto A, Jiang P, Takahashi M, Niwa T: Indoxyl sulphate induces oxidative stress and the expression of osteoblast-specific proteins in vascular smooth muscle cells. Nephrol Dial Transplant 2009, 24:2051–2058.

20. Namikoshi T, Tomita N, Satoh M, Sakuta T, Kuwabara A, Kobayashi S, Higuchi Y, Nishijima F, Kashihara N: **Oral adsorbent AST-120 ameliorates endothelial dysfunction independent of renal function in rats with subtotal nephrectomy.** *Hypertens Res* 2009, **32**:194–200.

21. Duranton F, Cohen G, De Smet R, Rodriguez M, Jankowski J, Vanholder R, Argiles A, European Uremic Toxin Work Group: **Normal and pathologic concentrations of uremic toxins.** *Am Soc Nephrol* 2012, **23**:1258–1270.

22

Self-reported adverse drug reactions and their influence on highly active antiretroviral therapy in HIV infected patients: a cross sectional study

Wondmagegn Tamiru Tadesse[1*], Alemayehu Berhane Mekonnen[2], Wubshet Hailu Tesfaye[2] and Yidnekachew Tamiru Tadesse[3]

Abstract

Background: Patients on antiretroviral therapy have higher risk of developing adverse drug reactions (ADRs). The impact of ADRs on treatment adherence, treatment outcomes and future treatment options is quiet considerable. Thus, the purpose of this study was to describe the common self-reported ADRs and their impact on antiretroviral treatment.

Methods: Cross-sectional study was conducted at antiretroviral therapy (ART) clinic of Gondar University Hospital. Semi-structured interview questionnaire was used to extract self-reported ADRs, socio-demographic, and psycho-social variables. Variables related to antiretroviral medication, laboratory values and treatment changes were obtained from medical charts. Chi-square and odds ratio with 95% confidence interval were used to determine the associations of dependent variables.

Result: A total of 384 participants were enrolled. At least one adverse drug reaction was reported by 345 (89.8%) study participants and the mean number of ADRs reported was 3.7 ($\pm$0.2). The most frequently reported ADRs were nausea (56.5%) and headache (54.9%). About 114 (31.0%) participants considered antiretroviral therapy to be unsuccessful if ADRs occurred and only 10 (2.6%) decided to skip doses as ADRs were encountered. Based on chart review, treatment was changed for 78 (20.3%) patients and from which 79% were due to documented ADRs (p = 0.00). Among them, CNS symptoms (27.4%) and anemia (16.1%) were responsible for the majority of changes. Around four percent of patients were non-adherent to ART. Non-adhered participants and those on treatment changes were not statistically associated with self-reported ADRs. Only unemployment status (AOR = 1.76 (1.15 - 2.70), p = 0.01) and ADR duration of less than one month (AOR = 1.95 (1.28-2.98), p = 0.001) were significantly associated with self-reported adverse effects of three or more in the multivariate analysis.

Conclusion: Self-reported ADRs to antiretroviral therapy are quite common. More of the reactions were of short lasting and their impact on adherence and treatment change were less likely. However, documented ADRs were the most prevalent reasons for ART switch. Moreover, the level of unemployment was a strong predictor of self-reported ADRs.

Keywords: Perceived adverse effect, Antiretroviral therapy, Self-report ADRs

* Correspondence: mail2wondm@gmail.com
[1]Department of Pharmacology, School of Medicine, Addis Ababa Science & Technology University, Addis Ababa, Ethiopia
Full list of author information is available at the end of the article

Background

Worldwide, 34 million people are living with HIV from which 22.9 million (67.4%) are in the Sub-Saharan African countries. In 2010, there were an estimated 2.7 million new HIV infections and 1.8 million deaths due to AIDS [1]. According to literatures, the overall prevalence of HIV/AIDS in Ethiopia is 2.1% in 2010 [2]. The use of effective antiretroviral therapy (ART) has dramatically improved the pattern of morbidity and mortality among HIV infected patients, changing the disease pattern to a chronic manageable infection [3,4]. Highly active antiretroviral therapy (HAART) is known to increase CD4+ lymphocyte cell count which enhances immune system in HIV patients. The clinical benefits of HAART is characterized by increased survival and longevity in HIV patients [5]. However, these clinical benefits are associated with aversive adverse drug reactions (ADRs). Edward and his colleague defined ADR as an appreciably harmful or unpleasant reaction resulting from an intervention related to the use of a medicinal product, which predicts hazard from future administration and warrants prevention or specific treatment, or alteration of the dosage regimen, or withdrawal of the product [6].

Antiretrovirals, like most chronically administered drugs, are reported to have adverse reaction and particularly higher occurrences are seen at the beginning of ART [4,7,8]. Moreover, long term adverse effects such as lipodystrophy and neuromotor disorders may be encountered in latter stages of treatment [4]. Not only this, studies also showed that ADRs could be a source for new co-morbidities and hospital admission [9,10]. ADRs due to antiretrovirals can range from mild gastrointestinal disturbance [11] to serious adverse effects including hematological disorders [10], hepatotoxicity [12,13] and lactic acidosis [12]. A study done in Brazil among patients initiating ART in the first six month of therapy showed that at least one adverse reaction was reported by 92.2% of the participants while 56.2% reported four or more different reactions [8]. Singh et al. reported that 86% of patients had at least one ADR, of which, the most common observed was peripheral neuropathy [14]. A prospective observational study by Nagpal et al. reported that about 90% of patients experienced ADR [11]. In this study, non-compliance due to ADRs was observed in 28.9% of patients. Clinical benefits from ART can only be achieved with strict adherence and life-long treatment [3,4]. However, ADRs are considered the most limiting factor that compromises patient compliance and adherence. A number of authors reported ADRs as reasons for non-adherence [4,11,15-17]. Moreover, meta-analysis and review studies reported that non-adherence to treatment is one of the factors that leads to treatment failure and poor prognosis [12,18]. ADRs leave fewer options to clinicians and practitioners and compromise antiretroviral

drug efficacy particularly if the intention is to withdraw and substitute the offending agent for the other. Furthermore, substitution is difficult in resource limited settings. Overall, ADRs become a concern and public health problem particularly in developing nations as adequate drug toxicity monitoring and reporting schemes barely existed. Lack of ADR monitoring and reporting system underestimates the burden of ART associated ADRs. Therefore, utilizing self-reported ADR studies could be one way of addressing such gaps. The aim of this study was thus, to assess the most common self-reported ADRs, determine associated factors and assess impacts of ADRs on treatment at ART clinic of Gondar University Hospital (GUH).

Methods

Cross-sectional study was conducted at Gondar University Hospital (GUH) which is located in Gondar town of the Amhara regional state, 738 km North-west of Addis Ababa. GUH is the first teaching and referral hospital for the region. The hospital opened the area's first ART clinic and began offering ART services in March 2002. At the time of the study period, GUH ART clinic was providing ART service to 6,163 HIV/AIDS patients. The study was carried out in ART clinic of GUH over three months period from April 1 to June 30, 2012. The study population was comprised of 4600 adult patients (18 years and above) who were active and on follow up at the ART clinic. Briefly, recruitment criteria were documented HIV positive status, at least 18 years of age, only those who had started only ART. Patients who were taking other medications along with ART, short-course ART for the sole purposes of prevention of mother-to-child transmission and post-exposure prophylaxis were excluded from the study.

Patients receiving ART treatment at GUH ART clinic were the sampling population for the study. The sample size was calculated based on a single proportion formula. The following parameters were used to calculate the sample size: total population of adult patients on ART 4600, proportion of patients who report at least one adverse reaction to ARTs 50% and 95% confidence interval with a marginal error of 5%. Additional 10% allowance for refusal to participate in the study was considered, which resulted in a total sample of 384. Using systematic random sampling method, patients were selected from the waiting room of ART clinic, on the day of their visit to refill ART medications. For data collection, a semi-structured interview questionnaire was used (Additional file 1). The questionnaire was first prepared in English, and then translated into Amharic. The questionnaire consisted of a list of common ART related symptoms, which were identified based on previously published studies [17,18] and pretested questionnaire. Before interviewing, patients were briefed about the definition pertaining to adverse drug reactions to ARTs. They were also asked if they had received any counseling about ADRs previously from physicians, pharmacists and nurses. In this study, adverse drug reaction refers to any undesirable symptoms reported by patients which they perceived it as a result of ART use. Respondents were asked whether they had experienced any of the range of options from the list. Additionally, patients were asked to report any other ADRs encountered during the course of therapy. In such a way, the outcome of interest was the number of adverse drug reactions which had occurred at least once since they had initiated ART.

Besides, socio-demographic, general health condition of the patient, questions related to impacts of self-reported ADRs on the treatment, social and psychological components were included. Patient medication chart review was also employed to extract information related to ART medications, ART treatment change, reasons for treatment change (documented ADRs, treatment failure, co-morbidity), baseline and current laboratory values. Recent self-reported antiretroviral medication adherence was assessed based on patients' report on missed doses of ART medications over the past three-days.

The textual data obtained were sifted, organized and coded; and then entered and analyzed using SPSS statistical software version 20. Descriptive analysis of participants and self-reported adverse drug reactions were carried out. Logistic regression was employed for bivariate and multivariate analysis. Variables with a p value of less than 0.2 were fitted to the final model. Median number of self-reported ADRs was considered as the cutoff point. Patients who reported three or more types of reactions were compared to those who reported fewer. The strength of associations between self-reported adverse drug reactions and selected variables was estimated by the odds ratio with a 95% confidence interval. Chi-square test was also carried out to measure the association of selected self-reported ADRs with those factors affecting ART treatment. Statistical associations were considered significant at p < 0.05.

The following operational definitions were used:

- Non-adherence – failed to take >95% or missing dose of the antiretroviral drugs prescribed in the last three days prior to the interview
- Healthy – asymptomatic, physical activity not affected and not confined to bed at the start of treatment
- Mild illness – mild symptoms, physical activity not affected and not confined to bed at the start of treatment
- Severe illness – recurrent illness with wide range of infections, frequent confinement to bed, marked physical activity limitation and/or hospitalized due to prevailing conditions.

Ethical consideration

The study was approved by the ethical review committee of School of Pharmacy, College of Medicine and Health Sciences, University of Gondar. Written informed consent was obtained from the respondents for the interview. Besides, confidentiality of the information was strictly maintained during data collection and data analysis process. Each interview questionnaire was assigned a study identification number. Respondents were also informed that their information would be used anonymously.

Result

A total of 384 participants were enrolled in the study. Descriptive socio-demographic variables indicated that 85.1% of the participants were below 40 years old, 66.9% were females, 55.2% were married and 38.8% were unemployed. Most study participants had some education, primary and above (74.7%) and 90.1% were from urban dwellings. With regard to clinical status, mean level of CD4 cells/mm at the initiation of ART was 165.68 ± 93.8 while at the time of data collection was 376.7 ± 181.3. The majority of participants (52.9%) CD4 level was over 350. Participants had received ART for a mean of 42.3 (± 24.1) months of treatment duration and had most recently been on ART triple regimen consisted of AZT/3TC/NVP (40.1%). Overall, only 3.6% of the participants taking ART medications indicated that they had skipped pills in the prior three days to result in less than 95% adherence. Initially, most patients were mild to severely ill. However, after the start of ART medication, most respondents' health status was improved in terms of body weight and CD4 level. In the contrary, social interaction of most participants was not changed (Table 1).

Based on the chart review, one out of five participants had changed their first ART because of ADRs (79%), treatment failure (13%), tuberculosis co-morbidity (5%) and pregnancy (3%). There were statistically significant association with these documented ADRs (p = 0.00). Central nervous system symptoms, anemia and peripheral neuropathy were among the major documented ADRs responsible for treatment change (Table 2).

At least one ADR was reported by 345 (89.8%) patients due to the use of ART and the mean number of ADRs reported was 3.7 (± 0.2). Most patients (94.6%) stated that they had received counseling regarding adverse reaction to ART from physicians, pharmacists or nurses before initiating and in the course of ART therapy. The most common self-reported adverse drug reactions were nausea (56.5%), headache (54.9%) and fever (40.9%) (Table 3).

Table 4 present results of the logistic regression analysis. In the bivariate analysis, unemployed status, urban residents, ART duration of more than four years, non-adhered patients and ADR duration of less than one

Table 1 Descriptive analysis of socio-demographic, clinical variables and health status of the participants, ART clinic, Gondar University Hospital, June 2012

Variables	n(%), N = 384
Socio-demographic	
Education (primary and above)	287(74.7)
Work status (unemployed)	149 (38.8)
Age (≤40 years)	327(85.2)
Gender (female)	257(66.9)
Marital status (married)	212 (55.2)
Residency (urban)	346 (90.1)
Clinical variables	
Duration of ART (≤4 years)	155(40.4)
Current CD4 level (cells/mm^3)	
< 200	47(12.2)
200-350	134(34.9)
>350	203(52.9)
Current ART regimens (triple)	
AZT/3TC/NVP	154 (40.1)
TDF/3TC/NVP	50 (13.0)
AZT/3TC/EFV	48(12.5)
D4T/3TC/NVP	44(11.5)
TDF/3TC/EFZ	42 (10.9)
D4T/3TC/EFZ	23(6.0)
Others	23(6.0)
Non adherence	14(3.6)
General profiles	
General health at the start of treatment	
Healthy	50(13.0)
Mild to severely ill	334 (87.0)
CD$_4$ count after treatment	
Increased	345 (89.8)
Decreased	9(2.3)
No change	30(7.8)
Health status after ART start	
Improved	344(89.6)
Not improved	40(10.4)
Body weight	
Increased	323(84.1)
Decreased	23(6.0)
No change	38(10.0)
Social interaction of patients after ART start	
Increased	81(21.1)
Decreased	10(2.6)
No change	293(76.3)

Table 2 Distribution of major reasons and documented ADRs responsible for treatment change (based on chart review), ART clinic, Gondar University Hospital, June 2012

Variables	n (%)*
Reasons for treatment change (N = 78)	
Due to ADRs	**62 (79.0)****
Due to treatment failure	10 (13.0)
Due to TB co-morbidity	4 (5.0)
Due to pregnancy	2 (3.0)
Documented ADRs responsible for treatment change (N = 62)	
CNS symptoms	**17 (27.4)**
Anemia	10 (16.1)
Peripheral neuropathy	9(14.5)
Skin rash	8 (12.9)
Lipodystrophy	7(11.3)
Weight loss	4(6.5)
Stomach ache	3 (4.8)
Hepatotoxicity	3 (4.8)
Dental illness	1 (1.6)

*Percent frequency out of the total number of patients (reasons for treatment change, N = 78; ADRs responsible for treatment change, N = 62). The most frequent reasons are highlighted in bold type.
**95% CI, 0.68-0.88; p =0.00.

Table 3 Most common self-reported adverse drug reactions of antiretroviral therapy, ART clinic, Gondar University Hospital, June 2012

Self-reported adverse drug reactions	n (%)*, N = 384
Nausea	217 (56.5)
Headache	211 (54.9)
Fever	157 (40.9)
Vomiting	147 (38.3)
Lethargy/fatigue	131(34.1)
Loss of appetite	130 (34)
Insomnia	102 (26.6)
Depression/stress	99 (25.8)
Skin rash	85 (22.1)
Night mare	72 (18.8)
Diarrhea	41 (10.7)
Oral ulceration/dry mouth	35 (9.1)
Anxiety	23 (6.3)
Others**	10 (2.6)

*number of frequency and percent proportions, total number of participants (N = 384).
**includes tingling in hands or feet, anemia.

Table 4 Logistic regression analysis of selected variables and adverse drug reactions to ART, ART clinic, Gondar University Hospital, June 2012

Variables	Total (N)[*]	Self-reported ADRs[**] ($\geq$3), n = 229	OR (95% CI)[***]	P value	AOR(95% CI)[†]
Age					
$\leq$ 40 years	327	192(58.7)	1		
>40 years	57	37(64.9)	1.28(0.69, 2.38)	0.44	
Gender					
Female	257	152(59.1)	1		
Male	127	77(60.6)	1.06 (0.69, 1.64)	0.78	
Education					
Illiterate	97	58(59.8)	1		
$\geq$primary	287	171(59.6)	0.92 (0.58, 1.46)	0.72	
Work status					
Employed	149	78(52.3)	1		1
Non-employed	235	151(64.2)	1.82 (1.17, 2.84)	<0.01	1.76 (1.15, 2.70)[a]
Marital status					
Married	212	121(57.1)	1		
Non- married	172	108(62.8)	1.16 (0.75, 1.82)	0.50	
Residency					
Urban	346	211(61.0)	1		
Rural	38	18(43.4)	0.58(0.28, 1.18)	0. 14	
Duration of ART					
$\leq$4 years	155	85(54.8)	1		
>4 years	229	144(62.9)	1.39 (0.92, 2.21)	0.11	
ART treatment change					
Yes	78	42(53.8)	1		
No	306	187(61.1)	1.35(0.82,2.22)	0.24	
Current CD4 level					
$\leq$350	181	107(59.1)	0.96(0.64, 1.44)	0.85	
>350	203	122(60.1)	1		
Current ART regimen					
AZT backbone	204	122(59.8)	1.01(0.67, 1.53)	0.94	
Non-AZT backbone	180	107(59.4)	1		
Adherence					
Yes	370	223(60.3)	1		
No	14	6(42.8)	0.50(0.17, 1.45)	0.2	
ADR duration (self-reported)					
$\leq$1 month	212	140(66.0)	1.81(1.20, 2.74)		1.95(1.28,2.98)[b]
>1 month	172	89(51.7)	1	<0.01	1

[*]Percent frequency that refers to the total number of patients (N = 384). [**]Number and proportion of patients' self-reporting 3 or more adverse drug reactions. [***]Values represent odds ratio (OR) at 95% confidence interval. [†]Values represent adjusted odds ratio (AOR) at 95% confidence interval, [a]p = 0.01, [b]p = 0.001.

month reported a high proportion of three or more different types of ADRs (p < 0.2). Among the variables assessed for further analysis, unemployment status (AOR = 1.76(1.15-2.70), p = 0.01) and ADR duration of less than one month (AOR = 1.95 (1.28-2.98), p = 0.001)

were significantly associated with self-reported adverse effects of three or more in the multivariate analysis.

Results of the impacts of self-reported ADRs showed that only 10 (2.6%) patients decided to skip doses as ADRs were encountered. But, none of the self-reported

ADRs were statistically associated with such dose skipping trend. As a measure of impact of ADRs on patients' perception regarding treatment, 114 (31.0%) of participants reported that they considered antiretroviral therapy to be unsuccessful due to the ADRs that they encountered. Moreover, it was found that such impacts of reported ADRs showed significant association with self-reported ADRs such as fever, vomiting, loss of appetite, diarrhea, insomnia, lethargy, dry mouth and depression. Similarly, various types of reported ADRs were significantly associated with the responses for questions linked with patients' social interaction (Table 5).

Discussion

This study was aimed at describing the commonly perceived ADRs, characterizing the impact on patients taking ART and associated factors with self-reported ADRs at ART clinic of Gondar University Hospital. Our findings indicated a high proportion of patients (89.8%) reported at least one adverse drug reactions because of antiretroviral therapy since they began ART. This finding is closely consistent with works of other studies that showed a high proportion of patients on ART reported at least one ADR to be as high as 86%-94% of the patients [8,11,14,19]. Almost, all these studies used a similar study design. This finding is relatively higher than the reports by Luma et al. [20] in Cameron and de Padua et al. [4] in Brazil. Our study assessed adverse reactions which were merely of patient self-report and thus, those symptoms perceived as adverse drug reactions to ARTs might be confounded with symptoms due to HIV. This is more evident as most patients reported fever as one of their ADR which is more likely to HIV and concurrent infections. In such occasions, this might lead to an overestimation of this outcome. On the other hand, this difference might be due to differences in the study design and lack of standardized definition of ADR among the different studies. Moreover, genetic and ethnic susceptibilities to ADR to a particular drug might also explain the difference.

In this study, the most common reported ADRs were from gastrointestinal symptoms; among which nausea was highly prevalent constituting more than half of all ADRs. In agreement with previous studies, gastrointestinal complaints were the reactions most commonly encountered [4,8,11]. In a Brazilian study of 406 patients, the most frequently reported adverse drug reaction was nausea where the occurrence was as high as 51.2% [8]. In the contrary, Singh et al. [14] and Luma et al. [20] reported that about a fifth of patients on ART developed peripheral neuropathy. Yet, a self-report by Melangu [19] in Pretoria, South Africa showed that sexual problems were the highest adverse effects reported. Few studies try to look the association between socio-demographic variables and adverse drug reactions, our study showed no difference in reported ADRs between age and sex differences. This finding is consistent with Eluwa et al. [7]. In this study, only unemployment status and ADR duration of less than one month were independently associated with self-reported ADRs of three or more. On top of the adverse drug reactions to ARTs, the level of unemployment in our study is a cause for concern because it results in a lot of psychosocial problems. Around one third of patients reported depression, stress and anxiety among the reported ADRs. Findings showed that unemployment is one of the causes of mental health problems [21,22]. We deduced that more of the reactions were of short lasting and their impact on adherence and treatment change were less likely. However, patient chart review showed that switching therapy was identified as major intervention used for the management of adverse reactions to ART in this population. Of those patients who had their ART regimen switched, 79% ascribed the change in regimen to the occurrences of adverse reactions due to ART. This is higher than the findings in 2007 in Brazil where ADR was found to account for 56.1% of all switches [4]. Unlike self-reported ADRs, the most documented reactions were more serious events like CNS symptoms, anemia and peripheral neuropathy. The patients' perception of adverse reactions would potentially attribute to non-adherence to medications. But this study showed no difference in reported ADRs between the adhered and non-adhered population. We observed that 3.6% of patients were non-adherent to ART. This result is lower than that of the report by Nagpal et al. who reported non-adherence in 28.9% of Indian patients due to ADRs to ART (11). Other reports also showed non-adherence rate of 13%-21% [15,16,23]. The differences can be attributed to variation in the adherence assessment method.

Only 2.6% of subjects skipped medications because of perceived ADRs. Different studies mentioned various reasons for missing doses; forgetting, being away from home and being busy were the most common [16,24]. The lower rate of missing doses indicates the strength of patient education system and competent follow up by the health practitioners. However, perceived medication side effects and ADRs influenced patients' perception on ART. Patients who considered ART as unsuccessful were significantly associated with the common ADRs including fever, GIT side effects, insomnia, lethargy and depression. Furthermore, these medication ADRs demonstrated significant influence on patient's social interaction behavior. For instance, 32.9% of the study subjects perceive that people would avoid them when ADRs encountered and some 32.2% tend to reduce social interaction. On contrary to these, most of the study groups (80.0%) would love to share their feeling about the ADRs with their family members. Specifically, the result indicated a significant family

Table 5 Impacts of self-reported ADRs on perception of treatment and social interaction, ART clinic, Gondar University Hospital, June 2012

Variables	n (%)	Association of variables with specific ADRs (chi-square or fisher test)										
		Nausea	Headache	Fever	Vomiting	Lethargy	Loss of appetite	Insomnia	Depression	Night mare	Diarrhea	OU/DM
Impacts on patients perception on treatment patients who:												
Decided to skip medication due to ADRs*	10 (2.6)	0.54	0.51	0.35	0.55	0.26	0.48	0.20	0.21	0.42	0.78	0.26
Consider ART unsuccessful due to ADRs**	114 (31.0)	1.43	0.10	7.42^b	5.00^a	29.53^c	25.93^c	14.47^c	24.43^c	1.43	13.63^c	13.70^c
Impacts of ADR on patients' social interaction patients who:												
Perceive that people avoid them due to observed ADRs**	21 (32.9)	5.68^a	0.76	11.97^c	12.7^c	28.13^c	26.67^c	18.28^c	23.15^c	3.19^a	8.45^b	14.94^c
Tend to reduce/avoid social interaction because of ADRs**	119 (32.2)	2.11	0.26	9.87^c	7.96^b	33.20	26.67^c	20.88^c	3.40^c	1.87	8.45^b	6.70^c
Perceive family members avoid them when ADRs occurred**	57 (15.4)	0.99	3.35^a	2.19	0.06	0.08	1.01	0.45	3.40^a	0.03	0.99	6.70^b
Talk to family members about ADRs as it appears**	296 (80.0)	14.32^c	10.24^c	5.92^b	7.73^b	4.34^a	2.84	0.61	2.21	0.31	0.01	0.62

n = 384. *Fishers exact test, **chi-square test was used to assess associations. ^{a}significant at a level of $p < 0.05$, ^{b}significant at a level of $p < 0.01$, ^{c}significant at a level of $p < 0.001$. OU/DM, oral ulceration or dry mouth.

interaction of patients when ADRs such as fever, headache, nausea, vomiting and lethargy had occurred.

This study has a number of limitations. The ADRs are self-report and there were no further investigation of laboratory tests and other diagnostic tests for ruling out for other possible causes which could lead to over-representation of ADRs. On the other hand, it might lead to under-estimation of ADRs which might have been detected clinically. Besides, the reporting could be influenced by the patient's ability to memorize events related to adherence assessment and the duration of time ADRs lasted.

Conclusion

Our study showed that perceived adverse drug reactions due to antiretroviral therapy are very frequent and prevalent in the studied population. More of the reactions were of short lasting and their impact on adherence and treatment change were less likely. Although treatment change and self-reported ADRs were failed to show statistical significance, documented ADRs were the most frequent reasons for ART switch. Unlike self-reported ADRs, documented ADRs were serious events. Moreover, the level of unemployment was a strong predictor of self-reported ADRs. Self-reported ADRs have a number of impacts on the patients' perception to ART and drug taking behavior. Specific self-reported ADRs showed their influences on the patients' perception to antiretroviral therapy and social interactions. Particularly, self-reported ADRs forced the patients to consider the antiretroviral therapy as if it was unsuccessful. In addition, self-reported ADRs demonstrated their potential threat to the patients social interaction as the patients considered people avoid them due to ADRs. Therefore, clinicians, caregivers and the patient himself/herself should actively collaborate for the better ART outcome because ADRs are a potential threat to the effectiveness of ART. ADR reporting, monitoring and management should further be strengthened to enhance better ART service. Patient education on ART associated ADRs should be an integral part of HIV care so as to facilitate reporting and management.

Additional file

Additional file 1: Annex 1. Study questioner used to collect variables and self-reported adverse drug reactions at ART clinic, Gondar University Hospital, April 2012.

Competing interests

The authors declare that they have no competing interests.

Authors' contributions

Data were collected by WTT and WHT. WTT, ABM and YTT contributed in statistical analysis. All authors were involved in manuscript write-up and correction. The final version of the submitted manuscript was approved by all authors.

Acknowledgements

Our appreciation extends to Gondar Hospital ART clinic staffs and to the study participants, supervisors and data collectors for their fullest participation. We also extend our appreciation to Mrs. Grum Zewdu, Department of Medicine and Health Sciences, Addis Ababa Science and Technology University for her relentless effort and help in the statistical analysis. A special word of thanks goes to Professor Peggy Soul Odegard, University of Washington, Seattle, USA for the language and grammar editing. Also, we thank Mr. Solomon Debebe, English department, Addis Ababa Science and Technology University for language and grammar editing.

Author details

[1]Department of Pharmacology, School of Medicine, Addis Ababa Science & Technology University, Addis Ababa, Ethiopia. [2]Department of Clinical Pharmacy, School of Pharmacy, University of Gondar, Gondar, Ethiopia. [3]Department of Internal Medicine, School of Medicine, University of Gondar, Gondar, Ethiopia.

References

1. WHO, UNAIDS and UNICEF: *Global HIV/AIDS Responses- Epidemic update and health sector progress towards universal access.* Geneva: WHO; 2011.
2. Federal Ministry of Health: *Report on Progress Towards Implementation of the UN Declaration of Commitment on HIV/AIDS.* Addis Ababa: Federal HIV/AIDS Prevention and Control Office; 2010.
3. Carrieri MP, Villes V, Raffi F, Protopopescu C, Preau M, Salmon D, Taieb A, Lang JM, Verdon R, Chene G, Spire B, APROCO-COPILOTE ANRS CO-08 Study Group: **Self-reported side-effects of anti-retroviral treatment among IDUs: a 7-year longitudinal study.** *Int J Drug Policy* 2007, **18**(Suppl 4):288–295.
4. de Pádua Menezes CA, César CC, Bonolo PF, Acurcio FA, Guimarães MDC: **High incidence of adverse reactions to initial antiretroviral therapy in Brazil.** *Braz J Med Biol Res* 2006, **39**(4):495–505.
5. Life expectancy of individuals on combination antiretroviral therapy in high-income countries. http://europepmc.org/articles/PMC3130543.
6. Edwards IR, Aronson JK: **Adverse drug reactions: definition, diagnosis, and management.** *Lancet* 2000, **356**:1255–1259.
7. Eluwa GI, Badru T, Akpoigbe KJ: **Adverse drug reactions to antiretroviral therapy (ARVs): incidence, type and risk factors in Nigeria.** *BMC Clin Pharmacol* 2012, **12**:7.
8. de Pádua CA M, César CC, Bonolo PF, Acurcio FA, Guimarães MC: **Self-reported adverse reactions among patients initiating antiretroviral therapy in Brazil.** *BJID* 2007, **11**(Suppl 1):20–26.
9. Mehta U, Durrheim DN, Blockman M, Kredo T, Gounden R, Barnes KI: **Adverse drug reactions in adult medical inpatients in a South African hospital serving a community with a high HIV/AIDS prevalence: prospective observational study.** *Br J Clin Pharmacol* 2008, **65**(Suppl 3):396–406.
10. Pulagam P, Rajesh R, Vidyasagar S, Varma D: **Assessment of hematological adverse drug reactions to antiretroviral therapy in HIV positive patients at Kasturba Hospital Manipal.** *BMC Infect Dis* 2012, **12**(Suppl 1):55.
11. Nagpal M, Tayal V, Kumar S, Gupta U: **Adverse drug reactions to antiretroviral therapy in AIDS patients at a tertiary care hospital in India: a prospective observational study.** *Indian J Med Sci* 2010, **64**:245–252.
12. Montessori V, Press N, Harris M, Akagi L, Montaner JSG: **Adverse effects of antiretroviral therapy for HIV infection.** *CMAJ* 2004, **170**(2):229–238.
13. Granta DA, Mngadib TK, van Halsemaa LC, Luttigb MM, Fielddinga LK, Churchyard JG: **Adverse events with isoniazid preventive therapy: experience from a large trial.** *AIDS* 2010, **24**(suppl 5):29–36.
14. Singh H, Dulhani N, Tiwari P, Singh P, Sinha T: **A prospective, observational cohort study to elicit adverse effects of antiretroviral agents in a remote resource-restricted tribal population of Chhattisgarh.** *Indian J Pharmacol* 2009, **41**(Suppl 5):224–226.
15. Wasti SP, Simkhada P, Randall J, Freeman JV, van Teijlingen E: **Factors influencing adherence to antiretroviral treatment in Nepal: a mixed- methods study.** *PLoS ONE* 2012, **7**(Suppl 5):e35547.
16. Alexander M, Violeta N-L, Rita Chung WY, Charlotte Lam SW, Patrick Li CK, Joseph Lau TF: **Factors associated with adherence to antiretroviral medication in HIV-infected patients.** *Int J STD AIDS* 2002, **13**:301–310.

17. Ammassari A, Murri R, Pezzotti P, Trotta MP, Ravasio L, De Longis P, Lo Caputo S, Narciso P, Pauluzzi S, Carosi G, Nappa S, Piano P, Izzo CM, Lichtner M, Rezza G, Monforte A, Ippolito G, d'Arminio Moroni M, Wu AW, Antinori A, AdICONA Study Group: **Self-reported symptoms and medication side effects influence adherence to highly active antiretroviral therapy in persons with HIV infection.** *Jf Acquir Immune Defic Syndr* 2001, **28**(Suppl 5):445–449.

18. Johnson MO, Charlebois E, Morin SF, Catz SL, Goldstein RB, Remien RH, Rotheram-Borus MJ, Mickalian JD, Kittel L, Samimy-Muzaffar F, Lightfoot MA, Gore-Felton C, Chesney A, NIMH Healthy Living Project Team: **Perceived adverse effects of antiretroviral therapy.** *J Pain Symptom Manage* 2005, **29**(Suppl 2):193–205.

19. Malangu NG: **Self-reported adverse effects as barriers to adherence to antiretroviral therapy in HIV-infected patients in Pretoria.** *SA Fam Pract* 2008, **50**(Suppl 5):49.

20. Luma HN, Doualla M, Choukem S, Temfack E, Ashuntantang G, Joko AH, Koulla-Shiro S: **Adverse drug reactions of Highly Active Antiretroviral Therapy (HAART) in HIV infected patients at the General Hospital, Douala, Cameroon: a cross sectional study.** *Pan Afr Med J* 2012, **12**:87.

21. Lin MW, Sandifer R, Stein S: **Effects of unemployment on mental and physical health.** *Am J Public Health* 1985, **75**:502–506.

22. Kessler RC, Turner JB, House JS: **Effects of unemployment on health in a community survey: main, modifying and mediating effects.** *J Soc Issues* 1988, **44**(4):69–85.

23. Filho BFL, Nogueira AS SA, Machado SE, Abreu FT, de Oliveira HR, Hofer BC EL: **Factors associated with lack of antiretroviral adherence among adolescents in a reference centre in Rio de Janeiro, Brazil.** *Int J STD AIDS* 2008, **19**:685–688.

24. Ajose O, Mookerjeeb S, Millsc EJ, Boulled A, Ford N: **Treatment outcomes of patients on second-line antiretroviral therapy in resource-limited settings: a systematic review and meta-analysis.** *AIDS* 2012, **26**(Suppl 8):929–938.

23

Exploiting high-throughput cell line drug screening studies to identify candidate therapeutic agents in head and neck cancer

Anthony C Nichols[1*], Morgan Black[1], John Yoo[1], Nicole Pinto[1], Andrew Fernandes[2], Benjamin Haibe-Kains[3], Paul C Boutros[4,5,6] and John W Barrett[1]

Abstract

Background: There is an urgent need for better therapeutics in head and neck squamous cell cancer (HNSCC) to improve survival and decrease treatment morbidity. Recent advances in high-throughput drug screening techniques and next-generation sequencing have identified new therapeutic targets in other cancer types, but an HNSCC-specific study has not yet been carried out. We have exploited data from two large-scale cell line projects to clearly describe the mutational and copy number status of HNSCC cell lines and identify candidate drugs with elevated efficacy in HNSCC.

Methods: The genetic landscape of 42 HNSCC cell lines including mutational and copy number data from studies by Garnett et al., and Barretina et al., were analyzed. Data from Garnett et al. was interrogated for relationships between HNSCC cells versus the entire cell line pool using one- and two-way analyses of variance (ANOVAs). As only seven HNSCC cell lines were tested with drugs by Barretina et al., a similar analysis was not carried out.

Results: Recurrent mutations in human papillomavirus (HPV)-negative patient tumors were confirmed in HNSCC cell lines, however additional, recurrent, cell line-specific mutations were identified. Four drugs, Bosutinib, Docetaxel, BIBW2992, and Gefitinib, were found via multiple-test corrected ANOVA to have lower IC_{50} values, suggesting higher drug sensitivity, in HNSCC lines versus non-HNSCC lines. Furthermore, the PI3K inhibitor AZD6482 demonstrated significantly higher activity (as measured by the IC_{50}) in HNSCC cell lines harbouring PIK3CA mutations versus those that did not.

Conclusion: HNSCC-specific reanalysis of large-scale drug screening studies has identified candidate drugs that may be of therapeutic benefit and provided insights into strategies to target PIK3CA mutant tumors. PIK3CA mutations may represent a predictive biomarker for response to PI3K inhibitors. A large-scale study focused on HNSCC cell lines and including HPV-positive lines is necessary and has the potential to accelerate the development of improved therapeutics for patients suffering with head and neck cancer. This strategy can potentially be used as a template for drug discovery in any cancer type.

Keywords: High throughput drug screening, Cell lines, Genomics, HNSCC, Mutations

* Correspondence: anthony.nichols@lhsc.on.ca
[1]Department of Otolaryngology Head & Neck Surgery, Western University, London, Ontario, Canada
Full list of author information is available at the end of the article

Background

Despite advances in multi-modal treatment of head and neck squamous cell carcinoma (HNSCC), mortality rates for advance disease remain high [1]. Thus there is an urgent need to identify novel chemicals with high activity in this disease. As with other tumor types, however, the time- and resource-intensive, multi-step clinical trial process remains a tremendous barrier to rapid drug development. Moreover, only specific molecular subtypes of tumors may respond to any given target agent [2], thereby decreasing the number of patients eligible for a particular study.

Targeted therapy has become an important method in personalizing treatment for cancer patients based on the genetic mutations present in their tumor(s). Such therapies enable the use of drugs to specifically target molecules within the tumor that are responsible for the malignancy. A search of the literature, as well as clinical trials that are currently underway in HNSCC, revealed a variety of agents being investigated that target various cellular molecules (e.g. epidermal growth factor receptor [EGFR], members of the phosphatidylinositide 3-kinase [PI3K] pathway, mammalian target of rapamycin [mTOR], cyclin-dependent kinases, vascular endothelial growth factor receptor [VEGFR], retinoblastoma protein [pRB], toll-like receptors and Aurora kinases) (clinicaltrials.gov). However, despite the multiple trials, only EGFR tyrosine kinase inhibitors and EGFR monoclonal antibodies (e.g. cetuximab) have been approved for clinical use and demonstrate only modest activity in a subset of patients [3]. New strategies are needed not only to identify active molecules, but also to define the target population that is most likely to benefit from therapy.

Cell lines are imperfect models of cancer: they tend to be generated from more aggressive, often metastatic tumors, can demonstrate genetic and epigenetic changes relative to the parent tumors, and lack interactions with the surrounding stroma and immune system [4-7]. However, they remain an invaluable discovery tool as they provide an unlimited source of self-replicating material, are easily manipulated and can be screened in a cheap and high-throughput way with large panels of drugs. Moreover, relationships between drug sensitivity and tumor genotypes observed in patient samples are also reflected in cell lines [8].

The advent of next generation sequencing has allowed complete, affordable and rapid genomic characterization of both patient samples and of cell lines. In parallel, the development of high-throughput robotic drug screening platforms has facilitated the rapid testing of a large number of drugs. Together these techniques provide the ability to correlate mutation status, copy number variation and expression levels with drug response. Two recent, large-scale studies, involving hundreds of cell lines of

different tissue types [8,9] have confirmed well known genetic markers of drug response (e.g. response to BRAF inhibitors in BRAF mutant cell lines) and identified novel associations such as the marked sensitivity of Ewing's sarcoma cells harboring the EWS-FLI1 gene translocation to poly(ADP-ribose) polymerase (PARP) inhibitors [8]. However, given the large volume of data generated, only a limited analysis of the HNSCC cell lines involved in either study was presented. We endeavoured to reanalyze the data presented in these studies to provide a mutational landscape of HNSCC cell lines and to identify markers of drug sensitivity and resistance in HNSCC.

Methods

Defining the mutational and copy number landscape of HNSCC cell lines

The study by the Broad-Novartis group (Barretina et al.) included 31 HNSCC cell lines (of 947 total), seven of which were screened with 24 anticancer agents [9]. The cell lines were characterized by sequencing of ~1500 genes, as well as with array-based copy number variation (CNV) analysis and using mRNA abundance microarrays. A second study, by Garnett and coworkers, evaluated 639 cell lines (22 HNSCC lines) treated with 131 agents and characterized by targeted sequencing of 60 cancer genes, as well as array-based assessment of CNVs and mRNA abundance [8]. Note that eleven identically named HNSCC cell lines were common to both studies yielding a total of 42 uniquely named cell lines when both studies were combined. We integrated the CNV and mutational analysis of the most commonly altered genes from the two studies into Figures 1 and 2 and correlated them with the changes reported from patient samples by Stransky et al. [10]. CNV levels from Garnett et al., were simply reported as 0 (deletion), between 0 and 8 (copy-number neutral), and greater than 8 (amplification). Barretina et al. reported CNVs as continuous variables, relative to control genes with 0 considered "non-amplified". We considered values greater than 2 (reflecting at least 2 extra gene copies) as amplifications and less than −2 (representing homozygous deletion) as this appeared to agree with the TCGA data from http://cbioportal.org and correspond best with the amplifications and deletions noted in the study by Garnett et al. (Additional file 1: Table S1).

Identification of biomarkers of chemotherapeutic sensitivity and resistance in HNSCC cell lines

Due to the small number of HNSCC cell lines that were treated with drugs in Barretina et al. (7 lines), we restricted drug sensitivity analysis to the data from Garnett et al. [8]. All statistical analysis was performed with the R statistical environment, version 2.15.2 (R Foundation

Legend: † Genes identified to be significantly mutated in tumors in Stransky et al., Science 2011, * copy number variation was not completed for these cell lines, CNV - copy number variation, Indel - insertion/deletion. Note: Cells containing more than one annotation indicate that multiple mutations are present in the gene.

Figure 1 Genetic landscape of head and neck cancer cell lines based on data from Barretina *et al.*, Nature 2012.

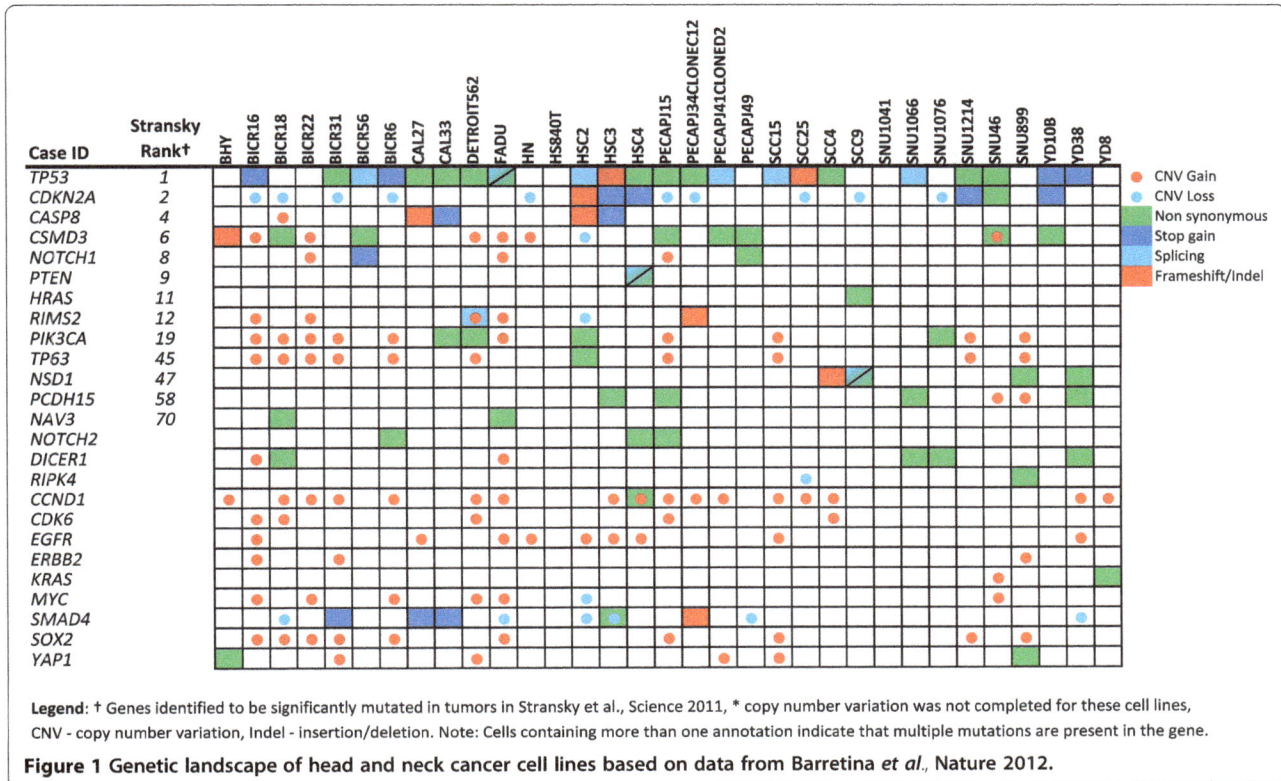

for Statistical Computing) with the fdrtool package [11] version 1.2.10, to control the rate of false discovery due to multiple testing. We compared the half-maximal inhibitory concentration (IC_{50} in μM) for each drug between HNSCC cell lines and non-HNSCC cell lines via one-way analysis of variance (ANOVA) as computed through t-tests. Specifically, for each drug i, cell lines were partitioned into two groups $j = \{\text{HNSCC, non-HNSCC}\}$ as per their cell-line type. Letting k denote replicate number, the linear model for each t-test was the standard $y_{ijk} = \mu_j + \varepsilon_{ijk}$, where y_{ijk} represents the observed $\log_2(IC_{50})$, μ_j represents the mean response of group j, and each ε_{ijk} represents a realization of $\varepsilon \sim N(0, \sigma_i^2)$. To control the false discovery rate, the "local false discovery rate" (LFDR) was estimated via computed p-values using Strimmer's fdrtool [11,12]. The LFDR has been championed by Efron and others for genomic studies

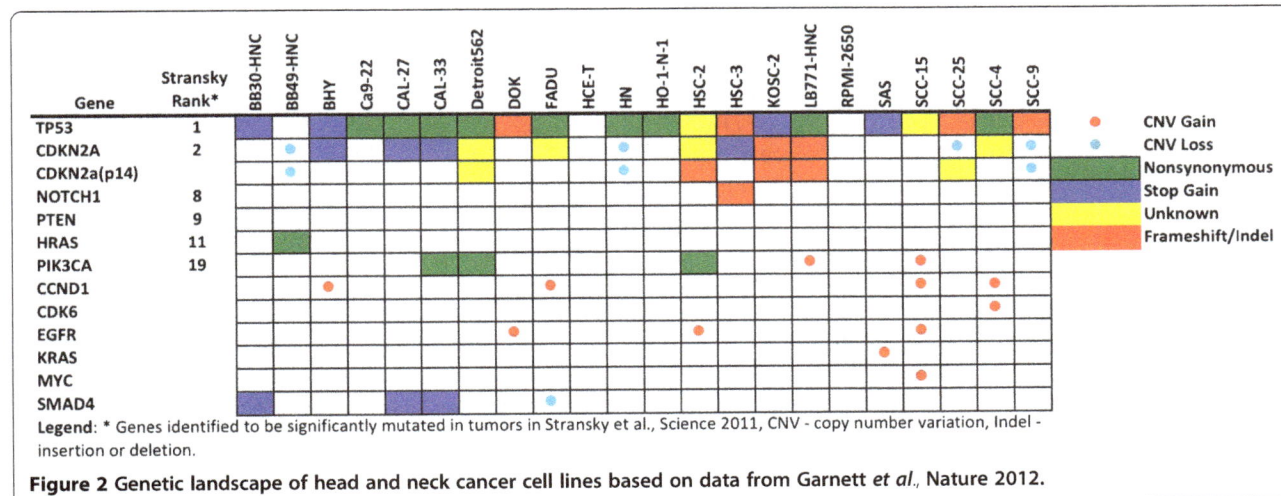

Legend: * Genes identified to be significantly mutated in tumors in Stransky et al., Science 2011, CNV - copy number variation, Indel - insertion or deletion.

Figure 2 Genetic landscape of head and neck cancer cell lines based on data from Garnett *et al.*, Nature 2012.

as it is directly interpretable as posterior probability, and not a "corrected *p*-value" [13,14]. A LFDR <0.05 was considered significant and a LFDR <0.1 was considered to be approaching statistical significance. We then looked for associations of copy number changes and mutations with response to drug treatment by two-way ANOVA including factor interaction, again using the LFDR to control false discovery rates. Specifically, the linear models used for the ANOVAs was $y_{ijk} = \mu + \alpha_i + \beta_j + \gamma_{ij} + \varepsilon_{ijk}$ where group i = {copy-number unchanged, copy-number changed}, group j = {wild-type, mutant}, and k again denotes replicate number. As per standard ANOVA, α_i and β_j represent the mean additive responses of their respective groups, γ_{ij} represents any non-additive interaction effect, ε_{ijk} represents a realization of $\varepsilon \sim N(0, \sigma^2)$, and μ represents the grand-mean effect. The standard constraints $\sum_i \alpha_i = 0$, $\sum_j \beta_j = 0$, and $\sum_{ij} \gamma_{ij} = 0$ were used to ensure that all parameters of each model were identifiable.

Results

The genetic landscape of HNSCC cell lines is similar to HPV-negative tumors

The mutational landscape of the 42 HNSCC cell lines, all of which were HPV-negative [7], demonstrated similarities with primary tumor samples from HPV-negative patients; including frequent mutations in tumor suppressor genes *TP53* (74% of cell-lines [9]; 62% of tumors [10]) and *CDKN2A*, and less frequent ones in *PTEN*, *SMAD4*, *NOTCH1* and *NOTCH2* (Figures 1 and 2). Other similarities were rare activating mutations in oncogenes *PIK3CA* and *HRAS*, deletions of *CDKN2A* and amplifications of *CCND1*, epidermal growth factor receptor (*EGFR*), *MYC* and *PIK3CA*. A complete listing of mutations identified in HNSCC cell lines in Barretina *et al.* is provided in Additional file 2: Table S2. However, there were multiple, recurrent mutations in genes rarely or not identified in the patient samples (Additional file 2: Table S2 and Additional file 3: Table S3). In fact, there were 22 genes more frequently mutated than *TP53*, which was the most commonly mutated gene found in tumor samples (Additional file 3: Table S3). Most of these mutations were identical in all cell lines, such as two 5′ UTR mutations observed in neural cell adhesion molecule 1 (*NCAM1*) (insertion of adenine at position 112832307 (dbSNP ID: rs117108942) and deletion of cytosine at position 112832340) in virtually every HNSCC cell line in Barretina *et al.* Of note, 11 cell lines with the same name were characterized in both studies. However, two of these lines had significant discrepancies in terms of mutations between the studies (BHY, SCC9) bringing the true identities of the lines into question (Additional file 1: Table S1). Personal correspondence with the authors of Barretina *et al.* and the methods section of Garnett *et al.*, have confirmed that the identification of their cell lines were confirmed with genotyping. The genotyping results are not provided in the supplementary data to allow direct comparison.

Chemicals with high and low activity in HNSCC cell lines

Four chemicals, Docetaxel (anti-mitotic chemotherapy), Bosutinib (combined SRC/ABL inhibitor), Afatinib (an EGFR and HER2 inhibitor), and Gefitinib (an EGFR inhibitor) were found to have significantly increased activity in HNSCC cell lines compared with the remainder of the cell line pool (Table 1, Figure 3). Two drugs, methotrexate and PD-173074 (an inhibitor of the fibroblast growth factor receptor [FGFR] and VEGFR) were found to have significantly lower activity in HNSCC lines (Table 1). A complete listing of the associations between drug response and HNSCC cell line type can be found in Additional file 4: Table S4.

Of note, there were five identically named cell lines in both studies that were tested with identical drugs (Additional file 5: Table S5), four of which had similar mutational profiles suggesting that they were indeed identical lines. SCC-9 was excluded due to discrepancies in the mutational profiles reported by Barretina *et al.* and Garnett *et al.* (Additional file 1: Table S1). We sorted the comparable IC50s into three groups, representing cell lines that were exquisitely sensitive (IC50 < 3 μM) to the drug, responders (IC50 3.1-7.9 μM) and resistant cell lines (IC50 > 8 μM). We found that the majority were comparable (Additional file 5: Table S5).

Activating PIK3CA mutations are correlated with response to the PI3K inhibitor, AZD6482

The complete listing of drug sensitivity and gene status can be found in Additional file 6: Table S6, with the significant findings summarized in Table 2. Only mutations and copy number changes in *EGFR*, *TP53*, *CDKN2A*, *PIK3CA* and *SMAD4* were present with sufficient frequency (>10%) in the cell lines to allow analysis. It should be noted that not all cell lines were treated with every drug and some genetic changes occurred in a very small number of cell lines, which resulted in exclusion of analysis of certain drugs with a particular genetic change. Of the 131 drugs tested, three were PI3K inhibitors including AZD6482, GDC0941, and the combined mTOR and PI3K inhibitor NVP-BEZ235. We calculated a robust increase in sensitivity to AZD6482, explainable by the interaction of *PIK3CA* mutation status and HNSCC cell-line type (*LFDR* <0.023, Figure 1). In addition, an increase in AZD6482 sensitivity was shared by all *PIK3CA* mutants (*p* <0.037, Figure 4A) regardless of cell line type. No association was observed for the other PI3K inhibitors, GDC0941 and NVP-BEZ235, and *PIK3CA* mutation status (LFDR ≈ 1). There were too few *PIK3CA* amplified cell lines to examine the effect of amplification alone on drug

Table 1 Drugs demonstrating significantly increased or decreased activity in HNSCC cell lines compared with non-HNSCC lines

Drug	p^*	LFDR**	Drug response relative to other cell lines	Effect (Log2(IC50(µM)))	95% CI (Log2(IC50(µM)))
Bosutinib	<0.0001	0.0015	Sensitive	−2.74	(−3.67 to −1.82)
Docetaxel	<0.0001	0.0161	Sensitive	−2.29	(−3.17 to −1.42)
BIBW2992	0.0002	0.0161	Sensitive	−3.12	(−4.53 to −1.71)
Gefitinib	0.0003	0.0258	Sensitive	−2.18	(−3.24 to −1.12)
PD-173074	0.0002	0.0183	Resistance	0.95	(0.50-1.40)
Methotrexate	0.0005	0.0258	Resistance	1.59	(0.77-2.42)

Legend: * - calculated by one way analysis of variance (ANOVA), LFDR - local false discovery rate, ** - calculated by the Strimmer method, IC50 - half maximal inhibitory concentration, CI - confidence interval.

response, however when these were pooled with the *PIK3CA* mutant lines, no drugs were found to be preferentially active when compared to *PIK3CA* wild-type cell lines (Additional file 6: Table S6).

When examining responses to inhibitors of upstream and downstream members of the *PIK3CA* pathway, the FAK inhibitor PF-562271 (upstream) demonstrated a trend towards selective inhibition of *PIK3CA* HNSCC mutant cell lines (LFDR = 0.079, Figure 4B), while no effect was observed for downstream inhibitors including three AKT inhibitors (AKT inhibitor VIII, MK-2206, A-443654) and four mTOR inhibitors (Rapamycin, Temsirolimus, JW-7-52-1, AZD8055).

There was a trend towards increased sensitivity to AZD6482 and JNK Inhibitor VIII in cell lines with EGFR amplifications (LFDR = 0.056, Figure 4C). The strongest association observed was increased activity of the retinoid receptor antagonist ATRA in *TP53* mutant lines (LFDR = 0.007, Table 2 and Additional file 6: Table S6).

Discussion

Following decades of active research, only one class of targeted molecular agents, epidermal growth factor receptor (EGFR) inhibitors, have been approved for use in head and neck cancers [15]. Despite a modest survival benefit when administered concurrently with radiation, response rates to EGFR inhibitors are low when given alone (13%) and of limited duration (2–3 months). More effective drugs are needed in order to improve outcomes and reduce treatment-induced morbidities for HNSCC patients.

By pairing next-generation sequencing of cell lines with high-throughput drug screening techniques, the impressive studies by Garnett *et al.* and Barretina *et al.* [8,9], confirmed, in multiple tissue types, known associations of genetic alterations with drug sensitivity and uncovered a multitude of new ones. Their sequencing findings were in agreement with preliminary data from The Cancer Genome Atlas (TCGA) HNSCC study, where a multitude of potentially druggable targets including

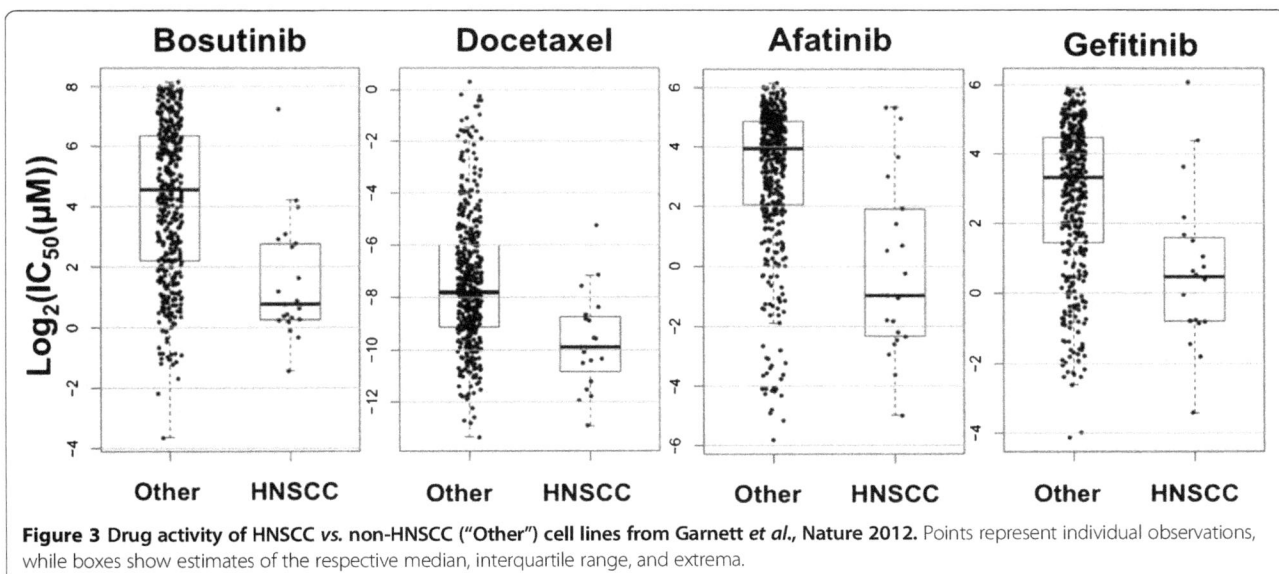

Figure 3 Drug activity of HNSCC *vs.* non-HNSCC ("Other") cell lines from Garnett *et al.*, Nature 2012. Points represent individual observations, while boxes show estimates of the respective median, interquartile range, and extrema.

Table 2 Significant associations of mutations and amplifications with drug response in HNSCC cell lines

Drug	Gene	Comparison	p	LFDR	Mean WT/NA log$_2$(IC50(μM))	Mut/Amp log$_2$(IC50(μM))	Effect Log2(IC50(μM)) [95% CI]
ATRA	TP53	wild-type vs mutant	<0.001	0.0069	9.96	7.15	2.81 [1.82-3.79]
AZD6482	PIK3CA	wild-type vs mutant	<0.001	0.023	4.87	0.689	4.18 [2.73-5.63]
JNK Inhibitor VIII	EGFR	non-amplified vs. amplified	<0.001	0.056	8.31	5.96	2.34 [1.49-3.20]
AZD6482	EGFR	non-amplified vs. amplified	<0.001	0.056	4.83	1.11	3.72 [2.17-5.26]
PF-562271	PIK3CA	wild-type vs mutant	<0.001	0.079	2.88	0.379	2.50 [1.55-3.46]

Legend: p – p value testing interaction, LFDR - local false discovery rate, WT - wild-type, NA - non-amplified, Mut – mutation, Amp – amplified, CI - confidence interval.

amplifications (e.g. *FGFR1*, *CCND1*, *MYC*, *EGFR*), deletions (e.g. *PTEN*), activating mutations (e.g. *PIK3CA*) and fusions (e.g. *FGFR3/TACC3*) were observed. Despite a relatively limited number of cell lines, our HNSCC-specific reanalysis of these studies shows that the spectrum of mutations observed in HNSCC cell lines is similar to that of primary HNSCC patient samples [10,16]. Overall, mutations in tumor suppressor genes, such as *TP53* are frequent, while activating mutations in oncogenes (*PIK3CA*, *HRAS*) occur at lower frequencies.

As mentioned, our analysis revealed 22 genes that are more frequently mutated than *TP53*, which is the most commonly mutated gene found in patient tumor samples (Additional file 3: Table S3). This discrepancy may be partially explained by the fact that mutations in introns and 5′ and 3′ untranslated regions (UTRs) were reported for the cell lines but not for the patient samples. In addition, there were multiple, identical mutations noted in cell lines, such the mutations observed in *NCAM1* [9]. Interestingly, *NCAM1* is known to signal through FAK, a direct target of PF-562271, which may contribute to its observed activity in *PIK3CA*-mutant HNSCC cell lines. However, we speculate that the near identical mutations found in these 22 highly mutated genes are germ-line variants and/or artifacts of cell line establishment. This inability to distinguish the cause of mutation(s) highlights the importance of comparing tumor sample or cell line DNA, to matched-normal tissue. Moving forward, it is crucial that matched-normal tissue and blood samples, representing the germ-line genetic profile are obtained when cell lines are established for improved sequencing analyses.

The most obvious directly druggable target in HNSCC appears to be the PI3K pathway, which was mutated in 8% of the patient samples examined by Stransky *et al.* [10]. We noted that activating *PIK3CA* mutations appeared to be more frequent in three HPV-positive tumors sequenced by Stransky *et al.*, and we confirmed this finding by sequencing the *PIK3CA* hotspots in a larger number of HPV-positive (46) and negative (43) oropharyngeal HNSCC samples [17]. We found that *PIK3CA* mutations occurred in 28% of the HPV-positive oropharyngeal tumors versus 10% of the HPV-negative

samples, confirming that this is an important therapeutic target in HNSCC. There is great interest in targeting PI3K as it is frequently either amplified or mutated in a large variety of human cancers [18], however the selection of the best possible drug is critical before moving forward with clinical studies. Selection of the appropriate agent is crucial because different drugs, which might target the same molecule, can display extremely variable potencies based on a variety of factors including a drug's binding site, delivery efficiency, half-life and metabolic interactions. An additional limitation of our analysis in terms of drug development progressing to routine patient care is the low number of drugs tested against the cell lines. Increasing the number of drugs tested, including drugs targeting identical molecules, would help ensure that potent drugs are identified and cellular targets further verified in the most appropriate patient population.

Cell lines are not perfect models of cancer due to their lack of three-dimensional stromal environment, lack of interactions with an immune system, and an inability to test drug delivery issues. Many of these concerns can be overcome in xenografts and human testing. The utility of cell line drug screening, given that poor correlation of drug testing in matched cell lines and patients have variably been observed [19,20] while patient derived xenografts appear to preserve nearly all the molecular feature of the original tumor. Emerging data suggests that while many cell lines may not recapitulate the molecular landscape of primary tumors, selecting cell line models with comparable genetic profiles will yield more accurate drug screening results [21-23]. With appropriate cell line models selected, cell line screening can be a robust, rapid and inexpensive preliminary screen before proceeding with more expensive and ethically-challenging animal and human studies. In our study, only molecules affecting the PI3K pathway (AZD6482 and PF-562271) were correlated with selective inhibition of *PIK3CA* mutant lines. However, it is somewhat surprising that AZD6482 was the most tightly correlated with *PIK3CA* mutation status as it has approximately an 87-fold higher affinity for PI3Kβ than PI3Kα [24]. It is noteworthy that AZD6482 appeared significantly more effective than the

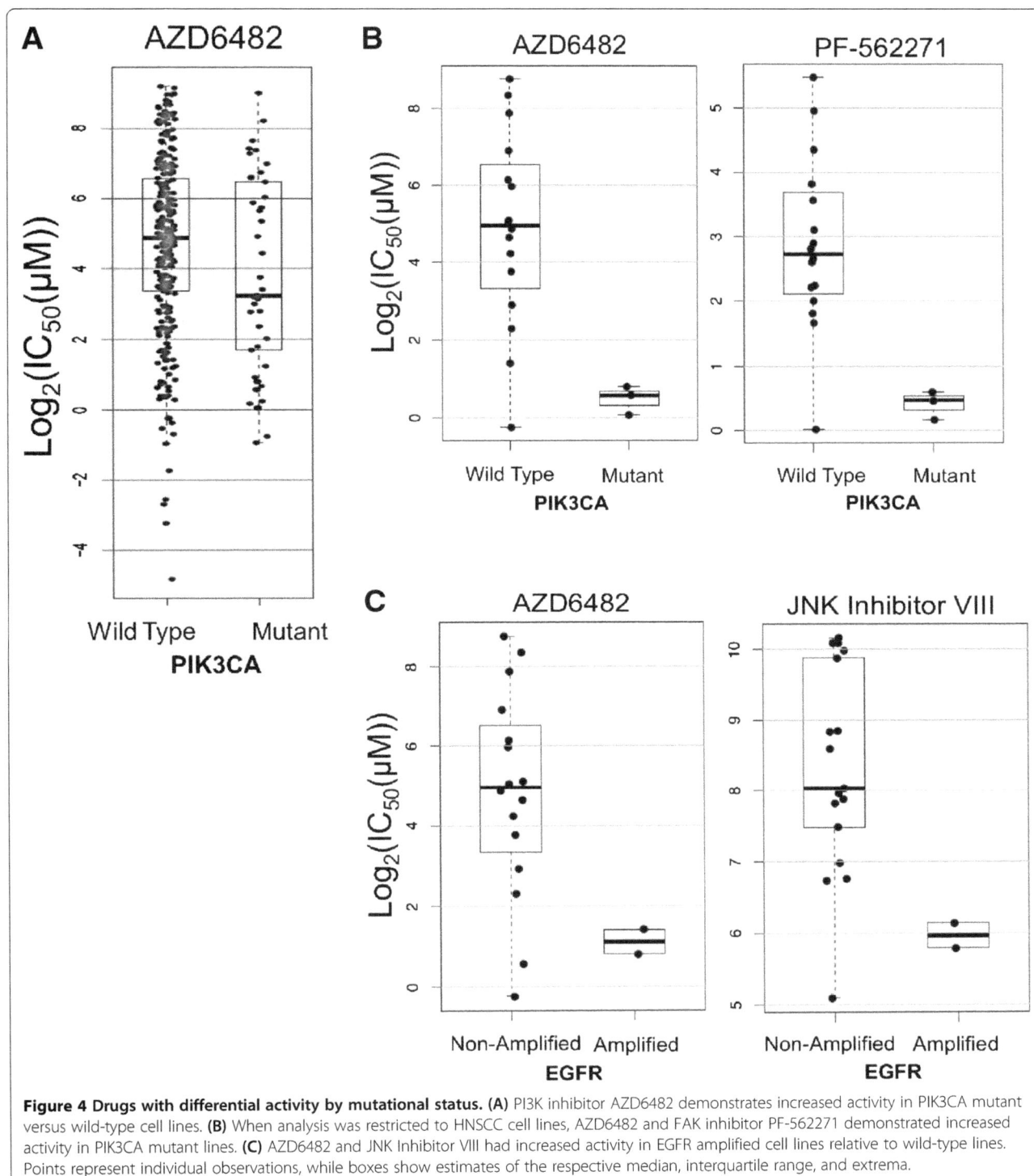

Figure 4 Drugs with differential activity by mutational status. (A) PI3K inhibitor AZD6482 demonstrates increased activity in PIK3CA mutant versus wild-type cell lines. **(B)** When analysis was restricted to HNSCC cell lines, AZD6482 and FAK inhibitor PF-562271 demonstrated increased activity in PIK3CA mutant lines. **(C)** AZD6482 and JNK Inhibitor VIII had increased activity in EGFR amplified cell lines relative to wild-type lines. Points represent individual observations, while boxes show estimates of the respective median, interquartile range, and extrema.

pan PI3K inhibitor GDC0941 (LFDR ≈ 1), which has a markedly higher affinity for PI3Kα [24,25] indicating that binding affinity may not be perfectly correlated with *in vitro* activity, much less *in vivo* efficacy. As well, compounds such as NVP-BEZ235, a PI3K/mTOR inhibitor have been previously found to have selective activity in *PI3KCA*-mutant HNSCC cell lines and patient-derived xenografts (PDX) [26]. However, NVP-BEZ235 activity did not correlate to *PI3KCA* mutant cell lines in these studies, reinforcing the importance of identifying the most promising preclinical candidates that have the strongest correlation with genomic changes to take forward into clinical trials.

There are two highly specific PI3Kα inhibitors, GDC-0032 (Genetech) and BYL719 (Novartis) that have demonstrated superior inhibition of *PIK3CA* mutant and amplified cell lines as well as tumor xenografts [27,28]. Indeed, BYL719 was screened against the CCLE cell line pool despite not being included in the report by Barretina *et al.* [28]. Given these promising preclinical studies, both compounds have been carried forward into phase I trials, and the study for BYL719 has been completed [27,28]. The trial included patients with solid tumors harboring *PIK3CA* amplifications and/or mutations including 8 HNSCC patients, six of which had stable disease and two had partial responses (25%) [28]. A phase II study in recurrent/metastatic HNSCC is already underway (http://clinicaltrials.gov/ct2/show/NCT01602315). BYL719 is an excellent example of a molecule initially identified in studies using cell lines, its efficacy confirmed in PDX models and results of the first Phase I clinical trials are now in the literature [29,30]. This process highlights the potential of this "bench to bedside" approach using high throughput platforms to identify effective anticancer agents. As targeted therapy for cancer treatment continues to develop, this bench to bedside approach will enable researchers to screen large numbers of drugs against a multitude of cancer cell lines with the goal of confirming successful agents in PDX models. Drugs that are found to be effective in both cell lines and in mice combined with NGS for biomarker prediction association, will better enable us to accurately treat patients.

EGFR inhibitors have been integrated into routine clinical care for HNSCC patients based on the landmark Bonner study [31]. EGFR is the only targeted therapy approved for the treatment of head and neck cancer. Perhaps it is not surprising that two of the four EGFR inhibitors that were tested demonstrated significantly higher activity in HNSCC lines versus the rest of the cell line pool (Table 1). However, only a subset of patients benefit from these agents [15]. To better illustrate this, Erlotinib was one of the EGFR inhibitors not found to have significantly increased activity in HNSCC cell lines compared with other cancer line types, further emphasizing the importance of accurate drug selection.

The mechanisms of sensitivity and resistance to EGFR inhibitors in HNSCC are poorly understood [15]. In lung cancer, EGFR response is tightly correlated with activating *EGFR* mutations, while resistance in colon cancer is mediated by downstream KRAS mutations [15]. These genetic changes essentially never occur in HNSCC [10], and EGFR inhibitor response has not been correlated with EGFR amplification or expression [15,31]. Indeed, in our study we failed to identify a genetic correlate of

EGFR inhibitor sensitivity. An expanded study including a larger number of molecularly characterized HNSCC cell lines could potentially address this important clinical issue.

While EGFR amplification was not correlated with EGFR inhibitor efficacy, it was associated with increased response to the PI3K inhibitor AZD6482 and JNK inhibitor VIII. EGFR signalling is mediated through several pathways including PI3K and JNK [32,33]. As EGFR amplifications do occur in HNSCC [10], this potentially relevant association should be explored further.

Ultimately our analysis is limited by the number of cell lines, which restrict the number of lines with any given genetic aberration(s) that could be tested. Another limitation is that not all drugs were tested in all cell lines. However, despite these limitations as well as discrepancies in drug responses described by Papillon-Cavanagh and colleagues [34], when comparing identical cell lines that were screened against the same compounds in the two studies, we found the results to be in agreement for many of the cell lines (Additional file 5: Table S5). There were 12 HNSCC cell lines displaying sensitivity to a compound (IC50 below 8 μM) in either or both of the studies. Of these 12 cases, ten were found to be very similar between the two studies (IC50 values within 3 μM) (Additional file 5: Table S5). In cases where cell lines displayed resistance, it was not possible for an exact comparison to be performed since Barretina *et al.* only screened drugs to a maximum of 8 μM, so many resistant cell lines are merely listed as having an IC50 of 8 μM. In contrast, Garnett *et al.* screened cell lines up to 3 orders of magnitude higher (10 mM). However, if we compare cell lines based on their characterization of resistance (IC50 above 8 μM) in their respective study, we find that the majority of cell line IC50 values were concordant between the two studies (Additional file 5: Table S5).

An additional limitation of our analysis is that all of the cell lines utilized were HPV-negative to the best of our knowledge [7]. Given the slow epidemic of HPV-related oropharyngeal cancer, this is a glaring omission as novel therapies for this patient cohort are of great interest to the head and neck oncology community. However, there are only 9 reported HPV-positive cell lines in the literature, all of which were derived from either recurrent tumors or smokers [35,36], and are thus less likely to recapitulate the treatment-sensitive HPV-positive tumors encountered in clinical practice. We suggest that the development of further HPV-positive cell lines and their incorporation into large-scale HNSCC cell line drug screening studies has the potential to identify novel effective agents and the mechanisms of drug sensitivity and resistance in HNSCC. Hopefully, this will lead to significant improvements in survival that has eluded us to date.

The disagreements noted in the cell line sensitivities and mutations between the two studies have significant implications for future work of this type. They are many factors that can explain these discrepancies, however the most likely is that the identically named lines are in fact different, despite the fact that genotyping was completed in both studies. Other possible sources of disagreements in the data are differences in screening techniques, different drug concentrations, and different statistical models to calculate IC50 values from the dose–response curves. Ideally, the genotyping data can be compared to determine the discrepancies and provide the definitive genotype for cell lines. We also suggest that a standard methodology of cell line drug screening needs to be developed to allow external validation of future findings.

Conclusions

High throughput drug screening of molecularly characterized HNSCC cell lines has the potential to rapidly identify promising agents to improve therapies for patients suffering with head and neck cancer. An expanded HNSCC specific study including HPV-positive cell lines has the potential to identify effective agents, as well as mechanisms of resistance and sensitivity to molecular agents.

Ethics approval

No ethics approval was required as this present work represents an investigation and analysis of publicly accessible data.

Additional files

Additional file 1: Table S1. Comparison of mutations noted in the studies by Garnett *et al.* and Barretina *et al.* Legend: CNV - relative copy number variation, Disagreements highlighted in bold.

Additional file 2: Table S2. Complete list of mutations found in the HNSCC cell lines in Barretina *et al.*, Nature 2012. Legend: Del - deletion, Ins - insertion, 5' UTR - 5' untranslated region, 3' UTR - 3' untranslated region, SNP - single nucleotide polymorphism.

Additional file 3: Table S3. Comparison of mutations noted in head and neck squamous cancer tumors and cell lines. Legend: *Significantly mutated genes found in patient tumor samples from Stransky *et al.*, Science 2011, **Most frequently mutated genes identified in cell lines in Barretina *et al.*, Nature 2012.

Additional file 4: Table S4. Associations of drug response and HNSCC cell line type versus non-HNSCC cell lines. Legend: t - t statistic calculated by ANOVA, p - p value calculated by ANOVA, LFDR - local falsed discovery rate, Effect - differences in the Log2(IC50(μM)) for HNSCC versus non-HNSCC cell lines, 95% lower limit and 95% upper limit delineate confidence intervals for the effect size.

Additional file 5: Table S5. Comparison of drug sensitivities in cell lines common to the studies by Garnett et al. and Barretina et al.

Additional file 6: Table S6. Associations of mutations and copy number alterations with drug response in HNSCC cell lines. Legend: wt - wild type, nor - normal (non-amplified), mt - mutation, amp - amplified, del - deletion, t - t statistic calculated by ANOVA, p - p value calculated by ANOVA, Wild-type: Log2(IC50(μM)) for wild-type cell lines, Other: Log2(IC50(μM)) for mutated and/or amplified cell lines, Effect: differences in the Log2(IC50(μM))

for WT/nor and mut/amplified cell lines, 95% lower limit and 95% upper limit delineate confidence intervals for the effect size, LFDR: Local false discovery Rate.

Abbreviations
HNSCC: Head and neck squamous cell carcinoma; HPV: Human papillomavirus; EGFR: Epidermal growth factor receptor; LFDR: Local false discovery rate; IC50: Inhibitory concentration, 50%; CNV: Copy number variation; UTR: Untranslated region; ANOVA: Analysis of variance.

Competing interests
The authors declare that they have no competing interests.

Authors' contributions
ACN conceived the study, and participated in its design and coordination, analyzed the data and helped to draft the manuscript. AF carried out some of the analysis. BHK and PCB participated in the design of the study and performed the statistical analysis. JWB participated in its design and helped to draft the manuscript. All authors read and approved the final manuscript.

Acknowledgements
This study was supported by a London Regional Cancer Program catalyst grant. This study was conducted with the support of the Ontario Institute for Cancer Research to PCB through funding provided by the Government of Ontario.

Funding
This study was supported by a London Regional Cancer Program catalyst grant. This study was conducted with the support of the Ontario Institute for Cancer Research to PCB through funding provided by the Government of Ontario.

Author details
[1]Department of Otolaryngology Head & Neck Surgery, Western University, London, Ontario, Canada. [2]Departments of Biochemistry and Applied Mathematics, Western University, London, Ontario, Canada. [3]Bioinformatics and Computational Genomics Laboratory, Institut de recherches cliniques de Montréal, Université de Montréal, Montreal, Quebec, Canada. [4]Department of Medical Biophysics, University of Toronto, Toronto, Canada. [5]Informatics & Biocomputing Platform, Ontario Institute for Cancer Research, Toronto, Canada. [6]Department of Pharmacology & Toxicology, University of Toronto, Toronto, Canada.

References
1. Argiris A, Karamouzis MV, Raben D, Ferris RL: Head and neck cancer. *Lancet* 2008, **371**(9625):1695–1709.
2. Baker SG, Sargent DJ: Designing a randomized clinical trial to evaluate personalized medicine: a new approach based on risk prediction. *J Natl Cancer Inst* 2010, **102**(23):1756–1759.
3. Burtness B, Bauman JE, Galloway T: Novel targets in HPV-negative head and neck cancer: overcoming resistance to EGFR inhibition. *Lancet Oncol* 2013, **14**(8):e302–309.
4. Gazdar AF, Girard L, Lockwood WW, Lam WL, Minna JD: Lung cancer cell lines as tools for biomedical discovery and research. *J Natl Cancer Inst* 2010, **102**(17):1310–1321.
5. Hennessey PT, Ochs MF, Mydlarz WW, Hsueh W, Cope L, Yu W, Califano JA: Promoter methylation in head and neck squamous cell carcinoma cell lines is significantly different than methylation in primary tumors and xenografts. *PLoS One* 2011, **6**(5):e20584.
6. Lacroix M, Leclercq G: Relevance of breast cancer cell lines as models for breast tumours: an update. *Breast Cancer Res Treat* 2004, **83**(3):249–289.
7. Zhao M, Sano D, Pickering CR, Jasser SA, Henderson YC, Clayman GL, Sturgis EM, Ow TJ, Lotan R, Carey TE, Sacks PG, Grandis JR, Sidransky D, Heldin NE, Myers JN: Assembly and initial characterization of a panel of 85 genomically validated cell lines from diverse head and neck tumor sites. *Clin Cancer Res* 2011, **17**:7248–7264.

8. Garnett MJ, Edelman EJ, Heidorn SJ, Greenman CD, Dastur A, Lau KW, Greninger P, Thompson IR, Luo X, Soares J, Liu Q, Iorio F, Surdez D, Chen L, Milano RJ, Bignell GR, Tam AT, Davies H, Stevenson JA, Barthorpe S, Lutz SR, Kogera F, Lawrence K, McLaren-Douglas A, Mitropoulos X, Mironenko T, Thi H, Richardson L, Zhou W, Jewitt F, *et al*: **Systematic identification of genomic markers of drug sensitivity in cancer cells.** *Nature* 2012, **483:**570–575.

9. Barretina J, Caponigro G, Stransky N, Venkatesan K, Margolin AA, Kim S, Wilson CJ, Lehar J, Kryukov GV, Sonkin D, Reddy A, Liu M, Murray L, Berger MF, Monahan JE, Morais P, Meltzer J, Korejwa A, Jane-Valbuena J, Mapa FA, Thibault J, Bric-Furlong E, Raman P, Shipway A, Engels IH, Cheng J, Yu GK, Yu J, Aspesi P Jr, de Silva M, *et al*: **The Cancer Cell Line Encyclopedia enables predictive modelling of anticancer drug sensitivity.** *Nature* 2012, **483:**603–607.

10. Stransky N, Egloff AM, Tward AD, Kostic AD, Cibulskis K, Sivachenko A, Kryukov GV, Lawrence MS, Sougnez C, McKenna A, Shefler E, Ramos AH, Stojanov P, Carter SL, Voet D, Cortes ML, Auclair D, Berger MF, Saksena G, Guiducci C, Onofrio RC, Parkin M, Romkes M, Weissfeld JL, Seethala RR, Wang L, Rangel-Escareno C, Fernandez-Lopez JC, Hidalgo-Miranda A, Melendez-Zajgla J, *et al*: **The mutational landscape of head and neck squamous cell carcinoma.** *Science* 2011, **333:**1157–1160.

11. Strimmer K: **Fdrtool: a versatile R package for estimating local and tail area-based false discovery rates.** *Bioinformatics* 2008, **24**(12):1461–1462.

12. Strimmer K: **A unified approach to false discovery rate estimation.** *BMC Bioinformatics* 2008, **9:**303.

13. Efron B, Tibshirani R: **Empirical bayes methods and false discovery rates for microarrays.** *Genet Epidemiol* 2002, **23**(1):70–86.

14. Aubert J, Bar-Hen A, Daudin JJ, Robin S: **Determination of the differentially expressed genes in microarray experiments using local FDR.** *BMC Bioinformatics* 2004, **5:**125.

15. Rabinowits G, Haddad RI: **Overcoming resistance to EGFR inhibitor in head and neck cancer: a review of the literature.** *Oral Oncol* 2012, **48**(11):1085–1089.

16. Agrawal N, Frederick MJ, Pickering CR, Bettegowda C, Chang K, Li RJ, Fakhry C, Xie TX, Zhang J, Wang J, Zhang N, El-Naggar AK, Jasser SA, Weinstein JN, Trevino L, Drummond JA, Muzny DM, Wu Y, Wood LD, Hruban RH, Westra WH, Koch WM, Califano JA, Gibbs RA, Sidransky D, Vogelstein B, Velculescu VE, Papadopoulos N, Wheeler DA, Kinzler KW, *et al*: **Exome sequencing of head and neck squamous cell carcinoma reveals inactivating mutations in NOTCH1.** *Science* 2011, **333:**1154–1157.

17. Nichols AC, Palma DA, Chow W, Tan S, Rajakumar C, Rizzo G, Fung K, Kwan K, Wehrli B, Winquist E, Koropatnick J, Mymryk JS, Yoo J, Barrett JW: **High frequency of activating PIK3CA mutations in human papillomavirus-positive oropharyngeal cancer.** *JAMA Otolaryngol Head Neck Surg* 2013, **139:**617–622.

18. Brana I, Siu LL: **Clinical development of phosphatidylinositol 3-kinase inhibitors for cancer treatment.** *BMC Med* 2012, **10:**161.

19. Gillet JP, Varma S, Gottesman MM: **The clinical relevance of cancer cell lines.** *J Natl Cancer Inst* 2013, **105**(7):452–458.

20. Shaw GL, Gazdar AF, Phelps R, Steinberg SM, Linnoila RI, Johnson BE, Oie HK, Russell EK, Ghosh BC, Pass HI, Minna JD, Mulshine JL, Ihde DC: **Correlation of in vitro drug sensitivity testing results with response to chemotherapy and survival: comparison of non-small cell lung cancer and small cell lung cancer.** *J Cell Biochem Supplement* 1996, **24:**173–185.

21. Domcke S, Sinha R, Levine DA, Sander C, Schultz N: **Evaluating cell lines as tumour models by comparison of genomic profiles.** *Nat Commun* 2013, **4:**2126.

22. Paez JG, Janne PA, Lee JC, Tracy S, Greulich H, Gabriel S, Herman P, Kaye FJ, Lindeman N, Boggon TJ, Naoki K, Sasaki H, Fujii Y, Eck MJ, Sellers WR, Johnson BE, Meyerson M: **EGFR mutations in lung cancer: correlation with clinical response to gefitinib therapy.** *Science* 2004, **304:**1497–1500.

23. Sharma SV, Haber DA, Settleman J: **Cell line-based platforms to evaluate the therapeutic efficacy of candidate anticancer agents.** *Nat Rev Cancer* 2010, **10**(4):241–253.

24. Nylander S, Kull B, Bjorkman JA, Ulvinge JC, Oakes N, Emanuelsson BM, Andersson M, Skarby T, Inghardt T, Fjellstrom O, Gustafsson D: **Human target validation of phosphoinositide 3-kinase (PI3K)beta: effects on platelets and insulin sensitivity, using AZD6482 a novel PI3Kbeta inhibitor.** *J Thromb Haemost* 2012, **10**(10):2127–2136.

25. Folkes AJ, Ahmadi K, Alderton WK, Alix S, Baker SJ, Box G, Chuckowree IS, Clarke PA, Depledge P, Eccles SA, Friedman LS, Hayes A, Hancox TC,

Kugendradas A, Lensun L, Moore P, Olivero AG, Pang J, Patel S, Pergl-Wilson GH, Raynaud FI, Robson A, Saghir N, Salphati L, Sohal S, Ultsch MH, Valenti M, Wallweber HJ, Wan NC, Wiesmann C, *et al*: **The identification of 2-(1H-indazol-4-yl)-6-(4-methanesulfonyl-piperazin-1-ylmethyl)-4-morpholin-4-yl-t hieno[3,2-d] pyrimidine (GDC-0941) as a potent, selective, orally bioavailable inhibitor of class I PI3 kinase for the treatment of cancer.** *J Med Chem* 2008, **51**(18):5522–5532.

26. Lui VW, Hedberg ML, Li H, Vangara BS, Pendleton K, Zeng Y, Lu Y, Zhang Q, Du Y, Gilbert BR, Freilino M, Sauerwein S, Peyser ND, Xiao D, Diergaarde B, Wang L, Chiosea S, Seethala R, Johnson JT, Kim S, Duvvuri U, Ferris RL, Romkes M, Nukui T, Kwok-Shing Ng P, Garraway LA, Hammerman PS, Mills GB, Grandis JR: **Frequent mutation of the PI3K pathway in head and neck cancer defines predictive biomarkers.** *Cancer discovery* 2013, **3:**761–769.

27. Ndubaku CO, Heffron TP, Staben ST, Baumgardner M, Blaquiere N, Bradley E, Bull R, Do S, Dotson J, Dudley D, Edgar KA, Friedman LS, Goldsmith R, Heald RA, Kolesnikov A, Lee L, Lewis C, Nannini M, Nonomiya J, Pang J, Price S, Prior WW, Salphati L, Sideris S, Wallin JJ, Wang L, Wei B, Sampath D, Olivero AG: **Discovery of 2-{3-[2-(1-isopropyl-3-methyl-1H-1,2,4-triazol-5-yl)-5,6-dihydrobenzo[f]imidazo[1,2-d][1,4]oxazepin-9-yl]-1H-pyrazol-1-yl}-2-methylpropanamide (GDC-0032): a beta-sparing phosphoinositide 3-kinase inhibitor with high unbound exposure and robust in vivo antitumor activity.** *J Med Chem* 2013, **56:**4597–4610.

28. Rodon J, Juric D, Gonzalez-Angulo A, Bendell J, Berlin J, Bootle D, Gravelin K, Huang A, Derti A, Lehar J, Würthner J, Boehm M, van Allen E, Wagle N, Garraway LA, Yelensky R, Stephens PJ, Miller VA, Schlegel R, Quadt C, Baselga J: **Towards defining the genetic framework for clinical response to treatment with BYL719, a PI3Kalpha-specific inhibitor.** In *American Association for Cancer Research.* Washington, DC, USA; 2013.

29. Juric D, Baselga J: **Tumor genetic testing for patient selection in phase I clinical trials: the case of PI3K inhibitors.** *J Clin Oncol* 2012, **30**(8):765–766.

30. Juric D, Argiles G, Burris HA, Gonzalez-Angulo A, Saura C, Quadt C, Douglas M, Demanse D, De Buck S, Baselga J: **Phase I study of BYL719, an alpha-specific PI3K inhibitor, in patients with PIK3CA mutant advanced solid tumors: preliminary efficacy and safety in patients with PIK3CA mutant ER-positive (ER+) metastatic breast cancer (MBC).** In *Thirty-Fifth Annual CTRC-AACR San Antonio Breast Cancer Symposium.* vol. 72. San Antonio, TX: American Association of Cancer Research; 2012. Supplement 3.

31. Bonner JA, Harari PM, Giralt J, Azarnia N, Shin DM, Cohen RB, Jones CU, Sur R, Raben D, Jassem J, Ove R, Kies MS, Baselga J, Youssoufian H, Amellal N, Rowinsky EK, Ang KK: **Radiotherapy plus cetuximab for squamous-cell carcinoma of the head and neck.** *N Engl J Med* 2006, **354:**567–578.

32. Takeuchi K, Shin-ya T, Nishio K, Ito F: **Mitogen-activated protein kinase phosphatase-1 modulated JNK activation is critical for apoptosis induced by inhibitor of epidermal growth factor receptor-tyrosine kinase.** *Febs J* 2009, **276**(5):1255–1265.

33. van der Heijden MS, Bernards R: **Inhibition of the PI3K pathway: hope we can believe in?** *Clin Cancer Res* 2010, **16**(12):3094–3099.

34. Papillon-Cavanagh S, De Jay N, Hachem N, Olsen C, Bontempi G, Aerts HJ, Quackenbush J, Haibe-Kains B: **Comparison and validation of genomic predictors for anticancer drug sensitivity.** *J Am Med Inform Assoc* 2013, **20**(4):597–602.

35. Tang AL, Hauff SJ, Owen JH, Graham MP, Czerwinski MJ, Park JJ, Walline H, Papagerakis S, Stoerker J, McHugh JB, Chepeha DB, Bradford CR, Carey TE, Prince ME: **UM-SCC-104: a new human papillomavirus-16-positive cancer stem cell-containing head and neck squamous cell carcinoma cell line.** *Head Neck* 2012, **34:**1480–1491.

36. Brenner JC, Graham MP, Kumar B, Saunders LM, Kupfer R, Lyons RH, Bradford CR, Carey TE: **Genotyping of 73 UM-SCC head and neck squamous cell carcinoma cell lines.** *Head Neck* 2010, **32**(4):417–426.

Permissions

List of Contributors

Mariëtte Hooiveld
NIVEL, Netherlands Institute for Health Services Research, Utrecht, PO Box 1568, 3500 BN Utrecht, the Netherlands

Tine van de Groep
Julius Center for Health Sciences and Primary Care, University Medical Center Utrecht, Utrecht, the Netherlands

Theo JM Verheij
Julius Center for Health Sciences and Primary Care, University Medical Center Utrecht, Utrecht, the Netherlands

Marianne AB van der Sande
Julius Center for Health Sciences and Primary Care, University Medical Center Utrecht, Utrecht, the Netherlands
Centre for Infectious Disease Control, National Institute for Public Health and the Environment, Bilthoven, the Netherlands

Robert A Verheij
NIVEL, Netherlands Institute for Health Services Research, Utrecht, PO Box 1568, 3500 BN Utrecht, the Netherlands

Margot AJB Tacken
IQ healthcare, Scientific Institute for Quality of Healthcare, Radboud University Nijmegen Medical Centre, Nijmegen, the Netherlands

Gerrit A van Essen
Julius Center for Health Sciences and Primary Care, University Medical Center Utrecht, Utrecht, the Netherlands

Zeina Nasr
Departments of Biochemistry, McGill University, Montreal, Quebec H3G 1Y6, Canada

Lukas E Dow
Memorial Sloan-Kettering Cancer Center, New York, USA

Marilene Paquet
Département de Pathologie et de Microbiologie, Faculté de Médecine Vétérinaire, Université de Montréal, Saint-Hyacinthe, Québec J2S 2 M2, Canada

Jennifer Chu
Departments of Biochemistry, McGill University, Montreal, Quebec H3G 1Y6, Canada

Kontham Ravindar
Départment de Chimie, Université Laval, Ste-Foy, Quebec G1V 0A6, Canada

Ragam Somaiah
Départment de Chimie, Université Laval, Ste-Foy, Quebec G1V 0A6, Canada

Pierre Deslongchamps
Départment de Chimie, Université Laval, Ste-Foy, Quebec G1V 0A6, Canada

John A Porco Jr
Center for Methodology and Library Development, Boston University, 590 Commonwealth Ave., Boston, MA 02215, USA

Scott W Lowe
Memorial Sloan-Kettering Cancer Center, New York, USA
Howard Hughes Medical Institute, New York, NY 10065, USA

Jerry Pelletier
Departments of Biochemistry, McGill University, Montreal, Quebec H3G 1Y6, Canada
Department of Oncology, McGill University, Montreal, Quebec H3G 1Y6, Canada
The Rosalind and Morris Goodman Cancer Research Center, McGill University, Montreal, Quebec H3G 1Y6, Canada

Vanessa Christe
Institute of Social and Preventive Medicine (IUMSP), Lausanne University Hospital, Bâtiment Biopôle 2, Route de la Corniche 10, 1010 Lausanne, Switzerland

Gérard Waeber
Department of Medicine, Internal Medicine, Lausanne University Hospital (CHUV) and Faculty of biology and medicine, Lausanne, Switzerland

Peter Vollenweider
Department of Medicine, Internal Medicine, Lausanne University Hospital (CHUV) and Faculty of biology and medicine, Lausanne, Switzerland

Pedro Marques-vidal
Institute of Social and Preventive Medicine (IUMSP), Lausanne University Hospital, Bâtiment Biopôle 2, Route de la Corniche 10, 1010 Lausanne, Switzerland

Shmeylan A Al Harbi
College of Pharmacy, King Saud bin Abdulaziz University for Health Sciences, King Abdulaziz Medical City, Riyadh, Saudi Arabia

Mohammad Khedr
College of Medicine, King Saud bin Abdulaziz University for Health Sciences, King Abdulaziz Medical City, MC 1425, PO Box 22490, Riyadh 1426, Saudi Arabia

Hasan M Al-Dorzi
College of Medicine, King Saud bin Abdulaziz University for Health Sciences, King Abdulaziz Medical City, MC 1425, PO Box 22490, Riyadh 1426, Saudi Arabia

Haytham M Tlayjeh
King Abdulaziz Medical City, Riyadh, Saudi Arabia

Asgar H Rishu
King Abdulaziz Medical City, Riyadh, Saudi Arabia

Yaseen M Arabi
College of Medicine, King Saud bin Abdulaziz University for Health Sciences, King Abdulaziz Medical City, MC 1425, PO Box 22490, Riyadh 1426, Saudi Arabia

Ngan N Lam
Department of Medicine, Division of Nephrology, Western University, London, ON N6A 3 K7, Canada
Department of Epidemiology and Biostatistics, Western University, London, ON N6A 3 K7, Canada
Kidney Clinical Research Unit, Room ELL-111, London Health Sciences Centre, 800 Commissioners Road East, London, ON N6A 4G5, Canada

Jamie L Fleet
Department of Medicine, Division of Nephrology, Western University, London, ON N6A 3 K7, Canada

Eric McArthur
Institute for Clinical Evaluative Sciences (ICES), London, ON N6A 5 W9, Canada

Peter G Blake
Department of Medicine, Division of Nephrology, Western University, London, ON N6A 3 K7, Canada

Amit X Garg
Department of Medicine, Division of Nephrology, Western University, London, ON N6A 3 K7, Canada
Department of Epidemiology and Biostatistics, Western University, London, ON N6A 3 K7, Canada Institute for Clinical Evaluative Sciences (ICES), London, ON N6A 5 W9, Canada

Keith A Candiotti
University of Miami–Jackson Memorial Hospital, 1611 NW 12th Avenue, Room 300, 33136 Miami, FL, USA

Syed Raza Ahmed
Becton, Dickinson and Company, 1 Becton Drive, 07417 Franklin Lakes, NJ, USA

David Cox
Eisai Inc., 100 Tice Boulevard, 07677 Woodcliff Lake, NJ, USA

Tong J Gan
Duke University Medical Center, 2100 Erwin Road, 27710 Durham, NC, USA

Thuc T Le
Nevada Cancer Institute, One Breakthrough Way, Las Vegas, NV 89135, USA
Desert Research Institute, 10530 Discovery Drive, Las Vegas, NV 89135, USA
Roseman University of Health Sciences, 11 Sunset Way, Henderson NV 89014, USA

Yasuyo Urasaki
Nevada Cancer Institute, One Breakthrough Way, Las Vegas, NV 89135, USA
Desert Research Institute, 10530 Discovery Drive, Las Vegas, NV 89135, USA
Roseman University of Health Sciences, 11 Sunset Way, Henderson NV 89014, USA

Giuseppe Pizzorno
Nevada Cancer Institute, One Breakthrough Way, Las Vegas, NV 89135, USA
Desert Research Institute, 10530 Discovery Drive, Las Vegas, NV 89135, USA

Vicent P Manyanga
Unit of Pharmacology and Therapeutics, Muhimbili University of Health and Allied Sciences, Dar Es Salaam, Tanzania

Omary Minzi
Unit of Pharmacology and Therapeutics, Muhimbili University of Health and Allied Sciences, Dar Es Salaam, Tanzania

Billy Ngasala
Department of Parasitology, Muhimbili University of Health and Allied Sciences, Dar Es Salaam, Tanzania

Jianchu Chen
College of Biosystems Engineering and Food Science, Fuli Institute of Food Science, Zhejiang Key Laboratory for Agro-Food Processing, Zhejiang University, Hangzhou 310058, China
College of Science, Technology and Mathematics, Alderson Broaddus University, Philippi, WV 26416, USA

Ashley Creed
College of Science, Technology and Mathematics, Alderson Broaddus University, Philippi, WV 26416, USA

Allen Y Chen
Department of Pharmaceutical Science, West Virginia University, Morgantown, WV 26506, USA

Haizhi Huang
College of Biosystems Engineering and Food Science, Fuli Institute of Food Science, Zhejiang Key Laboratory for Agro-Food Processing, Zhejiang University, Hangzhou 310058, China
College of Science, Technology and Mathematics, Alderson Broaddus University, Philippi, WV 26416, USA

Zhaoliang Li
College of Science, Technology and Mathematics, Alderson Broaddus University, Philippi, WV 26416, USA

Gary O Rankin
Department of Pharmacology, Physiology and Toxicology, Joan C. Edwards School of Medicine, Marshall University, Huntington, WV 25755, USA

Xingqian Ye
College of Biosystems Engineering and Food Science, Fuli Institute of Food Science, Zhejiang Key Laboratory for Agro-Food Processing, Zhejiang University, Hangzhou 310058, China

Guihua Xu
College of Biosystems Engineering and Food Science, Fuli Institute of Food Science, Zhejiang Key Laboratory for Agro-Food Processing, Zhejiang University, Hangzhou 310058, China

Yi Charlie Chen
College of Science, Technology and Mathematics, Alderson Broaddus University, Philippi, WV 26416, USA

Anne Polk
Departments of Cardiology, Herlev Hospital, University of Copenhagen, Herlev Ringvej 75, DK-2730 Herlev, Denmark
Departments of Oncology, Herlev Hospital, University of Copenhagen, Herlev Ringvej 75, DK-2730 Herlev, Denmark

Kirsten Vistisen
Departments of Oncology, Herlev Hospital, University of Copenhagen, Herlev Ringvej 75, DK-2730 Herlev, Denmark

Merete Vaage-Nilsen
Departments of Cardiology, Herlev Hospital, University of Copenhagen, Herlev Ringvej 75, DK-2730 Herlev, Denmark

Dorte L Nielsen
Departments of Oncology, Herlev Hospital, University of Copenhagen, Herlev Ringvej 75, DK-2730 Herlev, Denmark

Berhanu Geresu
Department of Pharmacy, College of Medicine and Health Sciences, Wollo University, Dessie, Ethiopia

Desye Misganaw
Department of Pharmacy, College of Medicine and Health Sciences, Wollo University, Dessie, Ethiopia

Yeshiwork Beyene
Department of Nursing, College of Medicine and Health Sciences, Wollo University, Dessie, Ethiopia

M Elle Saine
Department of Biostatistics and Epidemiology, Center for Clinical Epidemiology and Biostatistics, Perelman School of Medicine at the University of Pennsylvania, 423 Guardian Drive, Philadelphia, PA, USA
Department of Biostatistics and Epidemiology, Center for Pharmacoepidemiology Research and Training, Perelman School of Medicine at the University of Pennsylvania, Philadelphia, PA, USA

Dena M Carbonari
Department of Biostatistics and Epidemiology, Center for Clinical Epidemiology and Biostatistics, Perelman School of Medicine at the University of Pennsylvania, 423 Guardian Drive, Philadelphia, PA, USA
Department of Biostatistics and Epidemiology, Center for Pharmacoepidemiology Research and Training, Perelman School of Medicine at the University of Pennsylvania, Philadelphia, PA, USA

Craig W Newcomb
Department of Biostatistics and Epidemiology, Center for Clinical Epidemiology and Biostatistics, Perelman School of Medicine at the University of Pennsylvania, 423 Guardian Drive, Philadelphia, PA, USA

Melissa S Nezamzadeh
Department of Biostatistics and Epidemiology, Center for Clinical Epidemiology and Biostatistics, Perelman School of Medicine at the University of Pennsylvania, 423 Guardian Drive, Philadelphia, PA, USA
Department of Biostatistics and Epidemiology, Center for Pharmacoepidemiology Research and Training, Perelman School of Medicine at the University of Pennsylvania, Philadelphia, PA, USA

Kevin Haynes
Department of Biostatistics and Epidemiology, Center for Clinical Epidemiology and Biostatistics, Perelman School of Medicine at the University of Pennsylvania, 423 Guardian Drive, Philadelphia, PA, USA
Department of Biostatistics and Epidemiology, Center for Pharmacoepidemiology Research and Training, Perelman School of Medicine at the University of Pennsylvania, Philadelphia, PA, USA
HealthCore, Inc, Wilmington, DE, USA

Jason A Roy
Department of Biostatistics and Epidemiology, Center for Clinical Epidemiology and Biostatistics, Perelman School of Medicine at the University of Pennsylvania, 423 Guardian Drive, Philadelphia, PA, USA
Department of Biostatistics and Epidemiology, Center for Pharmacoepidemiology Research and Training, Perelman School of Medicine at the University of Pennsylvania, Philadelphia, PA, USA

Serena Cardillo
Department of Medicine, Perelman School of Medicine at the University of Pennsylvania, Philadelphia, PA, USA

Sean Hennessy
Department of Biostatistics and Epidemiology, Center for Clinical Epidemiology and Biostatistics, Perelman School of Medicine at the University of Pennsylvania, 423 Guardian Drive, Philadelphia, PA, USA
Department of Biostatistics and Epidemiology, Center for Pharmacoepidemiology Research and Training, Perelman School of Medicine at the University of Pennsylvania, Philadelphia, PA, USA

Crystal N Holick
HealthCore, Inc, Wilmington, DE, USA

Daina B Esposito
HealthCore, Inc, Wilmington, DE, USA

Arlene M Gallagher
Clinical Practice Research Datalink, Medicines and Healthcare Products Regulatory Agency, London, UK

Harshvinder Bhullar
Cegedim Strategic Data Medical Research, London, UK

Brian L Strom
Department of Biostatistics and Epidemiology, Center for Clinical Epidemiology and Biostatistics, Perelman School of Medicine at the University of Pennsylvania, 423 Guardian Drive, Philadelphia, PA, USA
Department of Biostatistics and Epidemiology, Center for Pharmacoepidemiology Research and Training, Perelman School of Medicine at the University of Pennsylvania, Philadelphia, PA, USA
Rutgers Biomedical & Health Sciences, Rutgers, the State University of New Jersey, Newark, NJ, USA

Vincent Lo Re III
Department of Biostatistics and Epidemiology, Center for Clinical Epidemiology and Biostatistics, Perelman School of Medicine at the University of Pennsylvania, 423 Guardian Drive, Philadelphia, PA, USA
Department of Biostatistics and Epidemiology, Center for Pharmacoepidemiology Research and Training, Perelman School of Medicine at the University of Pennsylvania, Philadelphia, PA, USA

Department of Medicine, Perelman School of Medicine at the University of Pennsylvania, Philadelphia, PA, USA

Sandrina Lambrechts
Division of Gynaecologic Oncology and Leuven Cancer Institute, University Hospitals Leuven, KU Leuven, Herestraat 49, 3000 Leuven, Belgium

Diether Lambrechts
Vesalius Research Center, VIB, Leuven, Herestraat 49, Box 912, 3000 Leuven, Belgium
Laboratory for Translational Genetics, Department of Oncology, KU Leuven, Herestraat 49, 3000 Leuven, Belgium

Evelyn Despierre
Division of Gynaecologic Oncology and Leuven Cancer Institute, University Hospitals Leuven, KU Leuven, Herestraat 49, 3000 Leuven, Belgium

Els Van Nieuwenhuysen
Division of Gynaecologic Oncology and Leuven Cancer Institute, University Hospitals Leuven, KU Leuven, Herestraat 49, 3000 Leuven, Belgium

Dominiek Smeets
Vesalius Research Center, VIB, Leuven, Herestraat 49, Box 912, 3000 Leuven, Belgium
Laboratory for Translational Genetics, Department of Oncology, KU Leuven, Herestraat 49, 3000 Leuven, Belgium

Philip R Debruyne
Oncologisch Centrum, Algemeen Ziekenhuis Groeninge, Loofstraat 43, 8500 Kortrijk, Belgium

Vincent Renard
Dienst Oncologie, Algemeen Ziekenhuis Sint Lucas, Groenebriel 1, 9000 Gent, Belgium

Philippe Vroman
Dienst Medische Oncologie, Onze-Lieve-Vrouwziekenhuis, Moorselbaan 164, 9300 Aalst, Belgium

Daisy Luyten
Dienst Medische Oncologie, Jessa Ziekenhuis, Stadsomvaart 11, 3500 Hasselt, Belgium

Patrick Neven
Division of Gynaecologic Oncology and Leuven Cancer Institute, University Hospitals Leuven, KU Leuven, Herestraat 49, 3000 Leuven, Belgium

Frédéric Amant
Division of Gynaecologic Oncology and Leuven Cancer Institute, University Hospitals Leuven, KU Leuven, Herestraat 49, 3000 Leuven, Belgium

Karin Leunen
Division of Gynaecologic Oncology and Leuven Cancer Institute, University Hospitals Leuven, KU Leuven, Herestraat 49, 3000 Leuven, Belgium

Ignace Vergote
Division of Gynaecologic Oncology and Leuven Cancer Institute, University Hospitals Leuven, KU Leuven, Herestraat 49, 3000 Leuven, Belgium

Luca Gallelli
Department of Health Science, University of Catanzaro, Catanzaro, Italy

Daniela Falcone
Department of Health Science, University of Catanzaro, Catanzaro, Italy

Monica Scaramuzzino
Department of Health Science, University of Catanzaro, Catanzaro, Italy

Girolamo Pelaia
Department of Medical and Surgical Sciences, University of Catanzaro, Catanzaro, Italy

Bruno D'Agostino
Department of Experimental Medicine-Section of Pharmacology, School of Medicine, Second University of Naples, via Costantinopoli 16, 80136 Naples, Italy

Maria Mesuraca
Department of Experimental Medicine, University of Catanzaro, Catanzaro, Italy

Rosa Terracciano
Department of Health Science, University of Catanzaro, Catanzaro, Italy

Giuseppe Spaziano
Department of Experimental Medicine-Section of Pharmacology, School of Medicine, Second University of Naples, via Costantinopoli 16, 80136 Naples, Italy

Rosario Maselli
Department of Medical and Surgical Sciences, University of Catanzaro, Catanzaro, Italy

Michele Navarra
Department of Drug Sciences and Health Products, University of Messina, IRCCS centro neurolesi "Bonino-Pulejo", Messina, Italy

Rocco Savino
Department of Health Science, University of Catanzaro, Catanzaro, Italy

Abeer Abuzeid Atta Elmannan
Al Neelain University, Steen Street, P.O. Box 7294, Code: 11123 Khartoum, Sudan

Khalid Abdelmutalab Elmardi
Federal Ministry of Health, Khartoum, Sudan

Yassir Ali Idris
Gezira State Ministry of Health, Wad Medani, Sudan

Jonathan M Spector
Harvard School of Public Health, 677 Huntington Avenue, Boston, MA 02115, USA

Nahid Abdelgadir Ali
Federal Ministry of Health, Khartoum, Sudan

Elfatih Mohamed Malik
Gezira State Ministry of Health, Wad Medani, Sudan

Maria Gustafsson
Department of Pharmacology and Clinical Neurosciences, Division of Clinical Pharmacology and Department of Community Medicine and Rehabilitation, Geriatric Medicine, Umeå University, Umeå, Sweden

Stig Karlsson
Department of Nursing, Umeå University, Umeå, Sweden

Yngve Gustafson
Department of Community Medicine and Rehabilitation, Geriatric Medicine, Umeå University, Umeå, Sweden

Hugo Lövheim
Department of Community Medicine and Rehabilitation, Geriatric Medicine, Umeå University, Umeå, Sweden

José C Álvarez
Universidad Nacional de Colombia, Facultad de Medicina, Bogotá, Colombia

Sonia I Cuervo
Universidad Nacional de Colombia, Facultad de Medicina, Bogotá, Colombia
(GREICAH): Grupo de Investigación en Enfermedades Infecciosas en Cáncer y alteraciones hematológicas, Bogotá, Colombia
Instituto Nacional de Cancerología, Bogotá, Colombia

Javier R Garzón
(GREICAH): Grupo de Investigación en Enfermedades Infecciosas en Cáncer y alteraciones hematológicas, Bogotá, Colombia

Julio C Gómez
(GREICAH): Grupo de Investigación en Enfermedades Infecciosas en Cáncer y alteraciones hematológicas, Bogotá, Colombia
Instituto Nacional de Cancerología, Bogotá, Colombia

Jorge Augusto Díaz
(GREICAH): Grupo de Investigación en Enfermedades Infecciosas en Cáncer y alteraciones hematológicas, Bogotá, Colombia

Departamento de Farmacia, Facultad de Ciencias, Universidad Nacional de Colombia, Bogotá, Colombia

Edelberto Silva
(GREICAH): Grupo de Investigación en Enfermedades Infecciosas en Cáncer y alteraciones hematológicas, Bogotá, Colombia
Departamento de Farmacia, Facultad de Ciencias, Universidad Nacional de Colombia, Bogotá, Colombia
Departamento de Medicina, Facultad de Medicina, Ciudad Universitaria, Carrera 30 No. 45-03, edificio 471, oficina 510, Bogotá A. A. 14490, Colombia

Ricardo Sánchez
Universidad Nacional de Colombia, Facultad de Medicina, Bogotá, Colombia
(GREICAH): Grupo de Investigación en Enfermedades Infecciosas en Cáncer y alteraciones hematológicas, Bogotá, Colombia
Instituto Nacional de Cancerología, Bogotá, Colombia

Jorge A Cortés
Universidad Nacional de Colombia, Facultad de Medicina, Bogotá, Colombia

Nathalie Eckel
German Institute of Human Nutrition Potsdam-Rehbrücke, Department of Molecular Epidemiology, Arthur-Scheunert-Allee 114-116, 14558 Nuthetal, Potsdam, Germany

Giselle Sarganas
Robert Koch-Institute, Department of Epidemiology and Health Monitoring, General-Pape-Str. 62-66 12101, Berlin, Germany

Ingrid-Katharina Wolf
Robert Koch-Institute, Department of Epidemiology and Health Monitoring, General-Pape-Str. 62-66 12101, Berlin, Germany

Hildtraud Knopf
Robert Koch-Institute, Department of Epidemiology and Health Monitoring, General-Pape-Str. 62-66 12101, Berlin, Germany

Suhashni Naiker
TB Research Unit, Medical Research Council, Durban, South Africa

Cathy Connolly
Biostatistics Unit, Medical Research Council, Durban, South Africa

Lubbe Wiesner
Division of Clinical Pharmacology, Department of Medicine, University of Cape Town, Cape Town, South Africa

Tracey Kellerman
Division of Clinical Pharmacology, Department of Medicine, University of Cape Town, Cape Town, South Africa

Tarylee Reddy
Biostatistics Unit, Medical Research Council, Durban, South Africa

Anthony Harries
International Union Against Tuberculosis and Lung Disease, Paris, France

Helen McIlleron
Division of Clinical Pharmacology, Department of Medicine, University of Cape Town, Cape Town, South Africa

Christian Lienhardt
WHO STOP Tuberculosis Programme, Geneva, Switzerland

Alexander Pym
TB Research Unit, Medical Research Council, Durban, South Africa

KwaZulu-Natal Research Institute for Tuberculosis and HIV (K-RITH), University of KwaZulu-Natal, Durban, South Africa

Qiang Sun
Center for Health Management and Policy, Key Lab of Health Economics and Policy Research of Ministry of Health, Shandong University, 250012 Jinan, Shandong, China

Oliver J Dyar
Medical Education Centre, North Devon District Hospital, Raleigh Park, Barnstaple, Devon EX31 4JB, UK

Lingbo Zhao
Center for Health Management and Policy, Key Lab of Health Economics and Policy Research of Ministry of Health, Shandong University, 250012 Jinan, Shandong, China

Göran Tomson
Department of Public Health Sciences, Department of Learning, Informatics, Management, Tomtebodavägen 18 A; Medical Management Centre (MMC), Ethics Karolinska Institutet, 171 77 Stockholm, Sweden

Lennart E Nilsson
Department of Clinical and Experimental Medicine, Clinical Microbiology, Faculty of Health Sciences, Linköping University, 581 85 Linköping, Sweden

Malin Grape
Antibiotics and Infection Control Unit, Public Health Agency of Sweden, 17182 Solna, Sweden

Yanyan Song
School of Public Health, Shandong University, Jinan, Shandong 250012, China

Ling Yan
Jinan Central Hospital, Jinan, Shandong 250013, China

Cecilia Stålsby Lundborg
Department of Public Health Sciences, Global Health (IHCAR), Tomtebodavägen 18 A, Karolinska Institutet, 1771 77 Stockholm, Sweden

Young-Hee Kim
Department of Microbiology, Soonchunhyang University Medical college, Cheonan, Korea

Kyung-Ah Kwak
Department of Microbiology, Soonchunhyang University Medical college, Cheonan, Korea

Hyo-Wook Gil
Department of Internal Medicine, Soonchunhyang University Cheonan Hospital, 31 Soonchunhyang 6gil, Dongnam-gu, Cheonan, Chungnam 330-721, Korea

Ho-Yeon Song
Department of Microbiology, Soonchunhyang University Medical college, Cheonan, Korea

Sae-Yong Hong
Department of Internal Medicine, Soonchunhyang University Cheonan Hospital, 31 Soonchunhyang 6gil, Dongnam-gu, Cheonan, Chungnam 330-721, Korea

Wondmagegn Tamiru Tadesse
Department of Pharmacology, School of Medicine, Addis Ababa Science & Technology University, Addis Ababa, Ethiopia

Alemayehu Berhane Mekonnen
Department of Clinical Pharmacy, School of Pharmacy, University of Gondar, Gondar, Ethiopia

Wubshet Hailu Tesfaye
Department of Clinical Pharmacy, School of Pharmacy, University of Gondar, Gondar, Ethiopia

Yidnekachew Tamiru Tadesse
Department of Internal Medicine, School of Medicine, University of Gondar, Gondar, Ethiopia

Anthony C Nichols
Department of Otolaryngology Head & Neck Surgery, Western University, London, Ontario, Canada

Morgan Black
Department of Otolaryngology Head & Neck Surgery, Western University, London, Ontario, Canada

John Yoo
Department of Otolaryngology Head & Neck Surgery, Western University, London, Ontario, Canada

Nicole Pinto
Department of Otolaryngology Head & Neck Surgery, Western University, London, Ontario, Canada

Andrew Fernandes
Departments of Biochemistry and Applied Mathematics, Western University, London, Ontario, Canada

Benjamin Haibe-Kains
Bioinformatics and Computational Genomics Laboratory, Institut de recherches cliniques de Montréal, Université de Montréal, Montreal, Quebec, Canada

Paul C Boutros
Department of Medical Biophysics, University of Toronto, Toronto, Canada
Informatics & Biocomputing Platform, Ontario Institute for Cancer Research, Toronto, Canada
Department of Pharmacology & Toxicology, University of Toronto, Toronto, Canada

John W Barrett
Department of Otolaryngology Head & Neck Surgery, Western University, London, Ontario, Canada

*9 7 8 1 6 8 2 8 6 1 6 6 0 *